New Approaches to Death in Cities during the Health Transition

International Studies in Population

Volume 12

The International Union for the Scientific Study of Population (IUSSP)

The IUSSP is an international association of researchers, teachers, policy makers and others from diverse disciplines set up to advance the field of demography and promote scientific exchange. It also seeks to foster relations between persons engaged in the study of demography and population trends in all countries of the world and to disseminate knowledge about their determinants and consequences. The members of the IUSSP scientific group responsible for this book were chosen for their scientific expertise. This book was reviewed by a group other than the authors. While the IUSSP endeavours to assure the accuracy and objectivity of its scientific work, the conclusions and interpretations in IUSSP publications are those of the authors.

International Studies in Population (ISIP) is the outcome of an agreement concluded by the IUSSP and Springer in 2004. The joint series covers the broad range of work carried out by IUSSP and includes material presented at seminars organized by the IUSSP. The scientific directions of the IUSSP are set by the IUSSP Council elected by the membership and composed for 2014–2017 of:

More information about this series at http://www.springer.com/series/6944

Diego Ramiro Fariñas • Michel Oris
Editors

New Approaches to Death in Cities during the Health Transition

Springer

Editors
Diego Ramiro Fariñas
Institute of Economics, Geography and Demography (IEGD-CCHS-CSIC)
Spanish National Research Council
Madrid, Spain

Michel Oris
Center for the Interdisciplinary Study of Gerontology and Vulnerability
NCCR LIVES
Genèva, Switzerland

Institute of Demography and Socioeconomics
University of Geneva
Genèva, Switzerland

International Studies in Population
ISBN 978-3-319-43001-0 ISBN 978-3-319-43002-7 (eBook)
DOI 10.1007/978-3-319-43002-7

Library of Congress Control Number: 2016951488

Printed on acid-free paper

This Springer imprint is published by Springer Nature
The registered company is Springer International Publishing AG Switzerland

Contents

1 **New Approaches to Death in Cities During the Health Transition: An Introduction** 1
Michel Oris and Diego Ramiro Fariñas

Part I Mortality Within the City: Historical Europe

2 **Understanding Infant Mortality in the City: Exploring Registration and Compositional Effects. Madrid, 1905–1906** 19
Bárbara A. Revuelta Eugercios and Diego Ramiro Fariñas

3 **Environment, Housing, and Infant Mortality: Udine, 1807–1815** 43
Alessio Fornasin, Marco Breschi, and Matteo Manfredini

4 **Residential Mobility and Child Mortality in Early Twentieth Century Belfast** 55
Alice Reid, Eilidh Garrett, and Simon Szreter

5 **Micro-Analysis of Mortality in Urban Areas. The Parish of Oliveira in Guimarães, in Northern Portugal Between the Eighteenth and Twentieth Centuries** 77
Maria Norberta Amorim, Antero Ferreira, and Luís Meira-Machado

Part II Urban Mortality in Transition

6 **Infant and Early Childhood Mortality in a Context of Transitional Fertility: Geneva 1800–1900** 97
Reto Schumacher

7 **A Slow Transition. Infant and Child Mortality Decline in a Sardinian Community: Alghero (1866–1935)** 115
Marco Breschi, Massimo Esposito, Stanislao Mazzoni, and Lucia Pozzi

8 The Democratization of Longevity: How the Poor Became Old in Paris, 1880–1913 137
Lionel Kesztenbaum and Jean-Laurent Rosenthal

Part III Urban Mortality in the Developing World

9 Estimating Area-Based Influences on Urban-Rural Inequalities in Health Outcomes: A Longitudinal Multilevel Epidemiological Investigation 157
Barthelemy Kuate Defo

10 Will Urban and Rural Mortality Converge in Africa? 181
Michel Garenne

11 Urban Mortality Transitions: The Role of Slums 197
Günther Fink, Isabel Günther, and Kenneth Hill

12 Health Disparities on the Periphery of Ouagadougou 217
Clémentine Rossier, Abdramane Bassiahi Soura, Bruno Lankoande, and Roch Modeste Millogo

Contributors

Maria Norberta Amorim CITCEM – Transdisciplinary Culture, Space and Memory Research Centre, Universidade do Minho, Guimarães, Portugal

Marco Breschi Department of Economic and Business, University of Sassari, Sassari, Italy

Massimo Esposito Department of Economic and Business, University of Sassari, Sassari, Italy

Antero Ferreira CITCEM – Transdisciplinary Culture, Space and Memory Research Centre, Universidade do Minho, Guimarães, Portugal

Günther Fink Global Health and Population, Harvard T.H. Chan School of Public Health, Boston, MA, USA

Alessio Fornasin Department of Economics and Statistics, University of Udine, Udine, Italy

Michel Garenne Institut de Recherche pour le Développement (IRD), Paris, France

Institut Pasteur, Epidémiologie des Maladies Emergentes, Paris, France

School of Public Health, Witwatersrand University, Johannesburg, South Africa

Eilidh Garrett Department of Geography, University of Cambridge, Cambridge, UK

Department of History, University of Essex, Wivenhoe Park, Colchester, UK

Isabel Günther Center for Development and Cooperation, ETH Zürich, Zürich, Switzerland

Kenneth Hill Global Health and Population, Harvard T.H. Chan School of Public Health, Boston, MA, USA

Lionel Kesztenbaum INED (Institut National d'Etudes Démographiques) and PSE (Paris School of Economics), Paris, France

Barthelemy Kuate Defo Public Health Research Institute, Department of Demography & Department of Social and Preventive Medicine, School of Public Health, University of Montreal, Montréal, Quebec, Canada

Bruno Lankoande Institut Supérieur des Sciences de la Population, University of Ouagadougou, Ouagadougou, Burkina Faso

Matteo Manfredini Department of Life Sciences, University of Parma, Parma, Italy

Stanislao Mazzoni Department of Economic and Business, University of Sassari, Sassari, Italy

Luís Meira-Machado Department of Mathematics for Science and Technology, Universidade do Minho, Guimarães, Portugal

Roch Modeste Millogo Institut Supérieur des Sciences de la Population, University of Ouagadougou, Ouagadougou, Burkina Faso

Michel Oris Center for the Interdisciplinary Study of Gerontology and Vulnerability, NCCR LIVES, Genèva, Switzerland

Institute of Demography and Socioeconomics, University of Geneva, Genèva, Switzerland

Lucia Pozzi Department of Economic and Business, University of Sassari, Sassari, Italy

Diego Ramiro Fariñas Institute of Economics, Geography and Demography (IEGD-CCHS-CSIC), Spanish National Research Council, Madrid, Spain

Alice Reid Department of Geography, University of Cambridge, Cambridge, UK

Bárbara A. Revuelta Eugercios Copenhagen Centre for Health Researh in the Humanities, Copenhagen, Denmark

Jean-Laurent Rosenthal Division of the Humanities and Social Sciences, Caltech (California Institute of Technology), Pasadena, CA, USA

Clémentine Rossier Institute of Demography and Socioeconomics, University of Geneva, Geneva, Switzerland

Institut National d'Etudes Démographiques, Paris, France

Institut Supérieur des Sciences de la Population, University of Ouagadougou, Ouagadougou, Burkina Faso

Reto Schumacher Secteur Prospective et aide à la décision, Statistique Vaud, Lausanne, Switzerland

NCCR Lives, Lausanne, Switzerland

Abdramane Bassiahi Soura Institut Supérieur des Sciences de la Population, University of Ouagadougou, Ouagadougou, Burkina Faso

Simon Szreter Faculty of History, University of Cambridge, Cambridge, UK

Chapter 1
New Approaches to Death in Cities During the Health Transition: An Introduction

Michel Oris and Diego Ramiro Fariñas

Cities are a world of differences and, consequently, of inequalities. We are no longer in the 1950s or 1960s, when the pioneers of historical demography thought peasant societies were uniform and immobile; many studies have demonstrated the existence of various and sometimes elaborate socioeconomic structures and dynamics in the rural world (see Bengtsson et al. 2004; Oris 2003). But cities remain, above all, the spaces of interactions among a variety of social groups, the places where poor, middle-class, and wealthy people, as well as elites, have coexisted in harmony or tension, from the past to the present, in the North and in the South. Urban areas also form specific epidemiological environments since they are characterized by population concentration and density. Inversely and coherently, cities develop answers in terms of sanitary policies and health infrastructures. This balance between risk and protective factors is, however, not at all constant across time and space and is especially endangered in periods of massive demographic growth, particularly periods of urbanization mainly led by immigration flows that transform both the socioeconomic and demographic composition of urban populations and the morphological nature of urban environments. Moreover, the stages of the epidemiological transition are also highly influential.

M. Oris (✉)
Center for the Interdisciplinary Study of Gerontology and Vulnerability, NCCR LIVES, Genèva, Switzerland

Institute of Demography and Socioeconomics, University of Geneva, 54 route des Acacias, Ch-1227 Genèva, Switzerland
e-mail: Michel.Oris@unige.ch

D. Ramiro Fariñas
Institute of Economics, Geography and Demography (IEGD-CCHS-CSIC), Spanish National Research Council, CCHS-CSIC, Albasanz 26-28, Madrid 28037, Spain
e-mail: diego.ramiro@cchs.csic.es

D. Ramiro Fariñas, M. Oris (eds.), *New Approaches to Death in Cities during the Health Transition*, International Studies in Population 12,
DOI 10.1007/978-3-319-43002-7_1

These topics have been widely studied, but they have attracted relatively less attention during the last 10 or 15 years. Therefore, we felt it necessary to promote new efforts and new approaches to improve our understanding of the evolution of health and mortality in urban environments in the long run, looking at transformations and adaptations during the process of rapid population growth. This long-run perspective is definitively crucial in our view, even more so when most of the challenges shown in this book are being faced in the present and will be faced in the near future by an increasingly urbanized world with a growing number of big cities, especially in less developed countries, which will need to combine population growth with urban sustainability.

These motivations were at the origin of a workshop that was organized in Seville on December 15–16, 2011, at the Institute of Statistics and Cartography of Andalusia. Some thirty participants discussed the abovementioned questions, and twenty communications were presented. This volume brings together a selection of eleven papers. We explicitly wanted, during the meeting and here, to go beyond the artificial division between past and present, as well as between previous and recent dynamics. Indeed, as will be shown in this book, similar problems were faced by European preindustrial and industrial cities and present cities in the developing world, in however largely different contexts (Günther and Harttgen 2012). To be clear, we do not accept an overly simplistic analogy between contemporary processes in the South and historical dynamics in the North. We are just convinced we have a lot to learn from each other in terms of both differences and similarities. The eleven contributions to this book all explore health and mortality differentials within urban spaces, the dynamics of change, and the differences between cities and rural areas.

In the following lines, we discuss first the data and methods and then the issue of social mortality differentials in urban areas, a topic that has been renewed by recent theoretical contributions. We also present the state of our knowledge on the so-called *urban penalty* and consider the interactions between places and classes in cities that are political and institutional constructions, with an emphasis on slums in the past and today. On that basis, we introduce the eleven chapters of this volume, emphasizing their empirical and theoretical contributions, which are summarized in the last section before we finish expressing our gratitude to those who made the meeting and this book possible.

1.1 Heuristic Challenges, Scientific Challenges

Working on health and death in cities is first a heuristic challenge: Which data do we use? Are the data reliable? What do we measure? How do we deal with mobility, which obviously affects the estimations of urban mortality? Whether we are looking to the past or to the present, in the historical North or in the contemporary South, does not really matter: Struggling with data and conducting rigorous critical evaluations of the material are absolute necessities for all researchers working to understand the differentials within dynamic populations that live in rapidly evolving environments. All contributors to this volume have dealt with differential frailty and heterogeneity, under-registration, *de jure* and *de facto* populations, strategies for participant recruitment for surveys or the effects of dropout, selection of immigrants but also of stayers, etc. The eleven chapters brought together here show very concretely how it is possible to deal with the heuristic challenges associated with the (re)construction of individual longitudinal data in chaotic urban spaces where highly mobile populations live(d).

Most of the time, historical demographers construct their own databases from various linked sources, whereas demographers tend to exploit data collected by others, typically *Demographic Health Surveys* (DHS). DHS are powerful sources with immense potential, thanks to their contents as well as their robust methodology, systematization, multiplication, and repetition. This treasure gave Barthélémy Kuate Defo, Michel Garenne, Günther Fink and colleagues the opportunity to look at the evolution of the mortality gap between urban and rural areas, as well as mortality differentials within the cities, at a world or continental level. They were also able to assess historical changes.

That said, making a distinction between historical demographers and demographers according to their type of sources and direct or indirect engagement in the data collection process is not fruitful. Indeed, for the past several years we have observed the development of what are called demographic observatories now associated in the *In-depth* network. They typically consist of panel data wherein a given geographically defined population is repeatedly surveyed to provide a longitudinal and detailed individual-level or micro-level perspective on changes.[1]

An excellent illustration is given by the *Ouagadougou Health and Demographic Surveillance System* in Burkina Faso, which is described and analyzed in this volume by Clémentine Rossier, Abdramane Soura, Bruno Lankoande, and Roch Millogo. Once again, we face a large capital city that has undergone significant demographic growth largely due to a hefty influx of immigrants. Since 2008, the Ouagadougou project has followed 80,000 people living in five neighborhoods on the periphery of the city, half of whom live in poor, informal settlements. A wealth of data has been diligently collected; we discuss the primary results later in this introduction.

Addressing the question of the causes of differentials in the levels of mortality, as well as the causes of changes in differential mortality, not only implies a careful reconstruction of individual life trajectories and population dynamics but also requires making some decisions about what constitutes a difference and what is regarded as an inequality. On this issue, Indian sociological studies are fascinating: Their discussion of the distinctions between castes and classes reminds us that social inequalities are not only economically rooted but are also culturally constructed, as are the processes of discrimination (Singh-Manoux et al. 2008). In this volume, the contributors defined a difference and assessed its impact on health and

[1] See http://www.indepth-network.org/

mortality using socioeconomic status, education, origin (migrants vs. natives), and religion.

There is also the need to take into account the urban environment whose details and differences interact with health and mortality in subtle and important ways. In all the studies presented here, the authors were aware of the classical redundancy between place of residence and social class. Impressive efforts have been made to record individual or household differences in urban spaces that are highly diverse. In historical Italy or Ireland, Alessio Fornassin, Alice Reid, and their colleagues used houses and housing conditions as a kind of total synthesis; others considered neighborhood characteristics. Regardless, the aim was not only to disentangle the two levels of explanation—inscription in socioeconomic structures and in urban structures—but also to identify the resulting accumulation of advantages or disadvantages.

Moreover, we must consider that the outcomes are also diverse—for example, dying in youth or in adulthood, from AIDS or from accidents—and, therefore, they do not necessarily result from the same causes.

1.2 Mortality Differentials Within Towns

Recently, Tommy Bengtsson and Frans Van Poppel (2011) proposed an in-depth assessment of our knowledge on the long-term changes in social mortality differentials. Till now, interpretations were essentially a story of convergence and/or divergence. For a long time, researchers thought social differences in mortality were modest during the Ancien Régime, increased in urban places during industrialization, then narrowed again thanks to the diffusion of modern hygienic infrastructures and the democratization of access to newly developed health services that culminated with the establishment of the welfare state.

Research coordinated by the same scholars, Bengtsson and Van Poppel (2011), have questioned these visions, as do all eleven chapters in this volume, adopting a newer perspective. Indeed, they all concern urban populations, not just by presenting long-term variations in the now-developed world but also by providing an in-depth assessment of the situation in low- and medium-income countries.

In that sense, they form a fruitful series for testing a theory on social inequalities in death that emerged in the mid-1990s and has rapidly gained large popularity. Elaborated by the epidemiologists Link and Phelan (1995; see also Phelan et al. 2004), this theory affirms that using a variety of indicators to assess the differentials within a population is not really useful since health and mortality inequalities can ultimately be reduced to a "fundamental cause": one's position in the socioeconomic hierarchy. From Link and Phelan perspective, the upper classes have higher-grade resources that they effectively use to cope with risks in terms of both anticipation and reaction. Moreover, those advantages are highly adaptive and are maintained regardless of the epidemiological regime. We consequently expect to observe this advantage of the elites, of the wealthy, everywhere—in the North and in the South—and always, in the past as well as today.

At the end of this introduction, we will show that the contributions of the researchers brought together in this volume both support and challenge this theory.

1.3 "Urban Graveyards," "Urban Penalty," or the Urban-Rural Mortality Gap from the Long-Term Perspective

Precisely because this book is about death in urban areas during the health transition, we also need to take into account the historical evolutions of the large mortality differentials between cities and the countryside, keeping in mind that both were (and are) connected by migration flows. From this point of view, Tony Wrigley (1967, 1969) proposed an "urban natural decrease model," characterizing early modern European cities as "urban graveyards," as early scholars such as Graunt, Malthus, and Weber had done previously (Graunt 1662; Woods 1989; Weber 1899). Wrigley observed that deaths were more numerous than births, with rural immigrants compensating for the population losses due to excess mortality, and concluded that the "city populations were only sustained due to migration" (Wrigley 1969).

In a paper published in 1978, Allan Sharlin reconsidered the question, defending an "urban migration model" in which migrants contributed to increased celibacy and age at first marriage and decreased birth rates in towns, all while substantially increasing the death rates since they came from relatively protected rural spaces and suddenly faced dangerous urban epidemiological environments characterized by more density and contacts and, generally, unhealthy conditions. While the models of Wrigley and Sharlin were theoretically consistent, their empirical assessment was deeply affected by the heuristic problems discussed above. Indeed, recent researchers have insisted on the impact of urban institutions, especially hospitals and foundling institutions, on urban death rates (Mooney et al. 1999; Ramiro Fariñas 2007). From a different perspective, Galley (1995) remembered that the motivations of rural migrants were not to compensate for urban losses but to find work and incomes, which depended on the urban economic dynamics.

From the eighteenth century in England and the nineteenth century in continental Europe and the United States, industrialization provoked massive flows of migrants. In its early days, modern economic growth produced the rapid urbanization of under-serviced neighborhoods. In the industrial British cities in the 1820s and 1830s; in Le Creusot, France, in the 1840s; in the booming East Belgian coal and steel towns in the 1840s–1860s; and as late as in 1900 in then-industrializing Bilbao, Spain, life expectancy at birth fell below 30 (Oris and Alter 2001).

In East Belgium, although the working conditions were dangerous and unhealthy, this epidemiological crisis in industrial cities during their initial phase of population explosion was associated with adult mortality below the national figures. This strange result is largely explained by the health selection of immigrants, which has been observed in other places, like Paris, for example (Alter and Oris 2005; Kesztenbaum and Rosenthal 2011).

Inversely, the same East Belgian industrial towns faced a terrible child excess mortality, especially after the age of weaning. From this observation confirming many testimonies by contemporary witnesses, it is easy to identify the culprits: the absence of safe water and milk, as well as the disruption of public hygiene and housing conditions resulting from the demographic explosion (Szreter and Mooney 1998). In nineteenth century Spain, we also observe a strong over-mortality not only of urban children aged 1–4 but also of adult males (Dopico and Reher 1998; Reher 2001; Pérez Moreda et al. 2004; Ramiro Fariñas 2008).

Several scholars consider that outmigration to industrial towns absorbed the demographic growth of most rural areas with a positive natural balance, which otherwise would have become overpopulated "rural slums," while at the same time the destinations of the rural migrants suffered much, including from the return of epidemics, especially cholera. This is the "paradox of growth," as cities that were the cradle of the economic expansion, of modern economic development, faced a terrible urban penalty over one or two generations (Szreter and Mooney 1998) while the countryside was untouched or even progressed. Quite probably, the urban–rural gap in life expectancy has never been so wide as during those times (Alter et al. 2004).

The pattern of advantageous mortality for adults and disadvantageous mortality for children was also observed in large, planned capitals. In Paris in the first half of the nineteenth century, massive flows of immigrants completely overpowered the city's sanitary infrastructures (see Preston and Haines 1991 or Kesztenbaum and Rosenthal in this volume). One question is whether Paris's size alone was a cause. At that time, the city was affected by serious excess mortality compared to France as a whole. Recently, Cain and Hong (2009) affirmed that the larger the city, the smaller one's chances of survival during the nineteenth century. Both the speediness of urbanization and the question of size can instruct our thoughts about recent changes in developing countries. Indeed, from the 1950s urban development in those parts of the world not only progressed at a rapid rate but also resulted in an explosion of large cities of one million inhabitants and over (Veron 2006).

Already in 1985, Paul Bairoch qualified these places as "Rome without empire" to describe their structural frailty. However, since at least the 1950s an "urban protective effect" has been obvious in the developing world, the main cause of which was the concentration of Western amenities, preventive programs, and medical facilities in towns. Although there is still a vivid debate on the timing of the transformation of Western urban areas from "graveyards" to "healthy places" (Kearns 1993; Reher 2001; Haines 2001), those elements explained that, in European populations, urban mortality declined more rapidly and the urban–rural mortality gap was closed in the 1920s or 1930s at the latest, followed by a long period of urban advantage or at least insignificant differences between urban and rural areas.

The classically accepted explanation is indeed that the diffusion of health and hygienic infrastructures in the urban space compensated for the inherently risky characteristics of the city, like density, contact, and pollution (Cain and Rotella 2001). In the newer epidemiological phase during which contagious diseases were replaced by chronic diseases as the main causes of death (Omran 1971; Caselli et al. 1999), the relative positions of cities have changed all across the world. Indeed, in the twentieth century, colonial and postcolonial cities benefited from Western technologies such that risk factors associated with rapid demographic growth and population size were managed by a combination of public health measures and urban planning structures (Woods 2003; Ramiro Fariñas 2008; Satterthwait 2011).

That urban advantage has significantly changed during the last few decades in developing countries, however. Indeed, since the mid-1980s, a process of convergence between cities and the countryside has appeared that is explained not by betterment in rural areas but mainly by the stagnation of progress in cities. It has been suggested that economic depression and adjustment policies limited the development of urban amenities while the population continued to grow (Philips and Verhasselt 1994). Even in a more accelerated manner with the continuous inflow of new citizens arriving from the countryside, especially in areas like Asia and Africa, in a process of rapid and chaotic urbanization, big cities will be the center of the political and population debate in the following years (UN-Habitat 2013). So, in the present and in the near future, we are and will be confronting themes regarding urban sustainability already experienced historically by other urban settlements in the past, such as how to build effective urban planning and management, how to deal with inadequate infrastructures, and how to solve the problem of the high incidence of slums and poverty (UN-Habitat 2013).

1.4 Slums in the Past and Today

In this context and in addition to demographic size and growth, recent research points to the horizontal extension and extensive land use associated with the impressive growth of slums everywhere in the developing world (except in China). Almost one-third of the urban population in the developing world is living in slums of one kind or another. Slums, as morphological forms of living environments, are the concrete manifestation in the urban landscape of the growing inequality in cities and the redistribution of poverty from the rural regions to towns, which is in opposition to the dominant view that—until recently—assumed better conditions for urban residents in terms of socioeconomic and human capital (Satterthwaite 2011; Kyu et al. 2013). We see here populations that are poorer, less endowed with resources, and obviously more vulnerable than their urban counterparts (Véron 2006), suggesting a growth of mortality differentials within the city that could be the cause of the stagnation of urban mortality as a whole that has been observed during the last decades (Konteh 2009; Rossier et al. 2014). This is a central concern in recent debates, and in this volume it is discussed in depth by Barthélémy Kuate Defo and Michel Garenne, while being a key point also in Fink et al.'s and Rossier et al.'s contributions. All four present original results that enrich our knowledge.

1.5 Eleven Contributions to Knowledge and Theories

Barbara Revuelta Eugercios and Diego Ramiro Fariñas's chapter provides an exemplary illustration of demographers' historical approaches and concerns. To understand infant mortality in a large capital city, Madrid, in the early twentieth century, they explored the deficiencies of registration and compositional effects, mainly due to the impact of a typical urban institution, the foundling hospital. Thanks to long and tedious work to develop linkages between various data sources, they identify causes of overestimation that are mainly due to massive migration flows. Revuelta Eugercios and Ramiro Fariñas demonstrate that part of the observed excess mortality can indeed be explained by factors that have to do with the production of the data used for estimating mortality, not with the actual environment of the city of Madrid. This lesson can be generalized beyond the case of the Spanish capital.

Indeed, in the nineteenth-century town of Guimarães, where both parish registers and *status animarum* have been used to construct a demographic–genealogical database through the parish reconstitution methodology, the impact of immigrants dying in the city hospital was much more limited than it would be in a huge, growing capital like Madrid. However, Norberta Amorin, Antero Ferreira, and Luis Machado show in their chapter the importance of right censoring, when young people avoided the risk of dying in Guimarães as a result of migrating to surrounding places or even to Brazil or the United States.

Along the same lines, Alessio Fornasin, Marco Breschi, and Matteo Manfredini offer a reconstruction of infant mortality precisely located in the urban space of Udine, the capital of Friuli in northeastern Italy, during the Napoleonic era, a period of modernization for the city's socioeconomic structures but of stagnation for its infrastructures. The authors explore an 1809 register listing 2100 houses and, for each, the number and rank of the soldiers who could potentially be lodged there, this information being a good indicator of housing quality. Each house was geo-coded, and this source was linked with the birth and death registers.

Using logistic regressions and a sophisticated geospatial analysis, Fornasin et al. identify a clear social gradient in infant mortality rates, that demonstrates the important negative impact of crowding on infant survival, and secondarily the role of housing quality. They find an important difference in infant mortality rates between a favorable area in the city center and two peripheral areas in which young children were at high risk. The latter presented an accumulation of four risk factors, two related to socioeconomic structures and two to the housing situation.

Working in depth on the physical urban environment, specifically assessing the quality of the house to measure its impact on child mortality, is also what Alice Reid, Eilidh Garrett, and Simon Szreter did with the capital of Northern Ireland, Belfast. In the early twentieth century, housing quality appears as a crucial variable since it is at this level that population density can be read as overcrowding and that we can consider the existence or absence of ventilation, facilities for cooking, access to water supplies, sewage, etc., as well as owner or renter status and the amount of rent. Housing quality reveals the inhabitants' position in both the socioeconomic and the urban structures. However, this variable is still often neglected because of a lack of data. Reid et al. tediously worked to link a sample from the 1911 census in Belfast with the 1901 census and the street directories. They located people and their moves from house to house in Belfast's urban spaces (see the maps in the appendix of their chapter).

Alice Reid, Eilidh Garrett, and Simon Szreter make very clear that internal mobility was so intense that it could significantly bias explanatory analyses that wrongly assume stability in a given environment. In their study of child mortality in early twentieth-century Belfast, they show, for example, that fewer than 20 % of household heads in 1911 had been living in the same house in 1901. Thus, using data from the 1911 census to assess the impact of environmental conditions on children's deaths during the previous 10 years consequently appears highly questionable. The authors linked various data sources at individual and family levels (see above and their chapter for more details). They show that mobility in the urban space was highly related to socioeconomic status (SES)—with clear signs of chronic insecurity for unskilled daily laborers—and at specific stages of family life, such as during the foundation of a new family. Moreover, they find that housing conditions were connected to wealth but had a distinct impact on child mortality even when controlling for parental SES, the quality of the house in 1901 being more informative than the same variable in 1911.

Reto Schumacher's chapter considers the variables that put individuals in a position of risk in urban social and economic structures: through a sophisticated statistical approach that combines hazard models and sequence analysis (an approach that is an important contribution in itself), he captures the interactions between reproductive behaviors and infant and child mortality at the family level. He observes death clustering in the context of nineteenth-century Geneva, which implies that a significant proportion of infant and child deaths came from a limited number of families, whereas some 60 % of the area's families did not experience child death at all.

Schumacher shows that the rhythm of childbearing did not systematically affect an infant's chances of survival until his or her first birthday. But upper-class families were underrepresented in the group with high infant or child mortality risk and overrepresented in the low infant mortality group. The migratory status of the parents, however, was not significant. Reto Schumacher not only disentangles the respective impacts of fertility behaviors and statuses but also demonstrates that the death of a previous sibling (and the timing of this death) sometimes negatively affected the survival chances of the index child, whereas it sometimes had a positive effect in families that shared similar characteristics. This between-family heterogeneity suggests differential parental behaviors, which are usually difficult to assess through historical data.

Marco Breschi, Massimo Esposito, Stanislao Mazzoni, and Lucia Pozzi reconstructed infant and child mortality in the town of Alghero (Sardinia) for cohorts born in 1866–1930. They show that urban children benefited from a clear advantage compared to their rural counterparts. This rare situation in the European context of that time can be explained by the high prevalence of malaria in remote areas.

Breschi, Esposito, Mazzoni, and Pozzi had the rare opportunity to contrast the old town of Alghero with a new area established in the early twentieth century and designed according to modern sanitary and hygienic principles. Multivariate modeling demonstrates the protective effect of the new environment in the post-weaning phase of children's lives. The impact was real but limited for the children of the well-off, while it was tremendous for children in unskilled/lower-skilled families, with a 60 % decrease in mortality risk.

Such results do not support the fundamental cause theory, which assumes members of the upper classes are systematically the first to benefit from improvements. However, more in line with Link and Phelan's vision, Marco Breschi and his colleagues demonstrate the existence of a social mortality differential that is more obvious in the post-weaning phase and presents more of a contrast between elites and others than a clear SES gradient.

The "fundamental cause" theory is central in Lionel Kesztenbaum and Jean-Laurent Rosenthal's study of the French capital, Paris, from 1870 to 1940. They demonstrate not only that the city was on average a more dangerous place to live than the country as a whole but also that it was the place where inequality in terms of death was by far the highest. Small-scale data on 80 neighborhoods for the period 1881–1911 indicate a gap of 14 years in life expectancy between the most and the least favored "quartiers" of Paris. Kesztenbaum and Rosenthal show the point at which those large differences can be explained by the spatial distribution of income and wealth. The latter, in their view, is not the only explanation but nevertheless the dominant one since, for example, the wealthiest were the first to benefit from the city's transformation, especially the construction of hygienic infrastructures. Indeed, the relationship between mortality and income was revealed to be stable across time, while mortality as a whole declined; it is this decline that leads to the democratization of longevity and gives the poor a chance to become old, not a reduction of social inequality in death. In this way, Kesztenbaum and Rosenthal's results clearly support the fundamental cause theory.

Moving through time and space, Barthélémy Kuate Defo exploits an impressive series of 217 Demographic Health Surveys from 86 countries nested within 13 regions on 4 continents, covering the period from 1985 to 2009. He explores the changes over time and space in covariates of infant mortality in urban and rural environments while addressing the issue of variability in exposure and outcome variables. First, the methodology is similar to that used by Kesztenbaum and Rosenthal, i.e., the transformation of repeated cross-sectional surveys in panel data. However, Kuate Defo additionally develops a multilevel approach specific to his contribution. The results show that, among urban populations, infant mortality is closely associated with low parental human capital (education) as well as access to public goods (specifically, health services and electricity). The appearance of an unmet need for family planning as a major determinant confirms the importance of access to health infrastructures and of considering babies' chances of survival in the framework of reproductive health. Barthélémy Kuate Defo strongly defends the importance of studying individuals within populations to carefully consider the impact of aggregates. In dangerous urban contexts, an individual behavior like long and exclusive breastfeeding is the best protection for young children.

Michel Garenne's contribution is centered on Africa. Using some 90 DHS for 37 countries, covering more than 90 % of the Sub-Saharan African population, he first reconstructed the mortality trends for children younger than 5 from 1950 to 2005. From the middle of the twentieth century until 1985, we can speak of a "rural penalty" because the progress in living conditions, education, preventive and curative health programs, and infrastructures were concentrated in towns. From the mid-1980s, however, the decline continued to be sustained in the rural world, while mortality levels stagnated in the cities.

To explain this new feature, which the experts had not anticipated, Garenne focused his second study on three countries where the mortality of children had recently become lower as an "urban penalty" reappeared: Tanzania, Zambia, and Sierra Leone. He assessed the respective impacts of the main determinants and concluded that health programs (especially vaccinations) were more beneficial to rural populations during the last two or three decades, while emerging diseases (especially HIV/AIDS) penalized the urban populations. As far as socioeconomic variables (wealth, education) are concerned, it is not that they have no effect on infant and child mortality, but they do not explain the urban–rural convergence, at least in the three countries studied.

Finally, when looking at the curves at the continental level, we can suppose the urban penalty will become a general feature of African demography. However, HIV is an important factor, and since 2005, infected people have benefited from important improvements in medical treatments. The future has yet to be written.

Günther Fink, Isabel Günther, and Kenneth Hill assessed the role of slums in the mortality transition. They started with an idea that has recently been advanced: in a context of rapid and chaotic urbanization, the development of slums slows down the mortality decline since infants and children face higher risks in those pockets of extreme poverty. This could be an explanation of the stagnation of the urban mortality of children under five in Africa, which was observed by Garenne (in this volume) and Bocquier (2011). Fink et al. considered low- and medium-income countries and used 72 DHS for 37 countries, half of them in Sub-Saharan Africa. They proposed an ad hoc definition of slums at a community, but not a household, level and established a distinction between rural areas, small towns, and large cities, as well as the slums within the latter two municipality types. Finally, they reconstructed neonatal mortality, post-neonatal mortality, and mortality from 1 to 3 years of age.

Their results show that, in this sample of countries, there is still a significant and large "urban protection effect." However, they also confirmed the existence of profound differences within towns and cities. Indeed, mortality risks for children from the slums are higher than for other urban children and similar to the levels observed in rural areas. Regarding the composition of the populations at risk in the different living environments, the educational level of mothers appears to be the most important variable contributing to observed mortality differentials. Once again, with a less-than-strict environmental effect, we see a combination of penalties acting to explain the variations in under-three mortality.

A comparison with pre- and post-2000 DHS by Fink, Günther, and Hill demonstrates that mortality in rural areas still benefits from a sustained decline that is two times faster than in urban areas. But, quite astonishingly, slum inhabitants do as well as rural dwellers, with more improvements than in the rest of the urban areas. Fink and his colleagues conclude that the pessimistic vision, the one suggesting that slums will have a negative impact on the mortality transition, is not justified.

The scale drastically changes when Clémentine Rossier, Abdramane Soura, Bruno Lankoande, and Roch Millogo explore the richness of the *Ouagadougou Health and Demographic Surveillance System.* Looking originally at the relationship between poverty and mortality in small children and adults, the authors first observed that children of poor and uneducated parents are twice as likely to die as others children. Their analyses considered the causes of death and suggested this large mortality differential in fact results from differences in access to preventive and curative health care. The unsanitary environment of informal areas produces a similar, significant impact on child mortality. The redundancies of institutional and environmental penalties are clear. However, adult mortality pattern seems to be inversed and counterintuitive: indeed, the risks are higher in the formal, wealthier neighborhoods. It seems adult health behaviors are similar across the city, but affluent adults are more often overweight and more likely to be HIV positive. However, education remains a protection because it is associated with a larger and more rapid use of medical care.

1.6 Death in Cities During Health Transitions

Death in cities is a crucial topic that transcends classical temporal and spatial boarders. Although nothing can be simply transposed, we demonstrate that historical demographers and demographers indeed have a lot to learn from each other. The eleven contributions that form this volume concretely show how researchers can face heuristic challenges through elegant articulations of data, methods, and theories. The potential of both historical and contemporary sources is demonstrated and will hopefully inspire new research. The assessment of housing quality and the measure of infrastructure accessibility proved to be especially fruitful. The same can be said of the many methodological developments proposed here to deal with the inscription of social positions and demographic behaviors in the urban spaces through mapping using geographic information systems or to cope with mobile populations by considering out-migrations, immigrations, or internal moves. The transformation of repeated panel data into (almost) longitudinal data and the combination of hazard models and sequence analysis should also be cited as important innovations.

Among the theories, the results accumulated in this volume sometimes support the perspective that socioeconomic inequalities are the fundamental cause of mortality differentials impacting the survival chances of urban populations with all other factors dependent upon the individual or family position in the social hierarchy. For example, the sources of evidence from nineteenth- and early-twentieth-century Paris and Geneva support this theory. However, the findings are more mixed in Alghero, where researchers were able to demonstrate that new urban amenities could benefit the lower classes more than the elites. And in Africa, contemporary data on Ouagadougou are simply not consistent with a "survival of the rich" and "disappearance of the poor" hypothesis (see Clark and Cummins 2009); our colleagues' results are more complicated, with the pattern of infant and child mortality supporting Link and Phelan's theory but the pattern for adults being exactly the opposite.

From a more empirical perspective, this volume provides repeated demonstrations that, even when one variable is dominant, identifying the redundancy of penalties is crucial not only for understanding death inequalities in the cities but also and consequently for properly designing policy answers. Any attempt to cope with the complexity of determinants and outcomes implies consideration of the interactions between places and classes in urban areas, which are also political and institutional spaces. Whether we approach the environmental effects on mortality through the urban–rural gap or through mortality differentials within the city, it systematically reveals the importance of institutions and policies, a point we did not anticipate when this collective research effort was initiated but that has clearly emerged from the results.

Cities have always pioneered collective answers to health changes. For example, until the early twentieth century urban hospitals were primarily used by disadvantaged populations, resulting in substantial effects on urban mortality estimates (see Revuelta and Ramiro here). But since the second half of the nineteenth century, the impact of public hygienic infrastructures has been recognized everywhere. Sanitary policies and their resulting programs explained the first closing of the urban–rural gap in the developed world, then the formation of an urban advantage in both wealthy and developing societies, and finally more recently the rural catch-up with the (relatively) low child mortality levels in the cities of the South. Kuate Defo's multi-continental perspective, Garenne's research on Africa, and Rossier and colleagues' in-depth analysis on one city, Ouagadougou, all consistently demonstrate that access to public goods as well as preventive and curative medicine is absolutely decisive, confirming the importance of a city's political and institutional management.

At the intersection of urban space, socioeconomic structures, and political management of cities, the situation in the slums of low- and medium-income countries is difficult, with redundant penalties. But at the same time, the expansion of the slums and of the population living in them does not appear to be a credible explanation for the urban–rural mortality convergence observed in the developing parts of the world since the mid-1980s.

Altogether, the data and methods elaborated by the authors of this volume, along with their results and theoretical discussions, represent a substantial step in our understanding of death in cities during the health transition, both yesterday and today. They contribute many elements to the crucial debates about sustainable city development in a world that is mostly driven by big urban areas.

*

**

As noted above, this volume is the result of a workshop organized in Seville, Spain, in mid-December 2011 by the IUSSP Panel of Historical Demography, the Spanish Council for Scientific Research, and the Andalusian Institute of Statistics and Cartography, with the support of the Institute of Statistics and Cartography of Andalusia (IECA), the European Social Fund, the Spanish National Research Council (CSIC), and the Ministry of Science and Innovation of Spain (MICINN) Grant CSO2011-15189-E. We want to express our gratitude to the organizing committee and the Institute of Statistics and Cartography of Andalusia for hosting this workshop, as well as to the anonymous reviewers of this volume whose comments were so useful.

References

Alter, G., & Oris, M. (2005). Childhood conditions, migration and mortality: Migrants and natives in 19th-century cities. *Social Biology, 52*(3/4), 178–191.

Alter, G., Neven, M., & Oris, M. (2004). Mortality and modernization in sart and surroundings. In T. Bengtsson, C. Campbell, & J. Lee (Eds.), *Life under pressure. Mortality and living standards in Europe and Asia, 1700–1900* (pp. 173–208). Cambridge, MA/London: The MIT Press.

Bairoch, P. (1985). *De Jéricho à Mexico. Villes et économies dans l'histoire*. Paris: Gallimard.

Bengtsson, A., & Van Poppel, F. (2011). Socioeconomic inequalities in death from past to present: An introduction. *Explorations in Economic History, 48*, 343–356.

Bengtsson, T., Campbell, C., Lee, J. Z., et al. (2004). *Life under pressure. Mortality and living standards in Europe and Asia, 1700–1900*. Cambridge, MA: The MIT Press.

Bocquier, P., Madise, N. J., & Zulu, E. M. (2011). Is there an urban advantage in child survival in Sub-Saharan Africa? Evidence from 18 countries in the 1990s. *Demography, 48*(2), 531–558.

Cain, L., & Hong, S. C. (2009). Survival in 19th century cities: The larger the city, the smaller your chances. *Explorations in Economic History, 46*(4), 450–463.

Cain, L., & Rotella, E. (2001). Death and spending: Urban mortality and municipal expenditure on sanitation. *Annales de Démographie Historique, 1*, 139–154.

Caselli, G., Meslé, Fr., & Vallin, J. (1999). Le triomphe de la médecine. In *Histoire des populations de l'Europe*. T. 3. *Les temps incertains, 1914–1988* (pp. 126–181). Paris: Fayard.

Clark, G., & Cummins, N. (2009). Urbanization, mortality, and fertility in Malthusian England. *American Economic Review: Papers & Proceedings, 99*(2), 242–247.

Dopico, F., & Reher, D. S. (1998). *El declive de la mortalidad en España, 1860–1930* (Monografias, Vol. I). Zaragoza: Asociación de Demografía Histórica.

Galley, C. (1995). A model of early modern urban demography. *Economic History Review, 48*(3), 448–469.

Graunt, J. (1662/1973). 'Natural and political observations and conclusions made upon the bills of mortality.' In P. Laslett (Ed.), *The earliest classics: John Graunt and Gregory King*. (Pioneers of demography series). Westmead: Gregg International.

Günther, I., & Harttgen, K. (2012). Deadly cities? Spatial inequalities in mortality in Sub-Saharan Africa. *Population and Development Review, 38*(3), 469–486.
Haines, M. (2001). The urban mortality transition in the United States, 1800–1940. *Annales de Démographie Historique, 1*, 33–64.
Kearns, G. (1993). Le handicap urbain et le déclin de la mortalité en Angleterre et au Pays de Galles, 1851–1900. *Annales de Démographie Historique*, 75–105.
Kesztenbaum, L., & Rosenthal, J.-L. (2011). The health cost of living in a city: The case of France at the end of the 19th century. *Explorations in Economic History, 48*, 207–225.
Konteh, F. (2009). Urban sanitation and health in the developing world: Reminiscing the nineteenth century industrial nations. *Health & Place, 15*(1), 69–78.
Kyu, H. H., Shannon, H. S., Georgiades, K., & Boyle, H. (2013). Association of urban slum residency with infant mortality and child stunting in low and middle income countries. *BioMed Research International, 2013*, 1–12.
Link, B. G.,& Phelan, J. C. (1995). Social conditions as fundamental causes of disease. *Journal of Health and Social Behavior, 35*, 80–94 extra issue.
Mooney, G., Luckin, B., & Tanner, A. (1999). Patient pathways: Solving the problem of institutional mortality in London during the later nineteenth century. *Social History of Medicine, 12*(2), 227–269.
Omran, A. R. (1971). "The epidemiologic transition. A theory of the epidemiology of population change". *The Milbank Memorial Fund Quarterly*, Vol. XLIX, 4, part 1, pp. 509–538.
Oris, M. (2003). The history of migrations as a chapter in the history of the European rural family. *The History of the Family. An International Quarterly, 8*(2), 187–215.
Oris, M., & Alter, G. (2001). Paths to the city and roads to death. Mortality and migration in East Belgium during the industrial revolution. *Revue Belge d'Histoire Contemporaine, 31*, 453–495.
Pérez Moreda, V., Ramiro Fariñas, D., & Sanz Gimeno, A. (2004). Dying in the city: Urban mortality in Spain in the middle of the health transition, 1900–1931. In C. Corsini & E. Sonnino (Ed.), *Living in the City (14th–20th Centuries)*. Rome: Centro Stampa d'Ateneo of the University of Rome "La Sapienza".
Phelan, J. C., Link, B. G., Diez-Roux, A., Kawachi, I., & Levin, B. (2004). 'Fundamental causes' of social inequalities in mortality: A test of the theory. *Journal of Health and Social Behavior, 45*(3), 265–285.
Philips, D. R., & Verhasselt, Y. (1994). *Health and development*. London: Routledge.
Preston, S. H., & Haines, M. R. (1991). *Fatal years. Child mortality in late nineteenth century America*. Princeton: Princeton University Press.
Ramiro Fariñas, D. (2007). Mortality in hospitals and mortality in the city in the nineteenth- and twentieth century Spain: The effect on the measurement of urban mortality rates of the mortality outsiders in urban health institutions. In J. Henderson, P. Horden, & A. Pastore (Eds.), *The impact of hospitals, 300–2000* (pp. 395–416). Oxford: Peter Lang AG.
Ramiro Fariñas, D. (2008). Il declino della mortalita durante l'infanzia nella Spagna urbana e rurale, 1860–1930. *Storia Urbana, 31*(119), 125–148.
Reher, D. S. (2001). In search of the urban penalty. Exploring urban and rural mortality patterns in Spain during the demographic transition. *International Journal of Population Geography, 7*, 105–127.
Rossier, C., Bassiahi Soura, A., Duthé, G., Lankoande, B., & Millogo, R. (2014). Are the urban poor really worse off? Socioeconomic differentials in adult cause specific mortality at the periphery of Ouagadougou, Burkina Faso. *Revue Quetelet, 2*(2), 61–80.
Satterthwait, D. (2011). Why is urban health so poor even in many successful cities? *Environment and Urbanization, 23*(1), 5–11.
Sharlin, A. (1978). Natural decrease in early modern cities: A reconsideration. *Past and Present, 79*(1), 126–138.

Singh-Manoux, A., Dugravot, A., Davey Smith, G., Subramanyam, M., & Subramanian, S. V. (2008). Adult education and child mortality in India: The influence of caste, household wealth, and urbanization. *Epidemiology, 19*(2), 294–301.

Szreter, S., & Mooney, G. (1998). Urbanization, mortality, and the standard of living debate: New estimates of the expectation of life at birth in nineteenth-century British cities. *Economic History Review, 51*(1), 84–112.

UN-Habitat. (2013). *State of the world's cities 2012/2013. Prosperity of cities*. New York: UN-Habitat, Routledge.

Véron, J. (2006). *L'urbanisation du monde*. Paris: La Découverte.

Weber, A. F. (1899). *The growth of cities in the nineteenth century: A study in statistics*. New York: MacMillan Company.

Woods, R. I. (1989). What would one need to know to solve the "natural decrease in early modern cities" problem? In R. Lawton (Ed.), *The rise and fall of great cities* (pp. 80–95). London: Belhaven Press.

Woods, R. I. (2003). Urban-rural mortality differentials: An unresolved debate. *Population and Development Review, 29*(1), 29–46.

Wrigley, E. A. (1967). A simple model of London's importance in changing english society and economy 1650-1750. *Past & Present, 37*(Jul.), 44–70.

Wrigley, E. A. (1969). *Population and history*. London: McGraw-Hill.

Part I
Mortality Within the City: Historical Europe

Chapter 2
Understanding Infant Mortality in the City: Exploring Registration and Compositional Effects. Madrid, 1905–1906

Bárbara A. Revuelta Eugercios and Diego Ramiro Fariñas

2.1 Introduction

The existence of the "urban penalty" in historical Europe, that is, an excess mortality in urban settings when compared with rural areas, has been explained by population housing and working conditions, social networks and living arrangements, as well as with higher exposure to infectious disease and ease of transmission that are typical of urban areas. However, some scholars have suggested that part of the excessive mortality could also be explained by other urban phenomena: registration inaccuracy and compositional effects in the computations. There could be large disparities between the numbers of individuals at risk and their corresponding events interfering with the proper computation of rates in a context with difficulties in maintaining an accurate registration system. Also, compositional effects could arise in a context of extensive migration where the presence of heterogeneous subpopulations with a different health composition or living in particular urban

This work comprises part of the results of two projects funded by the Spanish Ministry of Science and Innovation (SEJ–2005–06334, CSO2008–06130/SOCI and CSO2011-29970) undertaken at the Spanish National Research Council, as well as part of the program UCM–CSIC–UNED 2007/HUM–0517 and "Grupo de Estudios Dinámicas Demográficas del CSIC." This research was also supported by the Centre of Economic Demography at Lund University by means of postdoctoral research funding. We would like to acknowledge the work of A.B. Castillo Belmonte, B. Villuendas and S. Planta who helped with with the linkage of the Madrid dataset.

B.A. Revuelta Eugercios (✉)
Copenhagen Centre for Health Research in the Humanities, Copenhagen, Denmark
e-mail: barbara.revuelta@hum.ku.dk

D. Ramiro Fariñas
Institute of Economics, Geography and Demography (IEGD-CCHS-CSIC), Spanish National Research Council, CCHS-CSIC, Albasanz 26-28, Madrid 28037, Spain
e-mail: diego.ramiro@cchs.csic.es

D. Ramiro Fariñas, M. Oris (eds.), *New Approaches to Death in Cities during the Health Transition*, International Studies in Population 12,
DOI 10.1007/978-3-319-43002-7_2

environments could exert an excessive weight over the estimations. If these processes influenced urban mortality rates, it is very important to have a thorough comprehension of their impact, as mortality computations are crucial to understand urban environments.

All age groups show signs of excess mortality, but it was particularly important for working-age adults with more mobility whom are especially difficult to study. Conversely, infancy was an age group where urban-rural differences were rather narrow, as infant health and mortality are more influenced by family characteristics and behaviour and less sensitive to wider environmental or economic shocks as, for example, early childhood mortality. However, many studies have chosen to study urban-rural differentials for children as the infant mortality rate is considered a general measure of population health and is very straightforward to compute. Additionally, infant mortality measures are key, not only for understanding the environment of the city, but also for life-table computations and for studying later-life mortality or urban residents.

The aim of this chapter is to analyze whether factors associated with registration and compositional effects heavily affect our view of urban mortality for the city of Madrid around the turn of the century. Two sources of possible interference with mortality measures have been analyzed. First, we have studied the influence that inaccurate registration could have on infant mortality estimations with particular attention to the large number of migrants present in the city. And, secondly, we have assessed to what extent there were important compositional effects in the mortality estimations from two sub-groups. These are the children cared for in the main charity institution for children in the city, the compound Maternity Hospital-Foundling Hospital, which showed a very different mortality experience, and the children born to migrant mothers who were potentially affected by the difference in living conditions between their mother's place of origin and the city.

2.2 What Drives the Urban Penalty? Old and New Explanations

Until well into the twentieth century, Western cities were considered demographic sinks. There was an "urban penalty"[1] in terms of reduced survival probabilities for their residents (Woods 2003). Contemporaries noted the extreme mortality that characterized cities. Malthus referred to cities as graveyards in the eighteenth and nineteenth century (1826) and Weber emphasized that people died more rapidly in cities than in rural areas (1899). Local doctors and reformers also wrote about specific contexts, such as Revenga, who described Madrid as "the city of death" (1901). Aggregated and individual-level urban and rural data for several countries show that

[1] A good illustration of this debate can be found in Wrigley (1967, 1969), Sharlin (1978, 1981), Finlay (1981), Keyfitz (1980), Van de Woude (1982), Woods (1989), Hammel and Mason (1993), Galley (1995), Lee (1999), Ramiro Fariñas (2007, 2008).

these differentials were at work before and during the initial phases of the demographic transition (Kearns 1988; Woods et al. 1989; Preston and Haines 1991; Galley 1995; Williams and Galley 1995; Woods and Shelton 2000; Reher 2001; Bengtsson and Van Poppel 2011). Moreover, this penalty was also present when considering other health measures, such as height (Steckel and Floud 1997; Komlos and Baten 1998; Baten and Murray 2000) or when different age groups were taken into consideration.

This terrible image of cities can be explained, to a large extent, by two features: they were poles of attraction for the working-age population and functioned as administrative centres. The first occasioned a continuous inflow of rural population fleeing from the country, as cities boasted of larger and more diverse employment opportunities. When Sharlin (1978) developed his "urban migration" model, he considered that the arrival of migrants in the cities changed the balance between births and deaths, since the migrants, according to his theory, inflated the number of deaths, while contributing far less to the number of births than did the permanent residents. In terms of mortality, the obvious impact would be an increase in the number of deaths of persons of working age.

As administrative centers, cities had to sustain institutions, such as hospitals, prisons, retirement homes and foundling hospitals, which were characterized by high mortality rates. Their impact on urban mortality was accentuated because sections of the institutional population were not usually resident in the cities but in the contiguous rural areas (Ramiro 2007). An important unresolved issue is whether living conditions in the cities were really that bad and whether due allowance in the measurement of mortality has been accorded to the fact that the cities were the administrative centers and poles of attraction for migrants.

In general, however, only some aspects of life in the city have been deemed as responsible for this increased mortality. Poor and unsanitary conditions, along with deficient or insufficient public health measures or infrastructures created and maintained infection foci; high population densities and crowding facilitated the spread of infections; the close proximity of urban life implied more frequent and close contact with neighbors; and the shared use of resources, particularly food and water, increased the likelihood of contagion. The continuous arrival of individuals kept endemic diseases alive in the city, but it also brought new epidemics (Preston and Van de Walle 1978:278, Reher 2001:105). In short, the very poor quality of urban infrastructure and the large influx of poor migrants have been considered jointly responsible for most of the excess urban mortality in the past (Cain and Hong 2009).

The urban-rural differential in mortality was reversed during the early twentieth century as the mortality decline started earlier and gained momentum faster in urban areas. Public health measures, sanitation and sewage have been associated with a decreased prevalence of infectious disease and have been well documented in several cities (Preston and Van de Walle 1978). Additional factors that played a role in demographic modernization, such as increased education, higher wealth and improved living standards, also evolved earlier in cities than in rural areas (Reher 2001).

Evidence put forward by other scholars, however, suggest that processes behind the composition of urban populations and the registration of their vital events may also have helped to shape the observed excess mortality. Among them, two are particularly relevant: registration accuracy and compositional effects. Adequate accuracy in the registration of population and events is a key prerequisite for reliable mortality estimates as defective registration can distort our vision of urban mortality (Librero López et al. 1993; Librero López and Benavides 1995; Boyle 2004, Ocaña-Riola et al. 2009). Where no population registries were maintained, as in the city of Madrid, the inability to enforce complete vital registration may have produced underreporting or inaccuracy of the data used for estimating mortality levels. If deaths tended to be accurately reported but a sizeable proportion of individuals living in the city were likely to live unregistered, then mortality estimations could be severely overestimated. That could be very well the case of migrants (Remund 2010). This problem is not restricted to turn-of-the-century urban areas, as there is ample evidence of its effect in contexts with a high migration influx and a corresponding inability to enforce accurate registration, such as in contemporary Spanish touristic coastal areas until recently (Librero López et al. 1993; Librero López and Benavides 1995).

Attention has additionally been drawn to the compositional or selection effects that sub-groups of the population can have on general estimations. Clearly, the health of migrants was a combination of previous health and the consequences of integration (or lack thereof) in the city and these individual differences, aggregated, could have large effects on the measures of the destination area (Boyle 2002, 2004; Ocaña-Riola et al. 2009). For example, heavy out-migration of young and healthy individuals to a new area could “improve” the general mortality estimates of that place. The opposite effect would occur with the migration of sick or unhealthy people to urban areas in search of medical care.

The overall health effects of migrants in mortality estimations is impossible to generalize as there is mixed evidence for the effect of urban life on migrants’ health: some authors have found better health upon arrival in the city, as well as a progressive deterioration with time, as others have found worse health for different types of causes of death (Oris and Alter 2001; Alter and Oris 2005, 2008; Cain and Hong 2009; Kesztenbaum and Rosenthal 2011). As a result, the combined effect of those differences, when all inhabitants of the city are pooled together, is hard to anticipate. In any case, it probably it could have been very important, as in most European cities migrants accounted for large sections of the population (almost 50 % of the residents in Madrid in 1900).

A more localized compositional effect could arise from the presence of charity or health institutions in the city. Their role cannot be separated from their urban settings as they were institutions only found in urban areas that not only offered services to the city but to the surrounding hinterland (Ramiro Fariñas 2007). Two features, however, make them likely candidates to produce urban mortality miss-representation: they attracted individuals from the frailest end of the health distribution from both within and beyond the city; and the environments where inmates lived and the treatment received involved a set of risk factors different than that affecting urban dwellers (Revuelta Eugercios 2011).

The first issue is related to the role of cities as attraction poles of population from the hinterland. The presence of such migrants in the city would be expected to worsen urban mortality because only the more fragile individuals would resort to the city. Additionally, this phenomenon would be likely intertwined with the under-registration of migrants but also movers within the city (Mooney et al. 1999). The second feature is exemplified by the extreme mortality that characterized the population of foundlings, whose low survival probabilities were related to feeding practices and institutional environment that no urban babies faced (Revuelta Eugercios 2011).

It is unclear, however, to what extent the potential problems described above could significantly affect mortality estimations. On the one hand, infants are less mobile than young adults and the period that elapsed from birth to death should limit registration problems. On the other hand, institutions such as foundling hospitals cared for children who were characterized by extreme mortality, which could heavily influence aggregated computations.

Accordingly, a better grasp on the processes behind infant mortality rate computations is relevant for two reasons: on the one hand, it can help us to understand the differences between urban and rural mortality experiences when using more general measures, such as life expectancy, which are heavily affected by infant deaths. And, on the other hand, it can also help us to shed light on the later-life mortality of urban dwellers due to the impact of early life experiences on later life (Bengtsson and Lindström 2003; Bengtsson and Broström 2009; Gagnon and Mazan 2009).

2.3 The Longitudinal Historical Dataset for the City of Madrid and the Foundling Hospital of Madrid Database

We have used the Longitudinal Historical Dataset for the City of Madrid (LHISTDATA-MAD) and the Foundling Hospital of Madrid Database (FHMD). The LHISTDATA-MAD is an ongoing project linking census and vital statistics at the individual level with a linked Spatial Data Infrastructure (HISDI-MAD) for the city of Madrid around 1900.

We obtained birth information for 1905 and 1906 from the Civil Register of the City and its records include information on the date of birth, sex and name of the new-born; and the name and two surnames of the father and mother, as well as their age and place of birth. We also obtained death information from Civil Register records, which includes date of death and of death registration; cause of death; place of death and district; and the individual's personal details: name and two surnames, age, sex, occupation, marital status and place of birth. Total numbers amount to 32,695 births and 6659 infant deaths.

We only attempted to link infant deaths (children dying younger than 1 year of age) that occurred in 1905 and 1906 if their "computed birth" (death date minus age at death) had occurred in our period of observation (i.e., after January 1, 1905). Thus, from a total number of 3192 infant deaths in 1905, we only considered 1905 cases (60 % of the deaths). For 1906, we considered the full 3471 deaths. Lastly, we also excluded deaths belonging to infants reported as born outside of the city (2 and 4 % of cases), leaving 1861 deaths in 1905 and 3320 deaths in 1906. The total success rate of the linkage process was 88.46 %, slightly better for 1906 (90.48 %) than for 1905 (84.85 %).

The Foundling Hospital of Madrid Database is a source that has already been compiled from the archives of the Foundling Hospital of Madrid for the period between 1890 and 1935 that contains the life-histories until age 5–7 of all children ever institutionalized in that period, 59,301. We extracted information from the Admission Books (*Libros de Entrada*) and the Entries and Exits books (*Libros de Entradas y Salidas*). Jointly, they provide information on the characteristics of abandonment (specific means of admission to the institution and date), children's characteristics (sex, age and name), family information (name, surnames, age, marital status, place of birth and occupation of mothers) and information regarding their stay in the institution, placement in the countryside and death, if it took place.[2] We also linked these records to the Civil Registers for 1905–1906 and had a success rate of 97 and 99 % of cases.

We have computed aggregated mortality rates and rates derived from published and individual-level data to assess the differences in mortality estimations according to the quality and accuracy of the data used. For aggregated mortality rates, we have computed traditional cohort estimations, as well as real cohort estimations. In all estimations, in order to overcome the problems involved by under-registration of deaths during the first day of life, we have corrected neonatal and infant mortality estimations by adding an inflator factor used by Ramiro and Sanz (2000a, 2000b).[3]

We have classified the diagnostics of cause of death with the schema designed by Bernabeu et al. (2003) that codes causes of death following the classification Bertillon created in 1900 and a modified classification based on McKeown's work. The classification criterion used is aetiological in order to help us shed light on different environments and epidemiological patterns. Additionally, we have used logistic regressions to assess the validity of the linkage between births and deaths, explaining the probabilities of finding a corresponding birth to a given infant death according to a set of variables. We have also used event-history analysis (Cox regression) to model differences in infant mortality according to mother's place of origin.

[2] More information on the specifics of this dataset can be found in Revuelta Eugercios (2011).

[3] Deaths in the first day of life are estimated according to the formula 0.0043 + 0.023xIMR, which is added to the actual computed IMR. For additional explanation on this methodology, see Ramiro and Sanz 2000a, b.

2.4 Effects of Miss-Registration on the Estimation of Infant Mortality

There is ample evidence of an urban penalty on mortality and other health measures in Spain, both for the country as a whole but also for different regions and cities (Quiroga 2001; Reher 2001; Pérez Moreda et al. 2004; Martínez Carrión and Moreno-Lázaro 2007). However, the differences in Spain were not as clear cut as they were in other places. Mortality was worse in the biggest and smallest urban areas, the latter experienced the problems of big cities, such as being administrative and health and charity provision centers, but did not acquire the infrastructures that were being implemented in larger cities until very late.

Modern estimations for Madrid for the late nineteenth and early twentieth century confirm the poor population health described by contemporary doctors (Hauser 1902). The decline of infant and early childhood mortality had started in the last decades of the nineteenth century but, by 1900, Madrid still showed an excess of infant and early childhood mortality when compared with any other city or town (Pérez Moreda et al. 2004). However, urban-rural infant mortality differences were relatively small when compared with other indicators, such as early childhood mortality.

The inversion of the relationship between the capital and the rural areas took place in the mid-1920s as in many other parts of Europe. However, in this chapter we examine whether the difference between urban and rural areas has been, at all times, overestimated using data for Madrid. In this section, we have focused on understanding to what extent incomplete registration could play a part in this image of excess mortality in Madrid that we see in aggregated estimations by focusing on the presence of migrants and registration deficiencies.

Migrant Deaths

To study long-term trends of urban-rural infant mortality differences in Spain, the main source available for research is published aggregated data, not tabulated by key variables. Thus, indicators created from published statistics are not intended to accurately portray the health and mortality experience of urban cohorts, but a general measure of population health in the urban environment since they pool together different exchanges of individuals between cities and the countryside. On the one hand, they capture the excess mortality produced by the presence of infants born elsewhere who died in the city and, on the other hand, they lack the deaths of Madrid-born children that occurred outside of the city. For the case of infant mortality, these interferences should be expected to be quite modest, as migration and mobility for this age group would be expected to be quite small.

The advantage of using individual-level data is that we can start to make these distinctions. Migrant infant deaths are straightforward to identify, as place of birth is clearly stated in birth records. However, "missed" deaths of natives are unaccounted for because deaths were registered where they occurred. Thus, an estimation of their weight requires us to address different situations in which infants could leave the city: family migration, relocation to the neighboring municipalities or placement in the countryside with a hired wet-nurse.

The magnitude of these processes in the city of Madrid is hard to assess. While migration outside the city was probably not very important, mobility between the city and the neighboring places must not have been uncommon. There were several villages close to Madrid that, in fact, were later incorporated as part of the city (i.e., the municipalities of Vallecas, Tetuán de la Victorias, Chamartín, etc.). Also, as urbanization was also taking place in the cheaper suburban area of the city, the grey area between the end of the city itself and the municipality (Carballo Barral et al. 2008), relocation outside the city after childbirth or temporary visits to the city's institutions could have been quite common, making it possible that birth and infant deaths were registered in different municipalities.

However, the importance of child placement in the countryside is impossible to determine and we can only try to gather evidence of its prevalence. According to contemporary doctors, around the turn of the century, hiring mercenary wet-nurses to breastfeed infants was still a common practice in Madrid. Some of them suggested that up to 50 % of children were breastfed by wet-nurses instead of their mothers (Rodríguez Ocaña 1996), but that did not necessarily mean that they sent them outside of the city. The primary users of wet-nurses in the city, the upper classes, usually hired live-in wet-nurses and lower classes tended to hire urban wet-nurses who could be found through advertisements placed in daily newspapers (Del Amo 2008). In fact, Madrid was not an industrial town and most women gained employment in informal sectors that could be combined with child-rearing or the use of social networks, thus reducing the need for out-of-town solutions.

In Table 2.1, we have computed several alternative measures, including and excluding sub-groups, to test the effect of these potential interferences on infant mortality estimations. The starting point is the estimation of infant mortality for the city of Madrid in 1905–1906 computed in a normal way with aggregated vital statistics for Madrid: 216 per thousand. The same figure is obtained when replicating the estimation with the figures from our civil registration data on births and deaths in LHISTDATA-MAD. We also computed a lower bound of the city's mortality experience by excluding all migrant deaths of the computation and assuming that not a single native-born child died outside the city: 207 per thousand. This means that the maximum overestimation bias produced by deaths of "migrant infants" would be of 4 %.

For the upper bound, there are no concrete numbers on the amount of children leaving the city. We only have information on the percentage of children from the Foundling Hospital leaving the city within the first year of life (38 %), thanks to the linkage with the Foundling Hospital, but that figure is not representative of the city, as the institutional policy was to place all children when possible. Instead, we have included the deaths of foundlings that we are absolutely sure that happened outside of the city, according to the institution, which yields 216 per thousand, cancelling out the migrant overestimation.

Table 2.1 Estimation of infant and neonatal mortality according to the 1905–1906 data and for the 1905 cohort

	Estimation 1905–1906		Cohort 1905	
	Infant (‰)	Neonatal (‰)	Infant (‰)	Neonatal (‰)
Regular estimation	215	55	202	53
Excluding migrants	207	54	193	53
Excluding migrants + including foundlings	216	54	202	53
Excluding migrants + 10%placement	228	58	213	57
Excluding migrants + 20%placement	250	64	233	62

Source: LHISTDATA-MAD. Own elaboration

For the rest of placement, an estimation of 38 % of children nursed in the countryside seems excessive for the city (almost 4 out of 10 children), but it is impossible to set a number. Thus, in an attempt to establish an upper bound, we have computed theoretical estimations for two scenarios where 10 or 20 % of children was placed in the countryside and exposed to the same mortality than that of the city. This would increase urban mortality toward 228 and 250 per thousand.

In any case, it still seems unlikely that we can be missing that many infant deaths, as that level of placement would mean that more than 1600–3200 children left the city every year to be nursed in the neighboring villages, which would not have gone unnoticed in the record.

While these broad re-estimations suggest that migration alone could cause urban mortality for Madrid in 1905–1906 to range between 207 and 250 %, we need the use of a more robust sub-population to limit the number of children leaving the city (as it is the most difficult aspect to estimate). The estimation of neonatal mortality rates (deaths within the first month of life) helps us to limit the effect of missing deaths. The neonatal mortality rate that we estimate, 55 per thousand, falls within the range expected according to the infant and childhood mortality levels of Madrid at that time and shows a similar relationship to infant mortality, as estimations for other regions in the World have shown (Oestergaard MZ et al. 2011). The re-estimations suggest that the differences are not that large (around 55 per thousand, the regular estimation), which would suggest that this measure is quite robust to migration, so we will make use of it in the process of assessing the magnitude of different problems on infant mortality.

Other Sources of Miss-Registration

In order to gain further knowledge of the potential bias of registration, we focus the analysis not only on individual records but on linked events, focusing on the experience of an actual cohort. This procedure changes slightly the figures but the substantive results remain unchanged. When applied to the 1905–1906 dataset (results also shown in Table 2.1), the cumulative experience of death of the cohort born in 1905 through the years 1905 and 1906 yields an estimation of infant mortality of 202 per thousand (versus the 215 per thousand of the previous section). When migrants are eliminated, the result is 194 per thousand (versus 207 per thousand), which involves a similar decrease of 4 % as in the period measures. For the upper bound, including possible missing infant deaths, the figures change to 215–233 per thousand for 10–20 % of placement and 202 per thousand for the inclusion of foundlings.

For the rest of the paper, we will focus the analysis only on deaths that occurred in the city, as they are the only cases where we can have accurate data. However, the fact that they only show part of the mortality experience of the cohort should be always kept in mind.

To follow the experience of actual cohorts, we have used the linkage between births and deaths provided by the LHISTDATA-MAD to compute our estimations.

Part of the mortality difference between the period and the cohort mortality rate may be related to the results of our linkage because 15 % of infant deaths of Madrid-born children could not be matched to any of the birth records in 1905 or 1906. The common problem of the underestimation of deaths during the first day, found in any other historical and contemporary settings, cannot be responsible for this change. These cases, missing both birth and death registrations of babies who died in the first 24 h of life, have been already taken into consideration by including those unobserved births and deaths via the inflator factor described earlier.

As the 15 % of missing birth records can heavily affect the estimations, we have carefully analyzed its main features: we have checked the specific characteristics of infant deaths without corresponding birth records, we have described some processes that could be behind these results and we have illustrated their consequences on the estimation.

First, we have estimated logistic regressions in order to explore the processes behind the appearance of unmatched deaths and we have modeled the probabilities of finding the corresponding birth registration to a given death registration according to a small set of variables. The results from univariate- and multivariate-saturated models are displayed in Table 2.2. The results indicate no evidence of sex bias on the probability of birth registration, but a disproportionate excess of unmatched death records for deaths during the second semester of life. The districts of Hospicio, Hospital and Inclusa (the poorest districts) were those whose corresponding birth certificates were less likely to be found and this effect seems to be inherent to the districts (and the population living in them) as the removal of institutional births (which were clustered in those districts) or inclusion with a dummy variable did not alter results at all.

The year of death also appears to be relevant because birth records were more likely to be found for certificates registered in 1906. Part of that difference may be related to the smaller number of cases searched for in 1905 and a higher effect of the variations between theoretical birthdate (computed from age at death) and the actual birth date. As age at death was rounded up upwards, we may have considered that

Table 2.2 Results of logistic regressions for the probability of finding the corresponding birth registration for a given death record

	Sex	Year	Age	Place of death	District of death	Complete
Sex (ref.male)						
Female	0.91					0.91
Year of death (ref.1905)						
1906		1.80***				1.99***
Age in months (ref. < 1month)						
1–2 months			0.88			0.85
2–3 months			0.54***			0.48***
3–4 months			0.79			0.67**
4–5 months			0.98			0.81
5–6 months			0.86			0.71
6–7 months			0.90			0.67
7–8 months			0.90			0.65*
8–9 months			0.69			0.47***
9–10 months			0.79			0.53**
10–11 months			0.65*			0.43***
11–12 months			0.86			0.54**
Place of death (ref. Households)						
Institutions				0.75**		0.80
District (ref. Buenavista)						
Centro					0.74	0.79
Chamberi					0.74	0.74
Congreso					0.47	0.48**
Hospicio					0.51*	0.53*
Hospital					0.55*	0.55*
Inclusa					0.53**	0.56*
Latina					0.76	0.78
Palacio					0.92	0.87
Universidad					0.79	0.82

Source: LHISTDATA-MAD. Own elaboration
Significance: * p-value <0.05; ** p-value <0.01; ***p-value <0.001

some births should have occurred after January 1, 1905, when they had actually occurred before. Finally, there is no different structure of causes of death of matched and unmatched children (results not shown).

Accordingly, the linkage seems to be robust to some processes but not to others, which warns us that taking only the experience of the matched dataset is likely to underestimate the importance of families living in poorer areas and deaths in the second semester of life, which should be taken into account when drawing the big picture.

We can hypothesize three different explanations behind this 15 % of non-matched infant deaths. First, there could be problems inherent to nominative linkage: spelling and miss-registration problems may have prevented us from finding a true match for some of these unmatched deaths, whose linkage is impossible to perform with the information available in the records. Second, there could be a real problem of birth underestimation of newborns in the city, produced by a delay of birth registration until years after the birth or never performed if the death closely followed the birth. And, third, the possibility that the place of birth of some newborns has been miss-registered as "Madrid" when they had been born elsewhere.

As the linkage has been manually revised, to a large extent, and children had been searched individually to allow for a higher success rate, the possibility that the first option accounts for most of the 15 % is relatively small when compared to the other two.

Our hypothesis is that both the underestimation of births in the city and misreporting of place of birth may have been largely responsible for this mismatch. On the one hand, there were no penalties attached to lack of birth registration. On the other hand, we have found evidence that place of birth, in some cases, may have been mistaken with place of residence, so it is likely that the same occurred in death records.

We have estimated several alternative measures that are displayed in Table 2.3 to assess the potential effect of these factors on actual infant mortality computations. If all unmatched deaths had a corresponding birth in our data but we are just unable to find it, we should retain the 193 per thousand figure. If only birth under-registration was at work, adding "artificially" one birth for each unmatched death to the number of 1905 births, we would obtain an infant mortality rate of 189 per thousand. However, it is excessive to assume that the under-registration of births was limited to those children who died during the first year of life. Accordingly, a potentially better procedure would be to extract deaths without corresponding births, which would lower mortality to 170 per thousand. Finally, if the only reason for the mismatch was the incorrect imputation of the birth place, the figure would be also 170 per thousand; all of those unmatched deaths should be eliminated since they did not correspond to an urban birth.

While these estimations show us exclusive and independent effects, that is not a credible historical situation, so we have estimated three additional scenarios. If

Table 2.3 Estimates of the effects of different reasons for the mismatch on infant mortality cohort estimations for 1905

Linkage problems	193‰
Under-reporting births	
Adding births	189‰
Subtracting deaths	170‰
Wrong place of birth	170‰
75%linkage–25%rest	187‰
50%linkage–50%rest	181‰
25%linkage–75%rest	175‰

Source: LHISTDATA-MAD. Own elaboration

75 % of unmatched deaths were produced by linkage problems and only 25 % was provoked by either under-reporting of births or imputed birth as native, infant mortality would be 187 per thousand. If the proportions were 50–50 %, mortality would decrease to 181 per thousand. And, finally, if only 25 % of the mismatch was provoked by linkage and the remaining 75 % was caused by underreporting of births and birth outside of the city, then mortality would be 175 per thousand.

As our hypothesis minimizes the problems arising from linkage, we think that the more appropriate figure for the infant mortality experience for the 1905 cohort of Madrid-born children would likely be between 170 per thousand and 175 per thousand, rather than closer to the original 193 per thousand.

When the analysis is replicated for neonatal deaths, the difference between assuming that the mismatch is produced by the linkage problems exclusively or by one of the other potential explanations is a change from a neonatal mortality rate of 55 per thousand to one of 47 per thousand. That means an 11 % decrease compared to a 14 % decrease for infant mortality.

To sum up, we think that the mismatch suggests that there were problems of miss-registration of births (under-reporting or wrongly imputing place of birth) that could cause important variations in mortality estimations, both at for the infant and neonatal period.

2.5 Compositional Effects in Urban Infant Mortality: Migrants and Foundlings

The second part of our analysis focused on the contribution of the experience of particular sub-populations to urban mortality estimates, scrutinizing the striking sub-population of foundlings and migrants' reproductive behavior.

The Presence of Foundlings in the City of Madrid

Among the large number of both public and private charities that Madrid housed, given its role as capital and the center of the developing state welfare provision system (Gutiérrez Sánchez 1989), the Foundling Hospital of Madrid was the main institution devoted to care for the age group that interests us: the population under 1 year of age. The Civil Register in Madrid reported 6.79 % of live births taking place in institutions and almost 80 % of them pertained to births in one of the Foundling Hospital-related institutions. However, this small contingent was responsible for a disproportionate amount of deaths of children under 1 year of age in the city, 17.71 %, so we need to understand whether they were "urban deaths" in the sense that they were provoked by life in the city (only at a higher level of mortality) or they represented a different pattern of mortality very specific to the institution. If the latter is true, then the inclusion of the foundling population in aggregated rates could create a compositional effect that distorts our view of the experience of infant mortality of city children.

If we take the infant mortality rate of 170 per thousand that was estimated in the last section as starting point and we disaggregate it by home/institutional occurrence, we can immediately obtain the typical excessive foundling mortality (Pérez Moreda 1980; Viazzo et al. 1997). Mortality for children born in the Maternity Hospital-Foundling Hospital compound reached 396 per thousand, while mortality for children born in the city decreased to 146 per thousand. That is a 14 % decrease of mortality produced by a contingent of roughly 1000 births in a city with more than 15,000 births. The difference is even more dramatic when the equivalent neonatal rates are computed: from 48 per thousand of the cohort estimation in the absence of migrants, mortality estimations decline to 35 per thousand (a 27 % decrease) when excluding the institution. This level of neonatal mortality is slightly below the levels of what could be expected according to the overall childhood mortality levels of Madrid's the cohort-period comparisons.

On the other hand, the neonatal mortality of the infants born in institutional settings reaches a staggering 191 per thousand, which is, in fact, lower than the rates calculated from institutional records that placed neonatal mortality around 200–300 per thousand (Revuelta Eugercios 2011, 2013). This underestimation with individual data is related to a further case of miss-registration in the Civil Register, as we have discovered by using the linked records of both the FHM and the LHISTDATAMAD. While all children born or abandoned in the institution were registered in the Civil Registration system, we have found that this practice was far from accurate as children who had not been born in the premises (and, in some cases, were already some months or years old) were registered as newborns in the Civil Register. While 85 % of those birth inscriptions were reported the same day they were admitted at the Foundling Hospital, only 50 % of those cases corresponded within 6 days of the theoretical birth date as recorded at the Foundling Hospital. Thus, only 35 % of the total number of children abandoned through the Foundling Hospital had an appropriate date of birth. As older children were registered as newborns, the Civil Register finds less infant deaths (as they had already survived the riskiest period of life) and thus, produces an underestimation of the real death risk foundlings faced.

Thus, even if it was, in fact, under-estimated, foundling mortality was still quite influential on the city's aggregate estimations so it is key to understand whether we should consider the mortality of foundlings as an "urban" phenomenon in the sense of being generated by the same processes than for regular children. For doing that, it is helpful to consider the two explanations for foundling excess mortality: the selection produced by the circumstances around their admission and the environment and treatment they experienced inside.

The circumstances of admission reflected health differences but not necessarily in the same direction. First, being abandoned or delivered at the Foundling Hospital-Maternity Hospital compound implied selection for ill health. Women who abandoned children in the Foundling Hospital did so as a last resort. They were poor, in most occasions single, sometimes in extenuating pregnancy circumstances, (which could, among other things, involve prostitution), etc. and their children were possibly more likely to being born with congenital diseases, syphilis, or lower health at birth (preterm or low birth weight). Additionally, the Foundling Hospital also received children born elsewhere with very severe conditions, abandoned there at the as a last resort or as a way of avoiding treatment or burial costs (Revuelta Eugercios 2011:440).

However, all those children with ill health at admission were not necessarily of urban origin. Ten percent of women who delivered in the Maternity Hospital were not native Madrilenians and some of them could just have arrived in the city to abandon or deliver a child. In fact, independent of their original birth place, at least 20 % of mothers declared a neighboring village as their permanent residence. However, mobility was very high and even those women who declared a residence in the city were only found living in the same residence in that year's census in 20 % of cases (Revuelta Eugercios 2011). Thus, it is likely that the experiences of these children could be of a very heterogeneous nature and did not necessarily reflect an "urban pattern."

On the other hand, circumstances after admission could have played a more important role in producing mortality differentials through treatment inside the institution. The feeding system inside the institution was very poor: only some of the children were breastfed by internal wet-nurses at admission and the rest were bottle-fed with disastrous consequences for the newborn's health. Continuous bottle-feeding for more than 5 days proved fatal until the late 1920s, arising from the poor hygienic conditions in which it was delivered. However, children nursed by internal wet-nurses were not completely safe. Breastfeeding was not sufficient as two or more children sometimes had to share the same wet-nurse, in addition to requiring complementary artificial feeding, which also placed them at risk of infections related to artificial food (Revuelta Eugercios 2015). In fact, the sequels could also be seen among the survivors as contemporary doctors systematically described the level of stunting and under-development that most of the surviving children showed when they were sent to the countryside with external wet nurses (Bravo Frías and Alonso Muñoyerro 1923).

In order to further investigate which of these factors were most likely to explain the dramatic mortality observed, selection issues leading to admission or institutional treatment can be roughly associated with different patterns of causes of death structure. If the selection into the foundling hospital was the main reason for excess foundling mortality, the cause of death structure would probably be an acute version of the pattern of urban mortality or an excess of perinatal causes, as deaths would be more likely attributed to the mother's health and pregnancy. Conversely, if the treatment received (feeding inadequacy) was the main cause of excess mortality, we would expect to see an excess of causes related to that different environment and its treatment; that is, of an infectious nature.

Table 2.4 Distribution of causes of death for births in dwellings and institutions and probabilities of dying for the city of Madrid including and excluding institutions

	Percentages		Probabilities	
Cause of Death	Dwellings (%)	Institutions (%)	Including institutions (‰)	Excluding institutions (‰)
Not recorded/ ill-recorded	2.29	2.83	8.2	7.5
Water & food-borne	15.78	61.7	41.93	26.65
Air-borne	35.96	8.23	57.27	55.24
Other	13.53	0.77	23.66	23.47
Wasting diseases	2.88	0.51	8.50	8.37
Nervous system	8.27	1.8	16.46	16.02
Digestive system	1.12	0.26	5.96	5.89
Perinatal	1.39	1.29	6.59	6.27
Shaping vices	8.09	18.51	20.35	15.76
External	9.39	3.34	18.44	17.61
Other non-infectious	1.3	0.77	6.34	6.15
Total	100	100	170.74	145.97

Source: LHISTDATA-MAD. Own elaboration

In Table 2.4 we see that the distribution of causes of death lends some support to the second possibility: the position of the two main infectious disease groups (respiratory and water- or food-borne) is reversed in the two settings. For the city of Madrid, diseases transmitted through air accounted for a third of deaths and water and food-borne infections accounted for 15 %. In the foundling hospital, institutional mortality was comprised of 60 % of water and food-borne transmitted infections and those related with air transmission only accounted for less than 10 %.

However, as percentages may be affected by the prevalent mortality rates, which were so radically different between institutions and the urban environment, we have also computed proper mortality estimations including and excluding institutional mortality. Probabilities of dying at the Foundling Hospital have not been computed because of the small number of cases, but results by Revuelta Eugercios (2011) for the same period point to the same cause of death groups. Additional consistency tests with data for longer periods suggest that the 1905 cohort is representative of the pattern for the first decades of the twentieth century.

The exclusion of institutional deaths reduces the magnitude of two groups of causes of death: water-borne and shaping vices, which could be thought as the two indicators of the two processes discussed above (e.g., infection caused by environment and treatment), shaping vices and a higher selection of individuals in worse health.

If we look at neonatal rates to restrict the analysis to a more robust measure, the same picture arises and the magnitude of the importance of the institutional births increases because those were the ages where it was concentrated. Although the small number of cases prevents us from computing the full probabilities of dying by causes of death, we can see that up to 70 % of neonatal deaths of foundlings were caused by the treatment in the premises: water- and food-borne infectious diseases, which is further supported by foundling hospital cohort estimations indicating that the probability of dying from water- and food-borne infections during the first month of life was around 70 % and for dying from shaping vices was around 20 %.

The extraordinary number of deaths produced by water- and food-borne infections in the neonatal period (where most causes of death in general are more related to congenital aspects) suggests that the burden of the explanation falls on insufficient or improperly administered feeding (most of the literal diagnostics used were "enteritis," "diarrhea" and gastrointestinal disorders). No infant outside of the institution was subjected to this regime so, overall, it seems that the inclusion of foundlings pooled in general computations tends to incorporate an excess mortality that was not representative of the general population.

In spite of this, it would not be completely accurate to drop all of those births and deaths as they were a part of the city's births and, in fact, the frailest part: there was a clear role of selection of the frailest children into the Foundling Hospital, as only women in the worst situations attended institutions for delivery, which is a sign of a clearly "urban" experience. Thus, a further exercise can help us try to estimate how the mortality of the city would look if only the selective effects of mortality had been in effect. If, instead of having been exposed to the environment of the foundling hospital, foundlings had been exposed to the same mortality rates that the unhealthiest population in the city experienced (for illegitimate children from the worst district, 191 per thousand), the overall infant mortality for Madrid would be 158 per thousand (in comparison with total infant mortality, 169 per thousand and the figure excluding all foundlings 153 per thousand). Similar exercises have been done using other sub-populations characterized by ill health, but all of them provide estimates lower than 160 per thousand that leave the estimation very close to the figure excluding foundlings. Thus, it seems clear that pooling foundlings' mortality experience with the rest of the city indeed includes a very specific sub-population which has an excessive effect on the aggregate mortality estimations that do not reflect the life chances of the actual infants living in the city.

Migrant Women Delivering in the City: Health Selection or Worse Living Conditions?

A final compositional effect can be studied by looking at further signs of heterogeneity of the urban population, particularly regarding the large influx of migration. As migrants accounted for almost half of the population of the city, it is interesting to take a look at their offspring to test whether there were additional sub-populations with different mortality patterns that may have large impacts on mortality estimations. Significant better or worse health of new-borns delivered by migrant mothers could be driving the city's estimates, as Madrid-born women only accounted for 37 % of births in Madrid in 1905 (Pallol Trigueros 2009).

The effect of migration on reproductive outcomes in this context could operate in two ways. As has been pointed out before, prior research has found health advantages from birth in rural areas as well as detrimental effects of living in cities. Migrant women could be expected to deliver healthier children as they were (at least initially) healthier than natives. They could also deliver children with poorer health than natives because their own health may have been compromised by migration to the city (through the environment they had to endure or through the lower socio-economic status they held in the city).

In order to test the direction of this effect, we have first estimated cohort infant mortality rates for infants both of native Madrilenians and non-natives and then run multivariate models to account for possible confounding variables. To simplify the estimation, we have taken the measure for the city excluding institutions as the reference (145 per thousand).

Mortality rates do not seem to be radically different according to maternal place of birth, but there seem to be some differences: children born from natives had slightly higher mortality than the rest of children (159–150 per thousand). This could be related to the migration composition, as we have stated before, but also with issues of under-registration, so we use the linked dataset to control for this and model the probability of dying, which also allows for disaggregating the group of migrants by distance from the place of birth.

Table 2.5 shows the results of a set of logistic regressions that assess the effect of maternal place of birth on neonatal mortality. The univariate model (model A) confirms the relationship from the cohort estimations and shows that women born in distant provinces had lower probabilities that their children had died as infants. The inclusion of additional control variables: age, sex of the child and season of birth in model B does not change the picture.

Unfortunately, in this chapter we have not included the socio-economic status of either father or mother because it is not included in the data and we cannot control for it. As a distant proxy of their situation in the city, we have included the district of residence. When included (model C), the differences found for mother's place of birth disappear, suggesting that the differences found before were related not with migration per se, but with socio-economic status that led mothers to reside in the different places in the city. Accordingly, against our preconception, no clear advantage or disadvantage can be observed related to the migrant origin and, thus, no compositional effect in this sense was further altering our view of mortality in the city.

2.6 Conclusion

This chapter has contributed to the growing corpus of studies on urban development and mortality by exploring how a relatively less studied subset of factors contributed to explain the existence of an "urban penalty" for infants in the city of Madrid.

Table 2.5 Cox regressions studying the probability of dying in the first year of life, according to several maternal characteristics and contextual factors

	Model A	Model B	Model C
	Haz. ratio	Haz. ratio	Haz. ratio
Place of birth (ref.Madrid)	0.941	0.934	0.936
Distant provinces	0.924*	0.915*	0.938
Close	0.973	0.936	0.866
Unknown	0.775	0.775	0.843
Mother age (ref.20–35)			
<20 years		0.850	0.874
>35 years		1.008	1.031
Unknown		0.896	1.035
Sex of the child (ref.Male)			
Female		0.855*	0.856*
Season of birth (ref.Spring)			
Summer		0.954	0.950*
Winter		1.101*	1.107*
Autumm		0.948	0.947*
District (ref.buenavista)			
Centro			1.065
Chamberi			1.125
Congreso			0.958
Hospicio			0.994
Hospital			1.385*
Inclusa			1.441*
Latina			1.307*
Palacio			1.168*
Universidad			1.381*

Source: LHISTDATA-MAD. Own elaboration
Significance: * p-value <0.05; ** p-value <0.01; ***p-value <0.001

The LHISTDATA-MAD has allowed us to test whether registration inaccuracies and compositional effects arising from the presence of migrants and charity institutions had any impact at all in the computation of mortality estimations in a period when registration was occurrence-based.

Our results have shown that some of these factors indeed had substantial effects in modifying the estimations of infant mortality upwards, but they did not necessarily imply worse conditions for all inhabitants of Madrid. Infant deaths of children born outside the city did not greatly affect the estimation and neonatal deaths had an almost negligible effect. However, problems arising from the registration process were much more important. The deaths of migrants and natives not captured in the registration process affected strongly the estimation: the 15 % discrepancies between our matched 1905 cohort rates and the un-matched rates could affect infant and neonatal estimations between 11 and 14 % which, in turn, could affect life expectancy in

1–2 years. Among the different processes that could have been responsible for this mismatch we argue that under-reporting of births and incorrect imputation of the place of birth could be more important than the linkage problems and that this finding has important consequences on the estimates and the derived inference.

Our analyses have also shown a strong compositional effect produced by the inclusion of the foundling experience with the rest of the city's inhabitants. Deaths from institutional births account for 17–25 % of excess mortality when included in general estimations.

This excess mortality could be explained by the selection of the children from the city with poor survival probabilities, as their mothers were in a vulnerable state that made them resort there, their health at admission was drawn from the unhealthiest component of the urban distribution. However, cause of death analysis suggests that the most important group of causes of death for foundlings was that of food- and water-borne diseases, more related with the specific circumstances of the institution. This indicates that institutional deaths did not represent an acute version of urban mortality but predominantly represented a specific phenomenon. Finally, no compositional effect was found to be associated with the offspring of migrants.

Accordingly, we can conclude that the presence of registration inaccuracies and compositional effects produces substantive alterations to our vision of the experience of urban infant mortality when we use aggregated estimations for the city of Madrid. Unfortunately, our effort to identify and attempts to quantify these sources of bias in infant mortality estimation cannot give us a full picture as there are other sources of underestimation that we have not been able to fully address with our data at this moment. Migration out of the city and placement of infants in the countryside are two sources of loss to follow up that interfere with our mortality estimations. Speculative upper bounds of mortality have been estimated, and we have suggested that a placement of only 20 % of infants outside the city would cancel out the over-estimation of migrant deaths. However, it is unlikely that such extreme numbers of children were annually leaving the city to be nursed in the countryside.

In any case, by exploring the influence that inaccuracy, irregularities and compositional effects may have had in the estimation of infant mortality, we have been able to offer in-depth knowledge on the meaning of the indicator and the processes and populations that are behind them. While it is clear that we need aggregated and published data to reconstruct long-term national and regional patterns for most areas, it is important to bear in mind that our inference needs to be very careful. And, this is particularly important when we discuss the urban environment and the effects of public measures, which may not have been equally affecting all sub-populations.

These results have contributed to shed additional light on the urban history of Spain since it is likely that the picture we see in Madrid was common across the country. As the type of registration and the presence of similar charity and health institutions were common across the capital cities of Spain, it is likely that similar processes could be behind some of the most striking mortality differentials, such as the excess mortality found for towns with less than 20,000 inhabitants. And, more generally, it is a useful illustration of the implications of these widely known biases in contexts with high migration attraction, health institutions and deficient registration.

A full comparison of Madrid and its surrounding countryside is beyond the scope of this paper since we lack complete urban and rural data to undertake that task. However, we think that aggregated estimates of the city offer an amplified view of that mortality penalty that may lead us to believe that life in the city was unhealthier than it really was, at least for infants. In fact, the importance of these sources of bias challenges the existence of urban penalty for Madrid for those ages. And this finding opens the door for further research, regarding the extent to which this process was additionally at work for other age ranges and what other processes may have helped to amplify it.

References

Alter, G., & Oris, M. (2005). Childhood conditions, migration and mortality: Migrants and natives in 19th-century cities. *Social Biology, 52*(3/4), 178–191.

Alter, G., & Oris, M. (2008). Effects of inheritance and environment on the height of brothers in the nineteenth-century Belgium. *Human Nature, 19*(1), 44–55.

Baten, J., & Murray, J. E. (2000). Heights of men and women in 19th-century Bavaria: Economic, nutritional, and disease influences. *Explorations in Economic History, 37*, 351–369.

Bengtsson, T., & Broström, G. (2009). Do conditions in early life affect old-age mortality directly and indirectly? Evidence from 19th century rural Sweden. *Social Science & Medicine, 68*(9), 1583–1590.

Bengtsson, T., & Lindström, M. (2003). Airborne infectious disease during infancy and mortality in later life in southern Sweden, 1766–1894. *International Journal of Epidemiology, 32*, 286–294.

Bengtsson, A., & Van Poppel, F. (2011). Socioeconomic inequalities in death from past to present: An introduction. *Explorations in Economic History, 48*, 343–356.

Bernabeu Maestre, J., Ramiro Fariñas, D., Sanz Gimeno, A., & Robles González, E. (2003). El análisis histórico de la mortalidad por causas. Problemas y soluciones. *Revista de Demografía Histórica, XXI*(I), 167–193.

Boyle, P. (2002). Population geography: Transnational women on the move. *Progress in Human Geography, 4*, 531–543.

Boyle, P. (2004). Population geography: Migration and inequalities in mortality and morbidity. *Progress in Human Geography, 28*, 767.

Bravo Frías, J., & Alonso Muñoyerro, J. A. (1923). *La transformación de las Inclusas. Memoria presentada al Congreso Nacional de Pediatría de San Sebastián*. Madrid: Imprenta de Mario Anguiano.

Cain, L. P., & Hong, S. C. (2009). Survival in 19th century cities: The larger the city, the smaller your chances. *Explorations in Economic History, 49*, 450–463.

Carballo Barral, B., Pallol Trigueros, R., & Vicente Albarrán, F. (2008). *El Ensanche de Madrid. Historia de una capital*. Madrid: Editorial Complutense.

Del Amo Del Amo, M. C. (2008). *La familia y el trabajo femenino en España durante la segunda mitad del siglo XIX*. PhD Thesis, History, Universidad Complutense de Madrid.

Finlay, R. (1981). Natural decrease in early modern cities. *Past & Present, 92*(1), 169–174.

Gagnon, A., & Mazan, R. (2009). Does exposure to infectious diseases in infancy affect old-age mortality? *Social Science & Medicine, 68*(9), 1609–1616.

Galley, C. (1995). A model of early modern urban demography. *The Economic History Review, 48*(3), 448–469.
Gutiérrez Sánchez, M. (Ed.). (1989). *La beneficencia pública en Madrid durante el último tercio del siglo XIX*. Madrid: Alfoz.
Hammel, E. A., & Mason, C. (1993). My brother´s keeper. Modelling kinship links in early urbanization. In R. David & S. Roger (Eds.), *Old and new methods in historical demography* (pp. 233–247). Oxford: Clarendon Press.
Hauser, P. (1902). *Madrid bajo el punto de vista médico-social*. Madrid: Editora Nacional.
Kearns, G. (1988). The Urban Penalty and the Population History of England. In A. Brändström & L.-G. Tedebrand (Eds.), *Society, Health and Population During the Demographic Transition* . Umea: Umea universitets tryckeri: 231.
Kesztenbaum, L., & Rosenthal, J.-L. (2011). The health cost of living in a city: The case of France at the end of the 19th century. *Explorations in Economic History, 48*, 207–225.
Keyfitz, N. (1980). Do cities grow by natural increase or by migration? *Geographical Analysis, 12*(2), 143–56.
Komlos, J., & Baten, J. (Eds.). (1998). *The biological standards of living in comparative perspective*. Stuttgart: Franz Steiner Verlag.
Lee, R. (1999). Urban labour markets, in-migration, and demographic growth: Bremen, 1815–1914. *Journal of Interdisciplinary History, 30*(3), 437–73.
Librero López, J., & Benavides, F. G. (1995). La validez del municipio de residencia en las estadísticas de mortalidad: hallazgos a partir de la actualización de los padres municipales en los muncipios de la Comunidad Valenciana. *Gaceta Sanitaria, 49*(9), 232–236.
Librero López, J., García Benavides, F., & Godoy Laserna, C. (1993). Análisis de la mortalidad en áreas pequeñas: el problema de la residencia. *Gaceta Sanitaria, 37*(7), 169–175.
Malthus, T. R. (1826). *An essay on the principle of population*. London: John Murray.
Martínez Carrión, J. M., & Moreno-Lázaro, J. (2007). Was tehre an urban height penalty in Spain, 1840-1913? *Economics and Human Biology, 5*, 144–164.
Mooney, G., Lucking, B., & Tanner, A. (1999). Patient pathways: Solving the problem of institutional mortality in London during the later nineteenth century. *Social History of Medicine, 12*(2), 227–269.
Ocaña-Riola, R., Fernández-Ajuri, A., Mayoral-Cortés, J. M., Toro-Cárdenas, S., & Sánchez-Cantalejo, C. (2009). Uncontrolled migrations as a cause of inequality in health and mortality in small-area studies. *Epidemiology, 20*(3), 411–418.
Oris, M., & Alter, G. (2001). Paths to the city and roads to death. Mortality and migration in East Belgium during the industrial revolution. *Revue Belge d'Histoire Contemporeaine, XXXI*, 453–495.
Oestergaard, M. Z., Inoue, M., Yoshida, S., Mahanani, W. R., Gore, F. M., Cousens, S., Lawn, J. E., Mathers, C. D., & On behalf of the United Nations Inter-agency Group for Child Mortality. (2011, August 30). Estimation and the child health epidemiology reference group neonatal mortality levels for 193 countries in 2009 with trends since 1990: A systematic analysis of progress, projections, and priorities. *PLOS Medicine*. http://dx.doi.org/10.1371/journal.pmed.1001080
Pallol Trigueros, R. (2009). *El Madrid moderno: Chamberí (el Ensanche Norte), símbolo del nacimiento de una nueva capital, 1860–1931*. Phd Thesis, History, Universidad Complutense de Madrid.
Pérez Moreda, V. (1980). *Las crisis de mortalidad en la España interior. Siglos XVI-XIX*. Madrid: Siglo XXI.
Pérez Moreda, V., Ramiro Fariñas, D., & Sanz Gimeno, A. (2004). Dying in the city: Urban mortality in Spain in the middle of the health transition. In E. Sonnino (Ed.), *Living in the city (14th-20th centurie). Vivre en ville (XIV-XX siècles)* (pp. 617–654). Rome: University of Rome, La Sapienza.
Preston, S., & Haines, M. R. (1991). *Fatal years. Child mortality in nineteenth-century America*. Princeton: Princeton University Press.

Preston, S. H., & Van de Walle, E. (1978). Urban French mortality in the nineteenth century. *Population Studies, 32*(2), 275–297.
Quiroga, G. (2001). Estatura, diferencias regionales y sociales y niveles de vida en Espan˜a (1893–1954). *Revista de Historia Económica, 19*(1), 175–200.
Ramiro Fariñas, D. (2007). Mortality in hospitals and mortality in the city in the nineteenth- and twentieth century Spain: The effect on the measurement of urban mortality rates of the mortality outsiders in urban health institutions. In J. Henderson, P. Horden, & A. Pastore (Eds.), *The impact of hospitals, 300–2000* (pp. 395–416). Oxford: Peter Lang AG.
Ramiro Fariñas, D. (2008). Il declino della mortalita durante l'infanzia nella Spagna urbana e rurale, 1860–1930. *Storia Urbana, 31*(119), 125–148.
Ramiro Fariñas, D., & Sanz Gimeno, A. (2000a). Childhood mortality in Central Spain, 1790–1960: Changes in the course of demographic modernization. *Continuity and Change, 15*(2), 235–267.
Ramiro Fariñas, D., & Sanz Gimeno, A. (2000b). Structural changes in childhood mortality in Spain, 1860–1990. *International Journal of Population Geography, 6*, 61–82.
Reher, D.-S. (2001). In search of the urban penalty. Exploring urban and rural mortality patterns in Spain during the demographic transition. *International Journal of Population Geography, 7*, 105–127.
Remund, A. (2010). Refreshing the typology of migration systems. A reformulation based on the case of early nineteenth-century Geneva. European Social Sciece History Conference. Ghent, Belgium.
Revenga, R. (1901). *La muerte en Madrid*. Madrid.
Revuelta Eugercios, B. A. (2011). *Los usos de la Inclusa de Madrid: mortalidad y retorno a principios del siglo XX (1890–1935)*. PhD, History, Universidad Complutense de Madrid.
Revuelta Eugercios, B. A. (2013). Abandoned and illegitimate, a double mortality penalty? Mortality of illegitimate infants in the foundling hospital of Madrid, La Inclusa (1890–1935). *History of the Family, 18*(1), 44–67.
Revuelta Eugercios, B. A. (2015). ¿Qué pasa en la Inclusa? The role of press scandals, doctors and public authorities in the evolution of La Inclusa de Madrid, 1890–1935. *Dynamis, 35*(1), 107–130.
Rodríguez Ocaña, E. (1996). Una medicina para los niños. In J. M. Borrás Llop (Ed.), *Historia de la infancia en la España Contemporánea* (pp. 149–193). Madrid: Ministerio de Trabajo y Asuntos Sociales, Fundación Germán Sánchez Ruipérez.
Sharlin, A. (1978). Natural decrease in early modern cities: A reconsideration. *Past & Present, 79*(1), 126–138.
Sharlin, A. (1981). Natural decrease in early modern cities: A Rejoinder. *Past & Present, 92*(1), 175–180.
Steckel, R. H., & Floud, R. (Eds.). (1997). *Health and welfare during industrialization*. Chicago: University of Chicago Press.
Van de Woude, A. (1982). Population developments in the northern Netherlands (1500–1800) and the validity of the "urban graveyard effect". *Annales de Demographie Historique, 1*, 55–75.
Viazzo, P. P., Bortolotto, M., & Zanotto, A. (1997). A special case of decline: Levels and trends of infant mortality at the Florence foundling hospital, 1750–1950. In C. Corsini & P. P. Viazzo (Eds.), *The decline of infant and child mortality. The European experience: 1750–1990* (pp. 227–246). The Hague: Martinus Nijhoff.
Weber, A. F. (1899). *The growth of cities in the nineteenth century: A study in statistics*. New York: Macmillan Co.
Williams, N., & Galley, C. (1995). Urban–rural differentials in infant mortality in Victorian England. *Population Studies, 49*(3), 401–420.
Woods, R. I. (1989). What would one need to know to solve the "natural decrease in early modern cities" problem? In R. Lawton (Ed.), *The rise and fall of great cities* (pp. 80–95). London: Wiley.

Woods, R. (2003). Urban–rural mortality differentials: An unresolved debate. *Population and Development Review, 29*(1), 29–46.

Woods, R., & Shelton, N. (2000). Disease environments in Victorian England and Wales. *Historical Methods, 33*(2), 73–82.

Woods, R., Watterson, P. A., & Woodward, J. H. (1989). The causes of rapid infant mortality decline in England and Wales, 1861–1921. Part II. *Population Studies, 43*(1), 113–132.

Wrigley, E. A. (1967). A simple model of London's importance in changing English society and economy 1650–1750. *Past & Present, 37*(Jul.), 44–70.

Wrigley, E. A. (1969). *Population and history*. London: McGraw-Hill.

Chapter 3
Environment, Housing, and Infant Mortality: Udine, 1807–1815

Alessio Fornasin, Marco Breschi, and Matteo Manfredini

3.1 Introduction

Much research on differentials of mortality focuses on the links to social class and socio-economic status, but these links can also be influenced by the location and spatial distribution of a population in a given area. This effect is particularly evident when referring to areas that differ greatly in terms of climate and resources, but less so if the analysis is narrowed to more limited context, such as individual towns.

In many urban settings, the distribution of inhabitants follows a logical pattern because different functions are associated with certain areas. This process creates distinctive districts or sub-areas where the population appears relatively socially and economically homogenous. This means we need to look for associations between mortality and environmental and socio-economic factors. However, in some urban settings, the geographical distribution of the population is not so clearly differentiated by the socio-economic status of the family.

This analysis of Udine, a small town in north-east Italy, aims to examine the socio-economic factors that affected infant and child mortality levels in the early nineteenth century; investigate whether these levels were affected by environmental factors, such as housing quality; and determine if the spatial distribution of this mortality can be interpreted in the light of social and environmental factors.

A. Fornasin (✉)
Department of Economics and Statistics, University of Udine, Udine, Italy
e-mail: fornasin@uniud.it

M. Breschi
Department of Economics and Business, University of Sassari, Sassari, Italy
e-mail: breschi@uniss.it

M. Manfredini
Department of Life Sciences, University of Parma, Parma, Italy
e-mail: matteo.manfredini@unipr.it

D. Ramiro Fariñas, M. Oris (eds.), *New Approaches to Death in Cities during the Health Transition*, International Studies in Population 12,
DOI 10.1007/978-3-319-43002-7_3

3.2 Background

Research on the links between mortality differentials and socioeconomic status shows that upper SES groups generally had a higher than average life-expectancy (Vedrenne-Villeneuve 1961; Perrenoud 1975; Blum et al. 1990; Bengtsson and van Poppel 2011), but there is evidence that these differences were largely determined during childhood and early adulthood. Perrenoud (1975) estimates a 17 year difference in infant mortality between the poor and wealthy in seventeenth century Geneva, and Hollingsworth (1977) shows that the 7 year gap in life-expectancy between the English peerage and general population was largely determined in childhood.

Studies on rural populations, where social difference is less pronounced than in urban contexts, also show the same tendency. Families in the highest tax bracket had the lowest IMR in Weir's (1995) study of Rosny-Sous-Bois, and we see the same situation in Italian rural communities, where SES is based on household head's occupation (Breschi et al. 2004). Comparisons between rural and urban populations show that IMR differentials by SES are more pronounced in the latter (van Poppel and Mandemakers 1997).

Although housing is associated to mortality and health, very few studies address this issue for pre-transitional populations, due partly to the lack of reliable data. This study makes use of sources with information on the characteristics and quality of individual houses, making it possible to evaluate their impact on infant mortality.

Most studies examine urban settings and reveal the correlation between overcrowding and infant mortality, as in Glasgow and Edinburgh in the nineteenth century (Cage 1994; Cage and Foster 2002). The reason given for this relationship is a direct and positive association between overcrowding and poverty. Although there is a clear connection between housing quality and mortality, it is not always easy to demonstrate the causal link (Burnett 1991). The Healthy Cities Project, launched in the eighties by The World Health Organization (WHO), investigated the determinants, including housing, of mortality and health status of present-day, urban populations (Ashton et al. 1986).

Some of the findings from this project are also relevant to historical populations. For example, the relationship between asthma and dampness in homes (Jaakkola et al. 2011); infants exposed to high levels of fungi spores are more likely to develop asthma and suffer from respiratory problems (Gent et al. 2002). Another risk factor is indoor smoke from burning coal or wood (Desai et al. 2011). Studies in developing countries reveal a relationship between biomass fuel use and low birth-weight, stillbirth, perinatal death and acute lower respiratory infection (Desai et al. 2004).

Other findings show a correlation between temperature and old-age mortality (Rudge 2011; Wilkinson et al. 2004). We also see an increased risk in winter, especially in warmer rather than colder climates, known as the "paradox of excess winter mortality". This issue is well-known in historical demography (Healy 2003; Barnett et al. 2005) and many studies of the preindustrial period show that low winter temperatures in rigid climates also affected infant mortality from respiratory disease (Derosas 2009; Dalla Zuanna and Rosina 2011; Breschi et al. 2000). Another element to emerge, supported by studies from the early nineteenth century, is the link between death from tuberculosis and overcrowding (Baker et al. 2011; Stein 1950). A similar connection is found between measles and infant and child mortality in Stockholm between the nineteenth and twentieth centuries (Burström et al. 1999).

3.3 Sources

Housing Registers

House numbering was introduced in many Italian towns at the turn of the nineteenth century. Udine had its first numeration in 1801, which just referred to houses within the town walls (Mansutti 1984), and a later integration in 1809. One of the aims was to compile accommodation lists for passing military troops.

The 1809 register is the most detailed of the two (Breschi and Serio 1999), listing a total of 2100 numbered houses, although some were uninhabited, others made up more than one residence, and a few, even if identifiable, remained numberless (e.g. the town-wall towers). This source contains valuable information such as the number of residences for each number, the property owner and families that lived there, the profession of the household head, presence of domestic staff, and indication of the number and military rank of soldiers who could be accommodated. There is also separate documentation on male and female occupants. In addition to demographic information, this source also records the number of rooms, fireplaces and kitchens on each floor of every house, and the presence of outhouses or stables.

Despite this wealth of information, some gaps do remain that currently impede analysis. While the numeration system does include the majority of the town's buildings, it only regards private residences, so lacks information on the residents of all public and religious buildings such as prisons, military barracks, monasteries, convents and rectories. The same is true of people with no fixed abode, or beggars, who had a strong presence in urban settings.

These lists were in no way intended for the drafting of a town map, which was done decades later by the engineer Antonio Lavagnolo (1842–1850). *While there is no connection between the lists and this map*, we can note that the total number of street numbers and their position of remained unchanged, which means we can pin point them with precision.

The Napoleonic Civil Registers

The creation of the Kingdom of Italy in 1806 saw the introduction of the Napoleonic Civil Code across the country, which initiated the keeping of civil registers on all births, deaths and marriages. This study uses the birth and death registers for Udine, which span from January 1st, 1807 to December 31st, 1815. These record not only the name and surname of each newborn and deceased, but also socio-economic information, such as the profession of individual, parents and spouse (in the case of deaths), and the date, time and house number of the event. This means we can give a precise location to each of the 5956 births and 6572 deaths recorded between 1807 and 1815. Like all main Italian towns at the time, Udine had a hospital which also functioned as a place to leave foundlings. The number of children abandoned in this period results as 1477, which is around a quarter of all births. These children were often left with documentation of their baptism including the parish where the ceremony took place. The majority originated from other, at times quite distant, locations. Of the 696 foundlings we have birthplace records for, only 28 were baptised in Udine. The deaths recorded at the hospital also show a concentration of 'outsiders', which account for almost all most of the 162 beggars, those with no fixed abode and the 978 foundlings.

3.4 Udine at the Start of the Nineteenth Century

Although Udine was a relatively small town in the early nineteenth century, with around 13,000 inhabitants within the walls, it was the only urban centre in Friuli – the region that formed the eastern part of the Napoleonic Kingdom of Italy. It had many craft stores and shops which drew in clientele from all over Friuli to stock up on provisions, and was also the region's main market place for grain, even after trade was liberalised in 1806. There were numerous mills along the two canals that ran through the town that also functioned as iron workshops and tanneries. Textiles was one of the town's most productive sectors, which led to a large number of resident spinners and weavers.

Udine had a small but relatively varied population, with Friuli's most important families and landowners and modest farming families who cultivated the area within the town walls for small-scale market gardening and more extensive farming. Udine also had a strong presence of religious institutions with nine parishes and numerous monasteries and convents, and was also the seat of the Bishop, with all the economic benefits this entailed.

Udine was also an important administrative centre. This period saw an increase in central state bureaucracy, and much effort was given to collecting the many taxes needed to fuel the Emperor's war machine. There was also the first modern cadastre of north-east Italy, which created demand for professional surveyors and qualified estimators, and led to many white-collar workers migrating to Friuli from other areas.

Although Udine was the most socio-economically diverse location in all Friuli, there is a lack of historical documentation on housing quality since the local authorities appear to have been concerned with the aesthetics of facades rather than health and hygiene (Mansutti 1984). Nevertheless, we can assume that the living conditions in the majority of town houses in the early nineteenth century were similar to the poor state depicted in an 1877 report (Baldissera 1877).

3.5 Territorial Diffusion and Socio-Economic Characteristics of Infant Mortality

Although we have information on occupation, this data is at times poor and incomplete; the House register indicates the SES of household heads only, and the Birth register records that of fathers. The best depiction of the socioeconomic characteristics of the inhabitants of Udine is given by the Death register, due to its detailed spatial coverage and the universality of this event.

The socio-professional classification adopted here has a traditional scheme; as well as the usual productive sectors, such as agriculture, handicraft and trade, we also consider white-collar workers, domestic staff and the upper classes (namely proprietors and professionals). Clergymen are considered separately, and beggars and people with no recorded occupation are counted as a residual group.

Table 3.1 presents a preliminary account of Udine's occupational structure, taken from records of 4221 deaths. This analysis does not take account of the deaths outside the town, the 1733 in hospital, the 41 in other public institutions and the 21 lacking indication.

Table 3.2 shows infant mortality rates in relation to gender and occupation at the individual level. The denominator is the total number of births within the town walls between 1807 and 1814 (N=3870), and the numerator, infant deaths (0 years) from the same sample (N=999). We can see the typically high levels of infant mortality in an urban context, with significant SES differentials (the upper class presenting the lowest, and the categories 'other', which includes beggars, and 'handicraft' the highest), consistent with previous literature. The high levels of infant mortality for children of white-collar workers, and low levels for agricultural workers are, however, fairly surprising, and notably, male mortality exceeds female in all SES categories, except the upper class.

Table 3.1 Occupational structure in Udine at the beginning of the XIX century

	Registers of deaths	
Occupation	Deaths	% deaths
Agriculture	567	13.4
Handicraft	1595	37.8
Trade	648	15.4
White collar workers	217	5.1
Domestics & servants	494	11.7
Upper class	462	10.9
Clergymen	102	2.4
Other	136	3.2
Total	4221	100.0

Source: Napoleonic civil registers, registers of deaths 1807–1815

Table 3.2 Infant mortality rates by occupation and gender, Udine generations 1807–1814

Occupation	F	M	Total	N deaths
Agriculture	234.1	257.9	247.3	113
Handicraft	267.3	288.5	279.0	395
Trade	206.7	239.4	222.6	183
White collars	218.0	298.5	258.4	69
Domestics & servants	271.0	301.7	287.3	131
Upper class	235.3	220.7	227.5	91
Other	181.8	433.3	326.9	17
Overall	242.0	272.4	258.1	999

Source: Napoleonic civil registers, registers of births and deaths

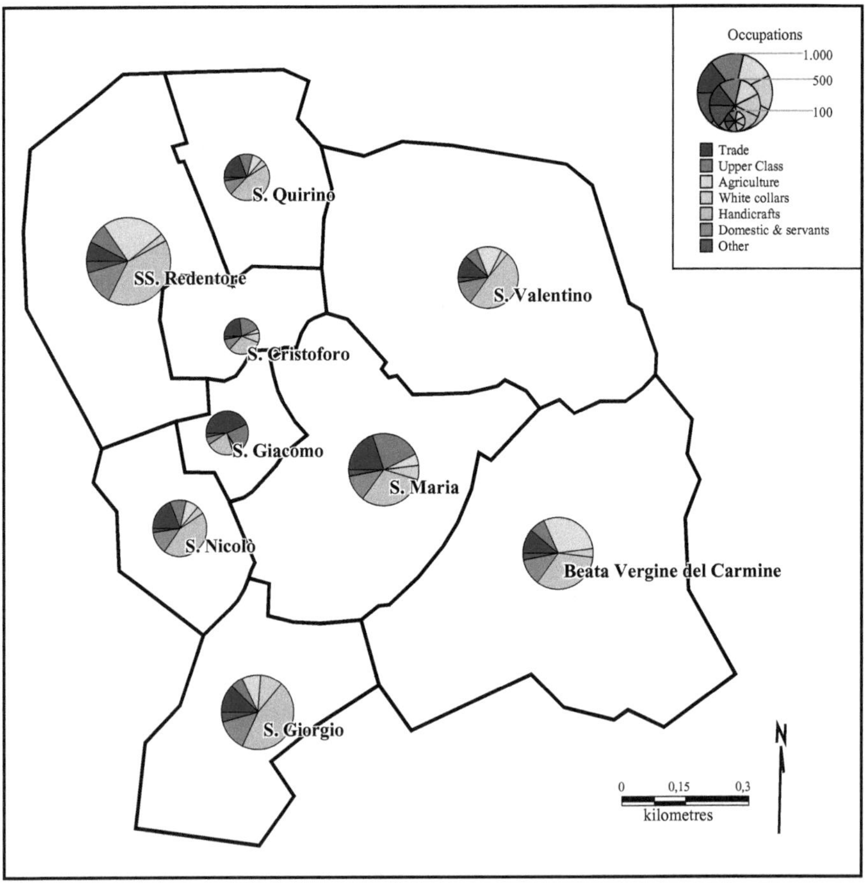

Fig. 3.1 Infant deaths by occupation. Udine (1807–1815) (Source: Napoleonic civil registers, registers of deaths)

Figure 3.1 presents territorial data on occupation and infant deaths within Udine. The territory has been subdivided into parishes since this partition reflects the socio-economic distribution of the population. Circle size is proportional to the number of infant deaths, and therefore, to some extent, population size. The coloured socio-professional categories clearly demonstrate the degree of occupational variety within each parish.

3.6 The Determinants of Spatial Distribution of Infant Mortality in Udine

Our findings show that the spatial distribution of infant mortality is linked to the geographic distribution of individuals and their related socio-economic status. This said, social difference only partly determined the population distribution in nineteenth century Udine. Occupation is only a rough indicator of the social status since one economic sector could include a wide range of social categories. The parish level is therefore insufficient to demonstrate the spatial relationship between SES and infant mortality. We need to analyse data on a smaller-scale, namely on the level of the individual house.

It may be possible to infer the socio-economic status of an infant who died from the characteristics of their home, although it is not easy to define the characteristics of a 'rich' or 'poor' house. The number of rooms, for example, is not a good indicator without information on their condition. The 1809 housing list provides information on the characteristics and quality of each residence, and specifies the suitability of each for different military ranks of guest soldiers. This makes it possible to examine the likelihood of infant death in a given residence in relation to this qualitative datum.

We devised four different regression logistic models with the dependent variable of 1 for houses where an infant death occurred and 0 otherwise (Table 3.3). Model 1 uses two explanatory variables: the number of births; and number of residents in each house. The first aims to capture the risk of infant death since a greater number of births implies a higher probability of these deaths. The second aims to detect any effects associated to crowding.

Models 3 and 4 include the variable of room density, estimated from the number of inhabitants in each house. Models 2 and 4 include the variable regarding house "quality", differentiating between lodgings deemed appropriate for officers and those for other military ranks. Variation in model fit was then estimated through a Likelihood Ratio test.

The only significant variable in model 1 is number of births. The risk of infant death doubles for each new birth within a house. A positive but not statistically significant association emerges between infant mortality and number of residents, although with model fit this link does become significant, suggesting an increased risk of death for infants living in crowded conditions. This is because the mean number of inhabitants per house is higher among the wealthy than the poor (9.59

Table 3.3 Logistic regression. Risk of at least one infant death in the house. Udine 1807–1815

	Model 1			Model 2			Model 3			Model 4		
	Odds ratio	Std. err.	P>z	Odds ratio	Std. err.	P>z	Odds ratio	Std. err.	P>z	Odds ratio	Std. err.	P>z
No of births	2.06	0.073	0.000	2.05	0.073	0.000	2.08	0.072	0.000	2.08	0.072	0.000
House inhabitants 1809/density per room	1.02	0.013	0.135	1.03	0.014	0.036	1.26	0.082	0.000	1.24	0.083	0.002
House assigned to officers (ref. All the other ranks)				0.68	0.114	0.022				0.85	0.141	0.335
Number of obs	2102			2102			2102			2102		
Log likelihood	−954.7			−952.0			−949.7			−949.2		
LR chi2(4)	772.5			777.9			782.5			783.4		
Prob>chi2	0.000			0.000			0.000			0.000		
Pseudo R2	0.288			0.290			0.292			0.292		
Likelihood-ratio test												
LR chi2(1)	5.4						0.9					
Prob>chi2	0.020						0.333					

versus 5.93), whereas infant mortality is higher for the latter (0.251 versus 0.210). In model 2, house "quality" has a statistically significant impact, with a lower risk of infant death in higher "quality" housing.

In line with previous studies on other European towns, room density is significantly and positively associated to the risk of infant death (model 3). House "quality" does not have a statistically significant impact in model 4, but the sign is consistent with model 2.

In short, a clear relationship emerges between crowding and infant mortality, and housing quality also appears to play a big role.

3.7 Infant Mortality Clusters

To examine how far these observations for IMR tendencies can be attributed to territorial location, we can look at "local dependence" conditions or spatial heterogeneity, which refers to the particular conditions that distinguish one territory from all others (Voss et al. 2006; Anselin 1992). This analysis aims at seeing if there are groups of civic numbers – i.e. clusters of houses – where residents assume similar behaviour. Local dependence is calculated using the LISA index (Cliff and Ord 1973; Upton and Fingleton 1985; Anselin 1995), obtained using GeoDa, a valuable and powerful spatial data analysis software tool (Anselin et al. 2006). This index calculation takes account of the variable under analysis, and a series of territorial weights applied at the house level. The choice of weights represents a "hypothesis on the part of the researcher regarding the interdependence of the places where the phenomena is observed and the extent to which these interdependent relations influence the phenomena itself" (Badaloni and Vinci 1988). These methods are described in more detail elsewhere (Zaccomer and Mason 2007; Anselin undated), but in short the analysis depends on the criteria for deciding the proximity threshold for two houses to be considered close. This can then be applied to every house in the analysis, resulting in the creation of a spatial weight matrix based on the distance between pairs. The proximity threshold used here is necessarily high, at 306 m, so as to be greater than the distance between the two most distant houses (81 m) and account for the houses which resulted as having no infant deaths. The values from the LISA index are shown below (Fig. 3.2).

The coloured circles indicate where the LISA index has a significance of at least 0.05. Dark blue represents spatially clustered houses with low levels of IMR, and red corresponds to those with high levels of IMR. The other colours represent outlier houses; those with an opposite tendency to neighbouring residences. Pink is for houses with high IMR values surrounded by low ones, and light blue for those with low IMR values surrounded by high ones.

This map clearly reveals three distinct clusters. The town centre is dominated by houses with low IMR values, whilst the south-west parish of S. Giorgio and that of SS. Redentore in the north-west, are characterised by houses with high levels.

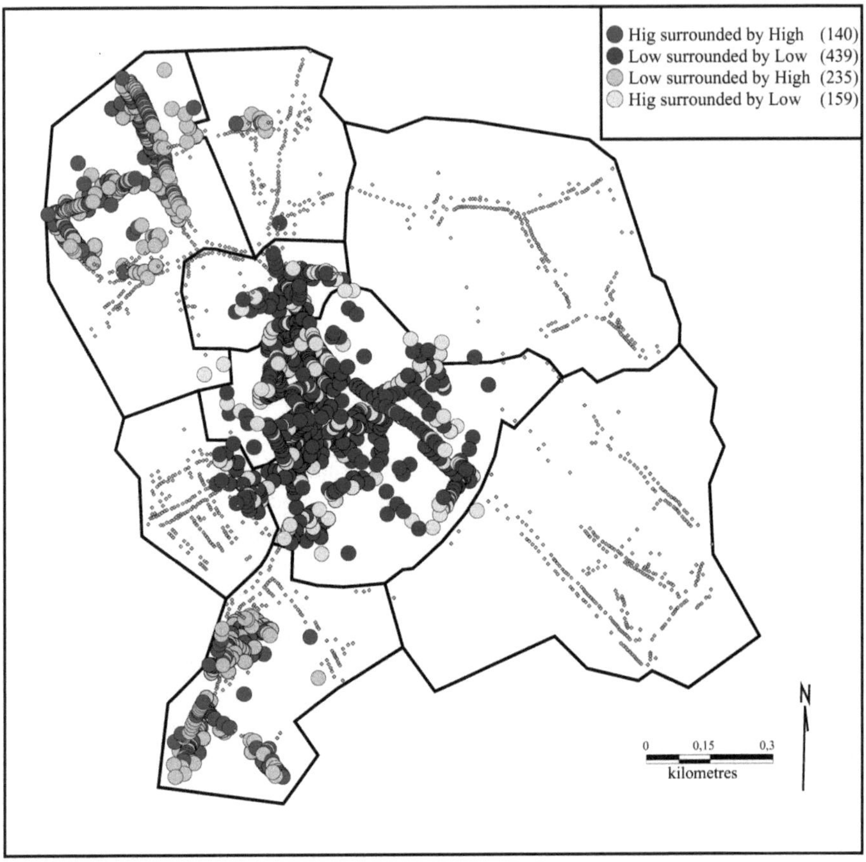

Fig. 3.2 LISA cluster map of the IMR figures of each house in Udine (1807–1815)

3.8 Conclusions

As seen in many other rural and urban contexts, there is a negative association between SES and IMR in Udine during the Napoleonic era. The link between poor socio-economic conditions and high infant mortality can be further explained when housing quality and overcrowding are taken into account.

Evaluation of the spatial distribution of infant mortality should also consider that some areas in a town are more prone than others, which is particularly important in cases like Udine, where there is no marked socio-economic distribution of the population.

In the case of Udine's central parishes, the greater presence of upper class families clearly did play a positive role, and the results from the LISA index reflect those from the descriptive analysis, but there is little correlation in the case of the outer parishes, and it remains unclear why two of them have a concentration of houses with high levels of IMR. It could be because S. Giorgio and SS. Redentore are the only parishes that have all-four of the following characteristics: (1) high density of artisans and craftsmen (linked to high infant mortality rates); (2) few trade workers (socio-professional group associated to low levels of infant mortality); (3) high number of overcrowded houses; (4) low number of high quality houses.

References

Anselin, L. (1992). *Spatial data analysis with GIS: An introduction to application in the social sciences*. NCGIA Technical Report. http://www.ncgia.ucsb.edu/Publications/Tech_Reports/92/92-10.PDF

Anselin, L. (1995). Local indicators of spatial association-LISA. *Geographical Analysis, 27*, 93–115.

Anselin, L. (undated). *Exploring spatial data with GeoDa: A workbook*. https://www.geoda.uiuc.edu/pdf/geodaworkbook.pdf

Anselin, L., Syabri, I., & Kho, Y. (2006). GeoDa: An introduction to spatial data analysis. *Geographical Analysis, 38*, 5–22.

Ashton, J., Grey, P., & Barnard, K. (1986). Healthy cities. WHO's new public health initiative. *Health Promotion International, 1*(3), 319–324.

Badaloni, M., & Vinci, E. (1988). Contributi all'analisi dell'autocorrelazione spaziale. *Metron, 46*, 119–140.

Baker, M. G., Venugopal, K., & Howden-Chapman, P. (2011). Household crowding and tuberculosis. In M. Braubach, D. E. Jacobs, & D. Ormandy (Eds.), *Environmental burden of disease associated with inadequate housing*. Geneva: WHO.

Baldissera, G. (1877). *Le strade e le case di Udine. Studio di igiene applicata*. Udine: Tipografia Jacob e Colmegna.

Barnett, A. G., Dobson, A. J., McElduff, P., Salomaa, V., Kuulasmaa, K., & Sans, S. (2005). Cold periods and coronary events: An analysis of populations worldwide. *Journal of Epidemiology & Community Health, 59*, 551–557.

Bengtsson, T., & van Poppel, F. (2011). Socioeconomic inequalities in death from past to present: An introduction. *Explorations in Economic History, 48*, 343–356.

Blum, A., Houdaille, J., & Lamouche, M. (1990). Mortality differentials in France during the late 18th and early 19th centuries. *Population (An English selection), 2*, 163–185.

Breschi, M., & Serio, N. (1999). Case e famiglie a Udine nell'anno 1809. In M. Breschi (Ed.), *Vivere in Friuli*. Udine: Forum.

Breschi, M., Derosas, R., & Manfredini, M. (2000). Infant mortality in nineteenth century Italy: Interactions between ecology and society. In T. Bengtsson & O. Saito (Eds.), *Population and economy. from hunger to modern economic growth*. New York: Oxford University Press.

Breschi, M., Derosas, R., & Manfredini, M. (2004). Mortality and environment in three Emilian, Tuscan and venetian communities, 1800–1883. In T. Bengtsson, C. Campbell, J. Z. Lee, et al. (Eds.), *Life under pressure: Mortality and living standards in Europe and Asia, 1700 – 1900*. Cambridge, MA: MIT Press.

Burnett, J. (1991). Housing and the decline of mortality. In R. Schofield, D. Reher, & A. Bideau (Eds.), *The decline of mortality in Europe*. Oxford: Clarendon.

Burstrom, B., Diderichsen, F., & Smedman, L. (1999). Child mortality in Stockholm during 1885–1910: The impact of household size and number of children in the family on the risk of death from measles. *American Journal of Epidemiology, 194*(12), 1134–1141.

Cage, R. A. (1994). Infant mortality rates and housing: Twentieth century Glasgow. *Scottish Economic and Social History, 14*, 77–92.

Cage, R. A., & Foster, J. (2002). Overcrowding and infant mortality: A tale of two cities. *Scottish Journal of Political Economy, 49*(2), 129–149.

Cliff, A. D., & Ord, J. K. (1973). *Spatial autocorrelation*. London: Pion.

Dalla Zuanna, G., & Rosina, A. (2011). An analysis of extremely high nineteenth-century winter neonatal mortality in a local context of north-eastern Italy. *European Journal of Population, 27*, 33–55.

Derosas, R. (2009). The joint effect of maternal malnutrition and cold weather on neonatal mortality in nineteenth-century Venice: An assessment of the hypothermia hypothesis. *Population Studies, 63*(3), 233–251.

Desai, M. A., Mehta, S., & Smith, K. R. (2004). Indoor smoke from solid fuels assessing the environmental burden of disease at national and local levels. (Environmental disease burden series, Vol. 4). Geneva: WHO. http://www.who.int/quantifying_ehimpacts/publications/en/Indoorsmoke.pdf

Desai, M. A., Rehfuess, E., Mehta, S., & Smith, K. R. (2011). Indoor smoke from solid fuel use. In M. Braubach, D. E. Jacobs, & D. Ormandy (Eds.), *Environmental burden of disease associated with inadequate housing*. Geneva: WHO.

Gent, J. F., Ren, P., Belanger, K., Triche, E., Bracken, M. B., Holford, T. R., & Leaderer, B. P. (2002). Levels of household mould associated with respiratory symptoms in the first year of life in a cohort at risk for asthma. *Environmental Health Perspectives, 110*, 781–786.

Healy, J. D. (2003). Excess winter mortality in Europe: A cross country analysis identifying key risk factors. *Journal of Epidemiology and Community Health, 57*, 784–789.

Hollingsworth, T. H. (1977). Mortality in the British peerage families since 1600. *Population, 32*, 323–352.

Jaakkola, M. S., Haverinen-Shaughnessy, U., Douwes, J., & Nevalainen, A. (2011). Indoor dampness and mould problems in homes and asthma onset in children. In M. Braubach, D. E. Jacobs, & D. Ormandy (Eds.), *Environmental burden of disease associated with inadequate housing*. Geneva: WHO.

Lavagnolo, A. (1842/1850). *Pianta della R. Città di Udine*. Ripamonti Carpano: Venezia.

Mansutti, V. (1984). Argomento introduttivo. In G. B. Della Porta (Ed.), *Memorie su le antiche case di Udine*. Udine: Istituto per l'Enciclopedia del Friuli Venezia Giulia.

Perrenoud, A. (1975). L'inégalité sociale devant la mort à Genève au XVIIe siècle. *Population, 30*(5), 221–243.

Rudge, J. (2011). Indoor cold and mortality. In M. Braubach, D. E. Jacobs, & D. Ormandy (Eds.), *Environmental burden of disease associated with inadequate housing*. Geneva: WHO.

Stein, L. (1950). A study of respiratory tuberculosis in relation to housing conditions in Edinburgh. I. The pre-war period. *British Journal of Social Medicine, 4*, 143–169.

Upton, G. J. G., & Fingleton, B. (1985). *Spatial data analysis by example*. New York: Wiley.

van Poppel, F., & Mandemakers, K. (1997). Differential infant and child mortality in the Netherlands, 1812–1912: First results of the historical sample of the population of the Netherlands. In A. Bideau, B. Desjardins, & H. P. Brignoli (Eds.), *Infant and child mortality in the past*. Oxford: Clarendon Press.

Vedrenne-Villeneuve, E. (1961). L'inégalité sociale devant la mort dans la première moitié du XIXe siècle. *Population, 16*(4), 665–698.

Voss, P. R., Curtis White, K. J., & Hammer, R. B. (2006). Explorations in spatial demography. In W. A. Kandel & D. L. Brown (Eds.), *Population change and rural society*. Dordrecht: Springer.

Weir, D. R. (1995). Family income, mortality, and fertility on the eve of the demographic transition: A case study of Rosny-Sous-Bois. *The Journal of Economic History, 55*, 1–26.

Wilkinson, P., Pattenden, S., Armstrong, B., Fletcher, A., Sari Kovats, R., Mangtani, P., & McMichael, A. J. (2004). Vulnerability to winter mortality in elderly people in Britain: Population based study. *British Medical Journal, 329*(7467), 647–651.

Zaccomer, G. P., & Mason P. (2007). *Progettazione e sviluppo di un software a supporto dell'analisi shift-share con struttura spaziale*. Nota di ricerca, 8, Department of Statistics, University of Udine.

Chapter 4
Residential Mobility and Child Mortality in Early Twentieth Century Belfast

Alice Reid, Eilidh Garrett, and Simon Szreter

4.1 Introduction

Despite several decades of research, and a general advancement of understanding, the precise influences on early age mortality during the demographic transition in the British Isles are still unclear. Woods, Watterson and Woodward's seminal two-part article (1988, 1989) on the causes of rapid infant mortality decline in England and Wales from around 1900 sets up the framework for analysis by discussing environmental conditions and overcrowding (particularly in urban areas) together with social class, occupation and income, and provides a good overview of the sources available to investigate the issue. Due to restrictions on the use of individual level data, analysis of these sources has had to be mostly at the aggregate level, being limited to the cross-tabulations and categorisations provided in the official publications of the Offices of the Registrars General who were responsible both for civil registration and the administration of the decennial censuses.[1] The published data tends to be available at either a regional level, or, rather less often, at a detailed occupational level (see for example 1911 Census of England and Wales, Vol. III, Part II).

[1] Britain had three Registrars General in the early twentieth century; one each for England and Wales, Scotland and Ireland.

A. Reid (✉)
Department of Geography, University of Cambridge, Cambridge, UK
e-mail: alice.reid@geog.cam.ac.uk

E. Garrett
Department of Geography, University of Cambridge, Cambridge, UK

Department of History, University of Essex, Wivenhoe Park, Colchester, UK
e-mail: eilidh.garrett@btinternet.com

S. Szreter
Faculty of History, University of Cambridge, Cambridge, UK
e-mail: srss@cam.ac.uk

D. Ramiro Fariñas, M. Oris (eds.), *New Approaches to Death in Cities during the Health Transition*, International Studies in Population 12,
DOI 10.1007/978-3-319-43002-7_4

Perhaps the broadest analysis using data from the Registrar General's Annual Reports was conducted by Lee (1991) who compared regional patterns in infant mortality over the second half of the nineteenth century, concluding that over half of all regional variation in infant mortality could be explained by industrial concentration and high density housing. Others have hypothesised about the means by which housing could be correlated with mortality: Cage (1994) maintained that overcrowding within individual dwellings was the crucial factor, and (Aaby et al. 1984) and Bernhardt (1994) suggested that congestion and the transmission of communicable diseases were crucial in increasing mortality from infectious diseases. Morgan (1993,2002) has suggested a different route to high mortality, arguing that the proximity of stables and dung heaps was crucial for the rapid breeding of flies in the summer, increasing mortality from diarrhoea among the occupants of surrounding houses (see also Buchanan 1985).

There was a clear hierarchy of housing quality in urban Britain, from damp, dark and airless cellar-dwellings, over-crowded tenements and back-to-backs, to through-terraces with a yard or garden and semi-detached and detached houses occupied by the better off (Burnett 1991: 161–6). Housing quality tended to go hand in hand with housing size and type, and the dangers of poor housing included overcrowding, unhygienic construction, a lack of ventilation, inadequate and impure water supplies, imperfect or absent sewerage, high rents, and poor facilities for cooking and food storage. It is difficult to find sources which allow the measurement of all or even some of these factors at an individual level.[2] Moreover because poor housing tended to combine cramped and overcrowded conditions with poor ventilation and sanitation, and to be occupied by the least wealthy in society, it is difficult to disentangle these factors.

Burnett (1991: 176) argues that 'It was beyond dispute that housing was one of the most important environmental factors which influenced disease and mortality. When housing conditions were at their worst in the early industrial towns, so also were mortality rates: when conditions improved during the later nineteenth century, mortality improved significantly'. However it should be recognised that infant mortality rates in the constituent countries of Britain did not see significant and sustained decline until the beginning of the twentieth century, as Fig. 4.1 shows. Rural areas however, tended to have worse housing but lower infant mortality rates and earlier declines, suggesting that the house itself was unlikely to be the principal determining factor in mortality.[3] Burnett goes on to assert that

> Although bad housing could clearly facilitate the transfer of communicable diseases, interfere with physiological needs, and cause injury to health and safety, so also could other factors, and it would be unwise to attempt to assign a quantifiable 'weight' to the specific influence of the house. … it is not possible to isolate the house as a physical structure from associated amenities such as water supplies and sewerage, from the external environment in which it was located, or from the wider social and economic environment of its occupants; poor housing almost always went with overcrowding, poor sanitation, poor diet, and a generally poor standard of living as part of the cycle of deprivation. (Burnett 1991, 176)

[2] The field books of the Valuation Office survey (carried out 1910–1915) offer some scope for work of this type, but they are neither easy to access nor easy to use (see Short 1997).

[3] On urban rural differences in morality see Williams and Galley (1995) and Woods and Shelton (1997) Table 4.5, p 54.

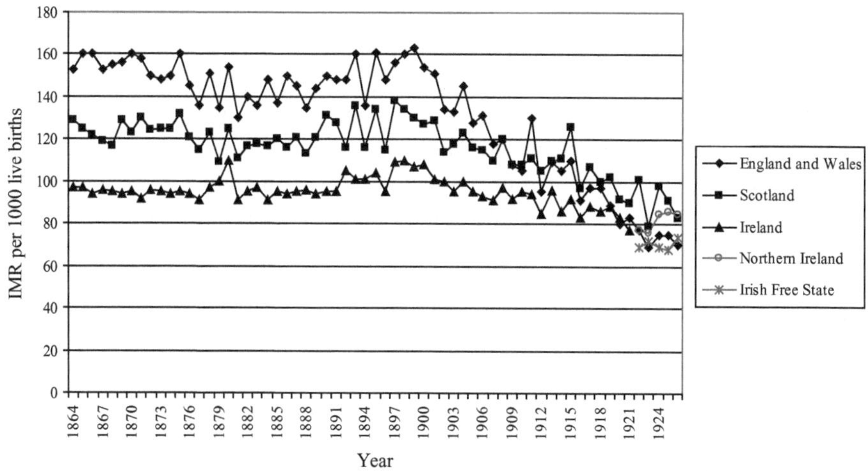

Fig. 4.1 Infant mortality rates England & Wales, Scotland and Ireland compared, 1864–1926 (Source: Annual Reports of the Registrars General)

As mentioned above, almost all data suitable for the investigation into the correlates of early age mortality over the British demographic transition is only available at aggregate level, rendering it all but impossible to look in more detail at the influence of housing on mortality. The emergence from the 100 year confidentiality clause of the individual level data from the 1911 census enumerators' books and their recent availability for academic use[4] will open up further possibilities for analysis of the influences in both early age mortality and fertility over the late nineteenth and early twentieth centuries. The value of this source is that, unlike previous British censuses, questions were directed to all currently married women about the duration of their marriage, the number of children born into that marriage and the number of those children still alive at the date of the census.[5] The analysis of the answers to these questions enables the estimation of early age mortality rates using the demographic techniques of indirect estimation (Brass 1975; Feeney 1980; Sullivan 1972; Trussell 1975).[6]

Although these data are newly available in this form, the aggregate results have been analysed by Watterson (1986, 1988) and Preston and Haines (1991). The latter used the data as a comparator for a more detailed analysis of parallel individual

[4] The individual level returns from the 1911 census of England and Wales, together with those from preceding censuses, are now available through the I-CeM project <https://www.essex.ac.uk/history/research/icem/>. However names and addresses are not routinely included in the I-CeM data sets, and the 1911 census of Scotland is not available.

[5] The census was taken across Britain on Sunday 2nd April in 1911. 1911 was the first time 'children ever born' and 'children dead' questions had been asked in censuses of the British Isles, but the United States had asked such questions in 1890 and 1900.

[6] A related set of techniques of indirect estimation uses questions on parental survival to estimate adult mortality and such techniques have been occasionally applied to developed populations (Luy et al. 2011; Luy 2012).

level data from the 1900 census of the United States of America and concluded that the size of families' accommodation was 'probably one of the most important pathways by which economic circumstances influence child mortality' (Preston and Haines 1991, 182). Garrett et al. (2001) analysed a sample of individual level data from the 1911 census of England and Wales obtained under special permission from the General Register Office of England and Wales (then known as the Office for Population, Censuses and Surveys) and concluded that the number of rooms was an important factor in explaining the social class differences in early age mortality, but pointed out that attempts to determine the significance of overcrowding as measured by people per room was problematic due to the fact that families who had experienced child deaths would have been in less crowded houses in 1911 than they would have been had they not suffered in this way (Garrett et al. 2001, 136–139).

Because the data from the 1911 census only provide numbers of children born and died, and not information about the precise age at death, cause of death or season of death, these data cannot provide conclusive evidence regarding precise age specific or cause specific mortality. Nevertheless, the fact that they are accompanied by socio-economic information about parental occupation and the number of rooms in the house, and that these houses can be located on maps and the neighbourhood circumstances can be assessed, will allow housing to be considered alongside other socio-economic information, and the relationship between them to be compared. It is anticipated that the availability of the 1911 data to the academic community will unleash a surge of interest in this type of analysis.

However before these sorts of questions can be answered, it is necessary to consider some of the methodological implications of working with data which combine both retrospective and cross-sectional information. For the most part, censuses are cross-sectional: they gather data which relate to the point in time the census is collected. The questions asked in 1911 regarding the number of children born and died, however, related to events which would have largely taken place in preceding years. This is a potential problem if the circumstances which are considered as possible influences on or correlates of early age mortality had changed between the time the children were young and at risk of dying and the time the census was taken. In other words, significant levels of residential mobility could undermine the consideration of housing- and location-related factors as influences on mortality. Previous studies indicate very high levels of residential mobility in Victorian and Edwardian cities and so this problem should be taken very seriously (Pooley 1979).

A similar problem has recently been identified in relation to the measurement of child mortality among migrants in African cities using recently collected DHS (Demographic and Health Survey) data (Bocquier et al. 2011). Housing and location related factors measured in the DHS are measured only at the time the survey is taken, but the survey also collects retrospective birth histories including information about mortality. Because the survey asks about the length of residence in the current location and place of previous residence, and additionally collects detailed information on the dates of birth and death of the children, the authors have been able to identify which children were at risk and died in which type of place, and to produce corrected mortality rates for urban and rural areas. As the majority of migrants went from rural to urban areas, and tended to have lower mortality than non-migrants in their rural places of origin even before they moved, correction for migration reduced urban-rural differences in mortality, although they were still significant.[7]

This chapter addresses a similar question, but instead of concentrating purely on migration between rural and urban areas (which was not inconsiderable in late nineteenth and early twentieth century Britain), it focuses on those individuals who moved between houses, however short a distance the move was, in order to capture the effect of moving between houses with different facilities and neighbourhoods. The 1911 census did not ask for length of residence or place of previous residence, rendering it impossible to tell from this source alone who had moved, when they had done so and from where they had migrated. To overcome this problem the members of 1911 census households have been linked backwards through time via street directories published in the intervening years, to locate them in the 1901 census, thus forming a longitudinal data source. The 1911 census also did not ask for birth and death dates of children, nor ages at death, so individual deaths cannot be assigned to particular places. Instead we are limited to the examination of the overall mortality experience of women. We can compare those who moved with those who did not move; for the movers we can compare the housing characteristics of the families before and after they moved and then correlate these factors with mortality. We have restricted the analysis to those married for more than 10 years in 1911 in order to be able to use housing details in the 1901 census to identify the housing that such women occupied when their children were small.

Before we examine mortality among movers and stayers and according to housing characteristics, it is instructive to describe the data set in more detail, and the patterns of residential mobility it reveals.

Although the 1901 and 1911 censuses, including names and addresses, for England and Wales and for Scotland are not yet available for systematic academic use, those for Ireland are not subject to the same restrictions and are freely available.[8] This project uses the census records of 37,643 people living in a selected sample of streets in Belfast, Northern Ireland in 1911. This dataset, covering about 10 % of the population of Belfast at that time, was drawn up by the BelFam project, under the guidance of Prof. Liam Kennedy at Queen's University, Belfast.[9] Details of the population of the same streets were also gathered from the census of 1901.[10] Furthermore the heads of household in the relevant streets were also identified in the

[7] However housing related facilities could still only be measured at the point of survey.

[8] The 1901 and 1911 censuses for Ireland are available free of charge from http://www.nationalarchives.ie/

[9] See www.belfastfamilyhistory.com

[10] The sample of streets collected by the BelFam project for 1901 and 1911 overlapped but were not identical. The current project has collected the additional streets to ensure that the same streets were included in both samples.

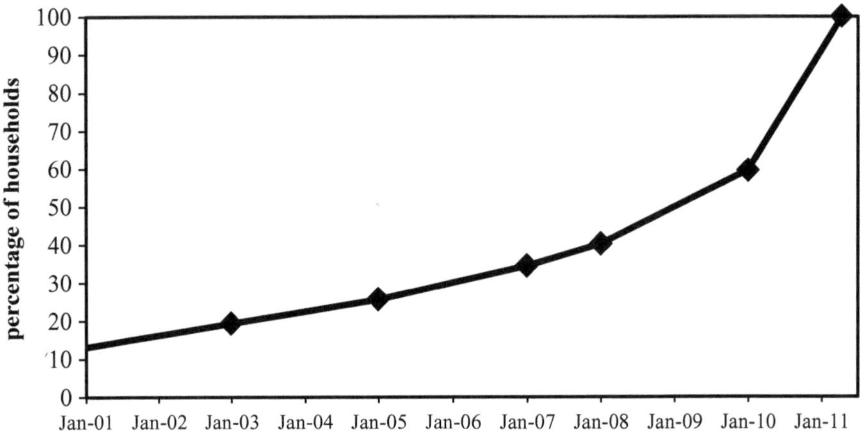

Fig. 4.2 Percentages of 1911 census households who had been in the same house in previous years (Source: Census of Belfast, 1911, BelFam sample. Belfast and Province of Ulster Street directories for 1901, 1903, 1905, 1907, 1908, 1910)

street directories for 1910, 1908, 1907, 1905, 1903 and 1901.[11] The sample streets were mainly chosen from within three distinct socio-economic and cultural areas: a working-class Protestant area (Shankill Ward), a working-class Catholic area (Falls Ward), and a more middle-class, mainly Protestant, area (Windsor Ward). The datasets have been described in more detail in Garrett et al. (2012).

Most studies of mobility have used prospective or forward-looking measures, identifying what percentage of people in a place was still living there the following year, or 10 years later. Because we are interested in the effect on retrospective measures, we have chosen to measure mobility in a retrospective way, and measure the percentage of those households in 1911 who had been in the same house at intervals of roughly 1, 3, 4, 6, 8 and 10 years previously.[12] We call this 'retrospective persistence', and the percentages are shown in Fig. 4.2.

This exercise highlights the highly mobile nature of the population: only about 60 % of household heads in 1911 were listed in the same house in the street directory of 1910, compiled about 15 months previously, and fewer than 15 % were listed as resident in the same house in 1901. These figures are very similar to those found for other British cities in this era (Pooley 1979).

Before proceeding to consider mobility in detail we should note that our initial analyses, as reported here, focus very much on the experience of married couples

[11] Late Victorian street directories usually contained comprehensive listings of the name and occupation of the head of household living at every street address in the city. This project uses *The Belfast and Province of Ulster Directory* (Garrett et al. 2012; Armstrong 2008). Some Belfast street directories are available from www.lennonwylie.co.uk

[12] The censuses were taken in early April, but the information in the street directories was probably collected in the final months of the year prior to the publication of the street directory, thus there is probably about 15–18 months in between the reference dates for the street directory of 1910 and the census of 1911.

Table 4.1 Number and percentage of women aged 20–49 by marital duration and co-residence with their husbands on census night, 1911, sample streets Belfast

Marital duration (years)	N of married women: husband present	N of married women: husband not present	% of married women husband not present
<5	1060	125	*11.8*
5–9	1000	94	*9.4*
10–14	869	71	*8.2*
15–19	655	63	*9.6*
20–24	502	64	*12.7*
25–29	207	27	*13.0*
30–34	38	5	*13.2*
Total	4331	449	*10.4*

Source: 1911 census of Belfast, BelFam sample

who reported their fertility and child survival in the census of 1911. This paper has neither considered married individuals living without their spouses, nor children living with only one parent or no parents at all. A married woman, living in a household where her husband was not resident, either because he was working elsewhere, was away on census night or because they had separated, would nevertheless report the number of her children and those who had survived, although of course they might not all be living with her. Such family groups might have had quite different housing trajectories, or fertility and infant and child mortality histories than those of co-resident married couples of the same marital duration, but they are much harder to trace in the street directories and the 1901 census. Thus, while they would have contributed to aggregate measures of fertility and child survival, they cannot be considered in a longitudinal study.

Table 4.1 shows the percentage of married women, aged 20–49 in the 1911 census, who were not resident with their husband on census night, by marital duration.

The table shows that over 10 % of married women in the 20–49 age group did not have their husband present with them on census night. As mentioned above, absent husbands may have been temporarily away from home, perhaps through work, or couples may have separated and been living apart. It is also possible that some women might have been erroneously reported as married: some, whose husbands had died, may have in fact been widowed, and others may have been reporting themselves as married when they were not, in order to hide the stigmatising evidence of an illegitimate child. The longer marital duration groups were slightly more likely to be without their husbands, possibly as they had grown-up children available to provide support. The shortest marital duration group also had a slightly elevated percentage of husbands away, which might reflect that many of these couples had not yet had children, making a father's absence rather easier.

Table 4.2 suggests that women at each marital duration who were living without a husband had both lower fertility and slightly higher child mortality than those who

Table 4.2 Children born per woman and the ratio of children who have died (cd) per 1000 children ever born (ceb) for married women aged 20–49 with and without co-resident husbands, by marital duration; Belfast 1911

	Husband present		Husband absent	
Marital duration (years)	Child/woman ratio	cd/ceb*1000	Child/woman ratio	cd/ceb*1000
<5	0.92	116	0.73	132
5–9	2.56	145	1.83	180
10–14	3.95	197	3.00	206
15–19	5.02	232	4.54	290
20–24	5.91	242	4.75	260
25–29	7.52	297	5.89	321
30–34[a]	8.39	395	6.40	93

Source: 1911 census of Belfast, BelFam sample
Note: For numbers of women in each category see Table 4.1
[a]Numbers in the marital duration category 30<35 are very small

Table 4.3 Logistic regression for the influences on the chance of having lived in the same house a year before the 1911 census, married heads of household only

	Exp(B)	Significance
Female	0.510	0.0000
Age	1.041	0.0000
Number of rooms in house	1.371	0.0000
Number of people in house	1.255	0.0000
People by rooms	0.965	0.0000
Labourer	0.660	0.0000
Married <1 year	0.079	0.0000
Married 1–4 years	0.393	0.0000
Children born	0.964	0.0102
Children born by married 1–4 years	1.283	0.0042

Source: 1911 census of Belfast, BelFam sample, linked to BPUD street directories
Note: interaction terms are italicised

were co-residing with their husband. By choosing to focus on married, co-resident couples in the analysis which follows, we therefore use a population which is not fully representative of the entire population.

It is also worth noting that only 80 % of the 8422 children aged less than 10 observed in the 1911 census were resident with both of their parents. Some 1244 (14.8 %) were resident with just their mothers, 219 (2.6 %) with just their fathers and 221 (2.6 %) with neither parent. Amongst the under-fives 83.9 % had both their parents resident with them, 12.5 % just had their mothers, 1.6 % just their fathers, and 2.0 % had neither parent. Thus the families we are observing in our analysis omit about one fifth of children in the youngest age groups, as well as those of their siblings who did not survive to be registered with them.

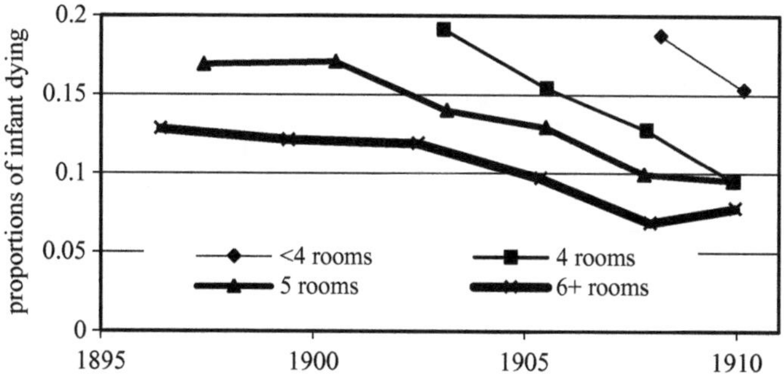

Fig. 4.3 Infant mortality estimates from the 1911 census, according to number of rooms occupied in 1911 (Source: 1911 census of Belfast, BelFam sample)

Table 4.3 shows a logistic regression model for married couples in 1911 for the influences on the chance of having been living in the same house a year earlier. The higher the coefficient, Exp(B), the higher the chance of having lived in the same house, and the lower the chance of having recently moved. The regression only shows statistically significant variables, the smaller the figure in the significance column, the more significant the result. The regression shows that older couples living in larger houses containing more people were more likely to have been living at the same address a year previously. However overcrowding (as indicated by the interaction term *people by rooms*) and reporting oneself as a labourer were linked to higher recent mobility. Thus mobility is shown to have been particularly high at the family building stages of the life-cycle, identified by Rowntree (1941: 459) in his seminal studies of town life in the early twentieth century as the period of greatest economic stress in a working man's life.

At this stage of the family life-cycle, especially among poor labourers, families would have been juggling the demands of a growing family at the same time as trying to establish a steady income (for more detail see Garrett et al. 2012). One of the strongest relationships in Table 4.3 is between recent stability and the number of rooms in the house. Those who lived in larger houses in 1911 were less likely to have moved recently. Such people are also likely to have experienced lower infant and child mortality, as shown by Fig. 4.3: the differences are large and fairly consistent and show that inhabitants of larger houses in 1911 had lower infant and child mortality, but it is important to remember that this is simply a correlation and does not imply a causal relationship. It is possible that small houses caused higher mortality through transmission of infectious diseases or via insanitary facilities, but it is also possible smaller houses were occupied by poorer people and that poverty affected mortality directly rather than indirectly via housing. Finally it is also possible that this relationship emerges because those who suffered higher mortality and therefore ended up with smaller families were able to remain in smaller houses.

If smaller houses were associated with both higher mortality and a higher chance of moving, we would also expect those who moved to have had higher mortality. This is demonstrated in Fig. 4.4, which shows indirect estimates of infant mortality

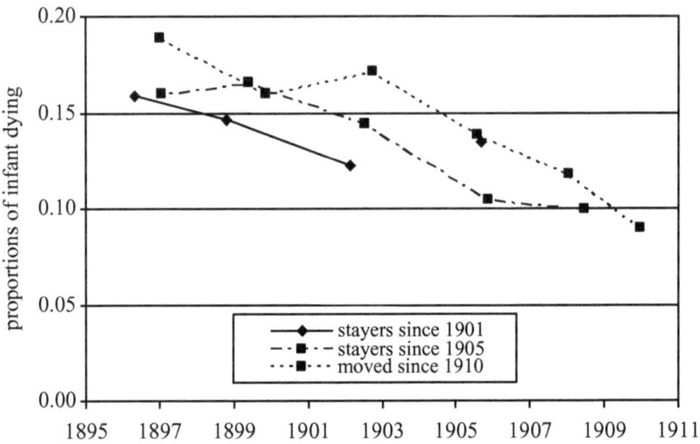

Fig. 4.4 Infant mortality estimations from Belfast 1911 census, according to mobility status (Source: 1911 census of Belfast, BelFam sample, linked to BPUD street directories)

for those who had lived in the same house since 1901 (stayers since 1901), those who had lived in the same house since 1905 (stayers since 1905) and those who had moved since 1910 (movers since 1910).

It might be supposed that the high mobility among the recently married was linked to a progression in housing from small houses with poor facilities in less salubrious neighbourhoods to larger houses with better facilities in more attractive neighbourhoods. Alternatively, job and income insecurity might have provoked frequent moves between similar housing: it has been argued that travel and employment conditions created a high demand for housing near to places of potential work but this caused rents to rise, and, to avoid eviction, many people chose the cheapest accommodation they could find (Rodger 1989: 12). For those whose income may have been fluctuating due to the chronic insecurities of unskilled labouring work in the city finding affordable accommodation suitable to their needs is likely to have been a particular problem.

The high rates of mobility mean that it should not be assumed that housing and neighbourhood characteristics measured in 1911 also applied in the preceding years, when the children were at highest risk of death. If the mortality risks for those who moved were similar to those amongst the residentially stable, this might not be a problem, but Fig. 4.4 shows that infant mortality rates for those who had been at the same address since 1901 (stayers since 1901) were lower than those who had been at the same address since 1905 (stayers since 1905), and markedly lower than those who had moved since 1910 (movers since 1910). In summary, recent mobility was associated with a higher risk of mortality in early childhood. However it is not clear whether mobility and mortality were causally connected to each other, or if they were both driven by a third factor, such as social class or job security.

If people moved around between houses with very similar characteristics and remained within the same neighbourhoods, then it might be legitimate to use housing characteristics in 1911 as indicators of these characteristics at an earlier date. However the fact that movement is strongly linked to life-cycle stages suggests that movement, in the early years at least, may have been between different types of housing in order to acquire improved facilities with each subsequent move. In order to explore this further the next section of this paper will examine people's housing trajectories over the 1901–1911 period.

4.2 Mobility and Housing

We wanted to compare household circumstances in 1911 with those in 1901 to see how different housing circumstances were at the two dates: did people move between houses of similar types and in similar surroundings or did they move through a particular trajectory of housing types or specifications.

Although we have census returns for our study areas for both dates, the high level of mobility means that many families moved to our sample streets from elsewhere in Belfast, Ireland or further afield. To generate a representative sample of 'movers' we needed to try to capture those moving to our areas from elsewhere in Belfast and beyond. This was a time-consuming task and therefore we restricted ourselves to those who were recently married in 1901, that is, those married 11–14 years in 1911. (We started off with those married 10–15 years, but it seems that considerable rounding of marital durations took place and many of those reporting in 1911 that they had been married for 10 years must have married after the census was taken in 1901 so they cannot be located, recorded as a married couple, at that date).

We started off with 623 couples from our sample streets where the wife was between 20 and 49 in 1911 and reported having been married for 11–15 years. We found 38 (6 %) of these had been living in the same house in 1901,[13] and a further 38 % could be readily identified as living at another address in the study areas, or the wards containing them, using automatic linking techniques.[14] Of the remaining 348 we chose to search for 186 in the census of Ireland and found 134. The 52 not found might have moved from other places within the British Isles, Europe or further afield. Alternatively they might not have been matched due to errors in reporting or transcribing.[15]

Table 4.4 shows these results, according to the distance moved over the 10 year period between 1901 and 1911. Of those moving, the majority moved just a short

[13] Six per cent is rather lower than the 15 % found for the whole database above, which can be explained by the fact that these couples were of a relatively short marital duration and consequently more mobile than the married population in general.

[14] We were able to search automatically though the census households in all the wards in which our census streets were located, but not elsewhere in Belfast or further afield. Manual searches through the on-line database (http://www.nationalarchives.ie/) were therefore undertaken for those we could not find automatically.

[15] 162 remain as yet unsearched for.

Table 4.4 Couples married 11–14 years and aged 20–49 in the BelFam sample of the 1911 census of Belfast

	Not moved	Automatically found in study area	Searched for	Not searched for	TOTAL	Total adjusted to include % of not searched for	%
Not moved	38				38	38	6.10
Moved within ward		174	28		202	226	36.34
Moved within Belfast		63	84		147	220	35.34
Moved within Ireland			22		22	41	6.61
Not found			52		52	97	15.62
Not in sample traced				162	162		
TOTAL	38	237	186	162	623	623	100

Source: Censuses of Belfast 1911 and 1901, BelFam sample, and 1901 census of Ireland, http://www.nationalarchives.ie/

distance, within the confines of the city of Belfast, although a small number moved from elsewhere in Ireland. The final columns show an adjustment to take account of the likely mobility pattern of those we did not search for, demonstrating that at least three-quarters of couples married between 11 and 14 years in 1911 had been resident in Belfast 10 years before although the majority of those had moved house at least once during that time.[16]

Among those who moved house, it was more common to move from a smaller house to a larger house: 55 % of couples moved from a smaller to a larger house and only 18 % moved from a larger to a smaller house, confirming a certain degree of progression in type or form. A large minority of couples, however, moved between houses of the same size, and about half of the sample moved between 4 and 5 roomed houses. A good deal of mobility, therefore, was apparently between similar houses. There are indications that different streets were attractive at different marital durations: some streets were extremely attractive to young couples: all of Ottawa Street's 65 households contained couples married for less than 10 years in 1911, compared to an average of 54 % of all households, and young couples were also well represented in a number of other street such as Oregon Street, Sandhurst

[16] The adjustment assumes that those not traced will be distributed in the same proportion as those searched for.

Gardens and Quebec Street.[17] Many of the young couples in these streets had not yet started to reproduce, but just around the corner there were other streets where there was an average or above average percentage of young couples, very few of whom had no children: such streets seem to have been places where those with young families congregated.[18] At the other end of the spectrum, there were streets where housing does not seem to have been available to young couples married less than 10 years, such as Wellesley Avenue and Wellington Park in Windsor Ward, where large houses may have priced out the newly married, but Rosebank Street in Shankill also had very few couples married for less than 10 years in 1911 with a similar average house size to Shankill ward as a whole.[19]

This suggests that couples moved around in quite a patterned way, which may have been connected to employment prospects, available housing, rents, neighbourhood character and individual facilities, supporting the filtering theory of household mobility. Filtering theory states that as people move up the social scale they move into more desirable housing and their former houses become occupied by lower-income groups (Gray and Boddy 1979). Thus homes slowly filter down the social scale and individuals filter up the housing scale in tandem with improvement in their wealth status. However the particularities of housing provision in Belfast in this period will also have played a part in housing trajectories and will determine how easy or hard it is to detect a clear progression in housing. Belfast developed relatively late as an industrial city, with a large building boom in the second half of the nineteenth century. Although in the mid-nineteenth century many houses had poor facilities and piped water was rare (McCracken 1967), the Health Act of 1875 required that all new houses be built with back yards, rear access, and piped water (Glasscock 1967; Collins 1983). The majority of newly built houses were ‘two up, two down’ – that is with two rooms on the ground floor and a further two upstairs. They were either ‘parlour houses’ the downstairs having a front parlour with a kitchen and a scullery (which was not counted as a room) behind, or ‘kitchen houses’ which had a front kitchen, a back bedroom and a scullery (Collins 1983; Fraser 1996: 63). Kitchen houses were both cheaper to rent and more popular due to the additional sleeping accommodation. It is plausible that they were particularly attractive to families with young children. Older houses often had only three rooms, and were less likely to have had the modern amenities of piped water and rear access. Finally, five roomed houses with an additional bedroom over the scullery were the most expensive houses available to the working classes.

[17] In all of these streets, each containing at least 50 households, at least 80 % of households were inhabited by a couple who had been married for less than 10 years. None of these streets appears to have been very recently built and the majority of houses were occupied in the 1901 census and street directory.

[18] For example Hawthorn Street, Earlscourt Street, Abyssinia Street and Utility Street.

[19] In these streets which contained 91, 64 and 56 households respectively, 22 %, 16 % and 18 % of those households contained couples married for less than 10 years, compared to an average of 54 % among all households.

Although newly built houses had to have piped water from 1878, working class houses did not have inside bathrooms, and the water supply was not reliable until the early years of the twentieth century (Glasscock 1967). Moreover it was some time before older houses reached the same standards; it is estimated that in 1898, 28 % of houses had no back access (Collins 1983), and that in 1914 about a third still had ash pits which were emptied every 7 or 8 weeks (Gribbon 1982). It is therefore plausible that houses which appear similar in terms of the number of rooms, or occupy a similar footprint on a map, enjoyed different facilities or states of repair. Overdevelopment of the housing sector due to speculative building meant that there was no pressure on the supply of houses in Belfast in this period: it is estimated that 10,000 (1 in 7) working class homes lay vacant in 1898 (Lynch 1998: 112). In such a renters' market, it is plausible that small changes in family circumstances and housing availability might have prompted a move, and additional rental-related features such as whether houses were furnished or un-furnished might have played a part. Smaller and poorer quality properties were more likely to have had very short term (weekly or monthly) tenancy agreements (Daunton 1983: 138), and this might also have increased the propensity of younger and poorer families to move often.

Moving trajectories can be illustrated by examples of residential histories for three different families. Appendix Fig. 4.5 shows the Scarrs, a family who did not move, but remained in the same house throughout the decade leading up to the 1911 census. Although it is possible that they had moved in their first 4 years of marriage, before 1901, much of the time their children were at risk of infant and child death will have been spent in the house at 179 Leopold Street. Appendix Fig. 4.6 shows the moves by the Skates family, who have been located in 7 of the 8 sources as living in Mossvale Street or Heather Street. Although they moved to and fro, the moves were incredibly short distances, and there does not seem to be much to choose between the housing: although there might have been differences in the condition of the houses they lived in, they stayed in the same neighbourhood and it might be reasonable to assume that the facilities were similar too. Appendix Fig. 4.7 shows the moves made by the Armour family who can be seen on the outskirts of Belfast in the 1901 census. By 1907 they had moved into the study area and they can be seen living in four different houses on three different, but nearby streets. Although these houses may have differed in internal layout, they all had four rooms, a small back yard with outhouse, and back alley. As was common with many of the frequently moving families, there was no clear progression in terms of ground floor area or number of rooms, although the final house we see them in has an L-shape rather than a square back, which is likely to have indicated it was a slightly more expensive 'parlour house'. In addition facilities or neighbourhoods may have differed in ways we cannot tell from the census, although large scale maps can give some indication of local amenities as well as potential hazards.

This aspect of our research indicates once again that residential mobility was very high in Belfast in the decade leading up to 1911. Only about 6 % of couples married for 11–14 years in 1911 had been living in the same accommodation since 1901. It is only for this small percentage of couples in this marital duration that it might be legitimate to assume that the housing characteristics in 1911 also reflect those when their children were at risk of death. A sizeable minority of other couples, however, appear to have lived in very similar housing despite moving frequently: although they have the same number of rooms at their disposal, the housing may differ in other ways not measureable using the census. A small proportion of couples moved into smaller houses, but the majority moved into larger ones, suggesting that life-course progression during the early years of marriage when children were young and at risk of death means that it should not be assumed that cross-sectional information gathered at the time of a census or survey can be assumed to represent conditions a decade or even a year or two earlier. The chances that they will be able to represent specific risk factors such as type of toilet facility or ventilation are slim. It is probable however that housing indicators can still reflect wealth or social-class and that they will show a correlation with mortality through this route. The next section examines mortality according to housing as measured in 1901 and 1911.

4.3 Early Age Mortality and Housing

Table 4.5 compares infant and child mortality among women married for 11–14 years and aged 20–49 in 1911. This is done using a simple 'children dead' to 'children ever born' ratio, as we are just interested in making comparisons within this marital duration and thus do not need to adjust the ratios to represent mortality to a particular age or at a particular point in time.[20] The table compares the mortality of those living in 3 or fewer rooms, 4 rooms, 5 rooms or 6 or more rooms at different dates. Although numbers in some of these categories are very small, those living in large houses in 1901 seem to be more consistently advantaged in terms of the survival of their children than those living in large houses in 1911: these are people who were already relatively comfortably off at the beginning of their married lives – even those who did not maintain this level of comfort in terms of the number of rooms they lived in were able to keep their children alive. Interestingly, however, children living in small houses in 1901 were not necessarily disadvantaged by this: for them what was important was their parents' subsequent housing trajectory (or the factors dictating the latter). Those children who had moved with their parents from a small (1–3) room house to a substantially larger one (with 6+ rooms) by 1911 had a distinct advantage in terms of survival – it is possible the factors which rendered their parents able to afford a larger house were able to confer an early advantage in terms of children's survival. The converse may be true for those who went from a medium sized house to a small one: although numbers are very small, such children appear disadvantaged, but it is also possible that families who had

[20] All these figures were adjusted by dividing by the same expected proportion dead for those married 10–14 years, which for this marital duration group (using the multipliers for indirect estimation from UN Manual X and the mortality levels from Coale-Demeny West Level 13) is 0.1901, thus transforming these ratios into estimates of under-five mortality (United Nations 1983).

Table 4.5 Children dead (cd) as a percentage of children ever born (ceb) to women who moved between 1901 and 1911, according to number of rooms at each date

		Rooms in 1911							
		1–3 rooms		4 rooms		5 rooms		6+ rooms	
		cd/ceb	# of women	cd/ceb	# of women	cd/ceb	# of women	cd/ceb	# of women
Rooms in 1901	1–3	14.29	*4*	24.49	*27*	18.29	*18*	15.91	*10*
	4	25.00	*4*	19.55	*52*	20.92	*64*	20.59	*17*
	5	42.86	*2*	23.53	*16*	21.60	*27*	21.88	*25*
	6+	0.00	*1*	10.71	*10*	12.66	*17*	5.67	*42*

Source: Censuses of Belfast 1911 and 1901, BelFam sample, and 1901 census of Ireland, http://www.nationalarchives.ie/

Table 4.6 OLS regression analysis of the influences on the proportion of children dead among women married 11–14 years in 1911

	Model 1		Model 2		Model 3	
	Coefficient	P>t	Coefficient	P>t	Coefficient	P>t
Small house 1911	0.0418	0.499			0.0347	0.569
Large house 1911	−0.0367	0.144			−0.0109	0.679
Small house 1901			0.0906	0.363	0.0285	0.368
Large house 1901			**−0.0562**	**0.000**	**−0.0893**	**0.002**
Overcrowded in 1901 (>2 people per room)			**−0.1081**	**0.030**	**−0.0497**	**0.030**
Social class I or II	−0.0421	0.118	−0.0405	0.478	−0.0161	0.562
Social class V	**0.0853**	**0.001**	**0.0884**	**0.002**	**0.0781**	**0.002**
Constant	**0.1604**	**0.000**	**0.1787**	**0.000**	**0.1845**	**0.000**
Number of observations		*381*		*381*		*381*
R-squared		*0.0803*		*0.1136*		*0.1149*
Adj R-squared		*0.0705*		*0.1018*		*0.0983*

Source: Censuses of Belfast 1911 and 1901, BelFam sample, and 1901 census of Ireland, http://www.nationalarchives.ie/

suffered many infant deaths chose to live in small houses as a result of their reduced family size.

Table 4.6 shows a regression analysis of the influences on the proportion of children dead to each woman married for 11–14 years in 1911.[21] Model 1 in the table examines the association of housing in 1911 with mortality: although living in a large house in 1911 was associated with lower mortality when no other variables were controlled, this was predominantly due to the fact that the lower social classes (class V) were less likely to live in large houses.[22] Once social class was controlled,

[21] Ordinary least squares regression is performed, and the analysis is at the woman level.

[22] On the well-known limitations of the RG's social classs cheme, see Garrett et al. 2001, 12, 197–200.

housing circumstances in 1911 had no effect on mortality. Model 2 shows the influence of housing measured in 1901, among exactly the same women. In this case social class does not account for all of the effect of housing: those who were already living in a large house in 1901 went on to have fewer child deaths than expected. Unexpectedly, those whose living conditions were overcrowded when their children were young also had a slight survival advantage.[23] Model 3 confirms that mortality was more sensitive to housing circumstances as measured in 1901 than 1911, and indicates that housing in 1911, although connected to wealth and opportunity, provides little additional insight into the factors linked to infant death. In comparison, housing in 1901 appears to have an independent effect on mortality and further research is needed into which particular facets of housing affected child health in the early twentieth century.

This chapter has offered tentative conclusions, but there are a number of reasons why these arguments may be even more compelling in other situations, both in the British Isles and elsewhere. The first is Belfast's housing stock: the majority of homes in Belfast were built very quickly in the second half of the nineteenth century, and were therefore relatively very homogenous with very few of the particularly insanitary and unhealthy back-to-backs found in English industrial cities such as Leeds (Daunton 1983: 26-6). Even in the working class district of Shankill, close inspection of contemporary large scale Ordnance Survey town plans shows that almost all houses had a back alley-way running behind their yards to facilitate the collection of refuse. In other towns and cities individuals' housing trajectories may therefore have been characterised by much greater differentiation than was true in Belfast. Secondly, Belfast's residential areas were strongly delineated along religious lines, restricting spheres of movement for particular groups.

The primary conclusion from this chapter must be that although housing, as measured by the number of rooms in the house, is correlated with child survival, indicators measured at the time a retrospective survey is undertaken must, if used as indicators of housing conditions when children were at risk of death, be treated with great caution. It is more legitimate to use them as proxies for wealth or stability of income, but it is clear that even in this role they are much more informative when combined in a longitudinal way with information from previous points in time. This is of importance not only for the likely burgeoning of research using the 1911 censuses of the British Isles and other historical census micro data which are increasingly available through projects such as IPUMS, NAPP and Mosaic, together with exciting developments in the more precise estimation of fertility and infant mortality,[24] but also for the use of cross-sectionally collected information in modern retrospective censuses and surveys.

[23] Overcrowding in 1911 is not included as it shows a strongly negative relationship with mortality, and it is suspected that low mortality families were more likely to be overcrowded in 1911 because they had lost few children. Thus causality runs from mortality to overcrowding, rendering it inappropriate to include this variable in the analysis. The negative relationship in 1901 might arise for the same reason, or because more overcrowded families had an incentive to move more quickly.

[24] See for example, new developments in indirect estimation by Goldstein et al. 2011.

Appendix

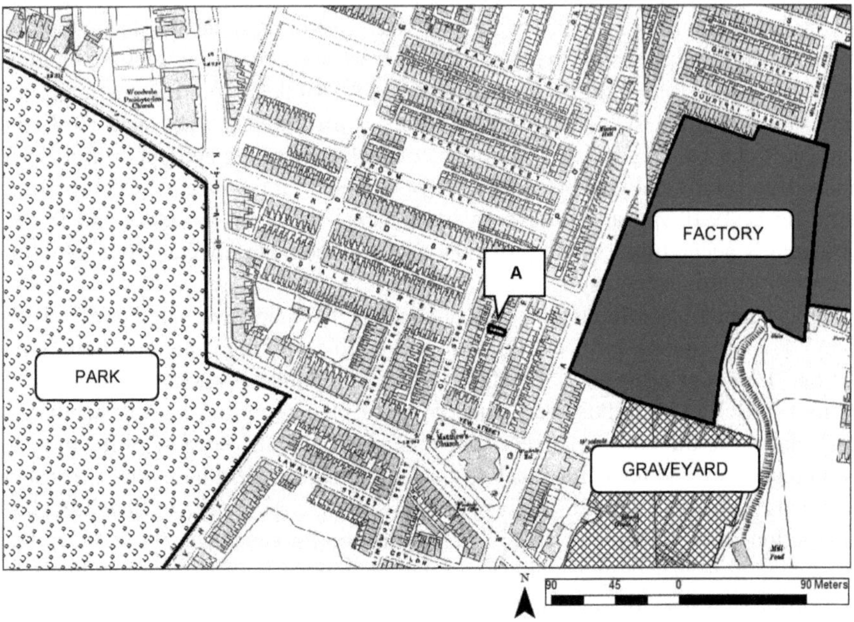

Fig. 4.5 Moves by the Scarr family, Belfast, 1901–1911. **A. 179 Leopold Street.** *1901 Census*: Elizabeth (aged 29) and Charles Scarr (31), iron turner, living at this address with 2 children. *1901, 1903, 1905, 1907, 1908 and 1910 Street Directories:* Charles Scarr, iron turner. *1911 Census:* Elizabeth (39) and Charles Scarr (40), iron turner, living with 3 children. Couple married for 14 years, 3 children, 0 dead. (Sources: for appendix figures: Census: 1901 and 1911 census returns: BelFam project, http://www.belfastfamilyhistory.com and National Archives of Ireland: http://www.census.nationalarchives.ie. Belfast Street directories: Belfast Street Directories online; http://www.lennonwylie.co.uk for 1901, 1907, 1908 and 1910 and The Belfast and Province of Ulster Directory 1903 and 1905. Base maps drawn from digital maps supplied by Ordnance Survey of Northern Ireland: Large Scale Town Plans, 5th Edition, 1901–1903)

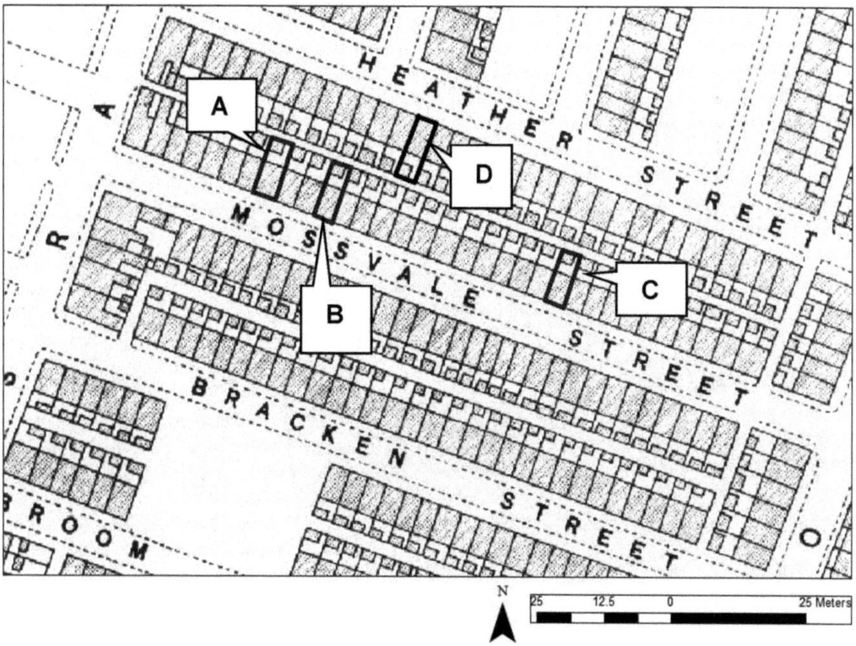

Fig. 4.6 Moves by the Skates family, Belfast, 1901–1911. **A. 51 Mossvale Street** *1901 Census:* Florence Skates (25), damask weaver, married with 2 children living with her parents, William (54) and Sarah (56) Donaldson. Matthew Skates not listed anywhere in Ireland. *1903 Directory:* Family cannot be located. **B. 45 Mossvale Street** *1905 Directory:* M. Skates, carter. **C. 21 Mossvale Street** *1907, 1908, 1910 Directories:* Matth. Skates, carter. **D. 42 Heather Street** *1911 Census:* Matthew (35), carter and Florence Skates living with 5 children. Couple married 12 years, 6 children, 1 dead. (For sources see Fig. 4.5)

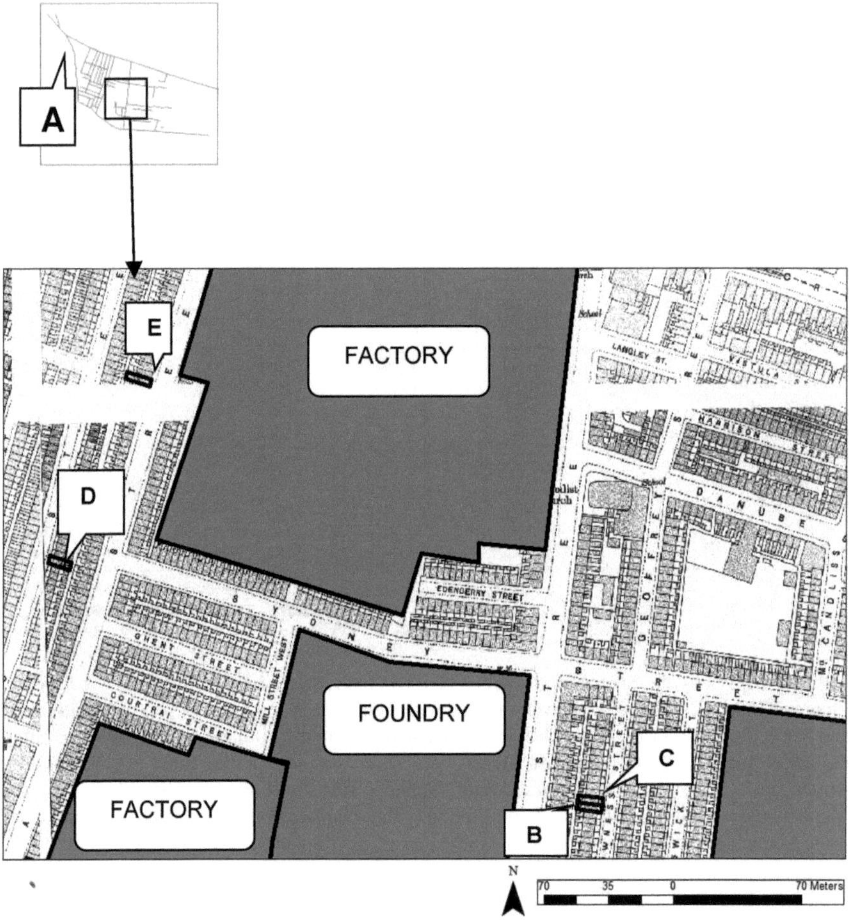

Fig. 4.7 Moves by the Armour family, Belfast, 1901–1911. **A. 5 Ligoniel Street (outskirts of Belfast)** *1901 Census:* Mary (26) and Simon Armour (28), quarry labourer living with 2 children and sharing house with Richard Proudfoot (44, widower, gardener) and his 5 children aged 4–16. *1901, 1903 and 1905 directories:* Family cannot be located. **B. 29 Bowness Road** *1907 Directory*: S. Armour, wood turner. **C. 31 Bowness Road** *1908 Directory*: S. Armour, wood turner. **D. 130 Leopold Street** *1910 Directory*: S. Armour, wood turner. **E. 59 Cambrai Street** *1911 Census*: Simon (38, wood turner) and Mary (35) Armour, living with 7 children. Couple married 14 years, 10 children, 3 dead. (For sources see Fig. 4.5)

References

1911 Census of England and Wales, 1923, Vol. XIII *Fertility of Marriage* Part II, HMSO: London.

Aaby, P., Bukh, J., Lisse, I., & Smits, A. (1984). Overcrowding and intense exposure as determinants of measles mortality. *American Journal of Epidemiology, 120*, 49–63.

Armstrong. D. (2008). *Belfast and ulster street directories 1805–1914: Guide and directory.* Library and Information Services Council (NI), Local History Panel. http://www.liscni.co.uk/docs/Belfast_and_Ulster_Street_Directories.pdf

Bernhardt, E. (1994). Overcrowding and mortality from airborne infectious disease: The case of Stockholm, 1895–1925. *Stockholm Research Reports in Demography, 83*, 27.

Bocquier, P., Madise, N. J., & Zulu, E. M. (2011). Is there an urban advantage in child survival in Sub-Saharan Africa? Evidence from 18 countries in the 1990s. *Demography, 48*, 531–558. doi:10.1007/s13524-011-0019-2.

Brass, W. (1975). *Methods for estimating fertility and mortality from limited and defective data.* North Carolina: Chapel Hill.

Buchanan, I. (1985). Infant feeding, sanitation and diarrhoea in colliery communities. In D. J. Oddy & D. S. Miller (Eds.), *Diet and health in modern Britain* (pp. 148–177). Beckenham: Croom Helm.

Burnett, J. (1991). Housing and the decline of mortality. In R. Schofield, D. Reher, & A. Bideau (Eds.), *The decline of mortality in Europe* (pp. 158–176). Oxford: Clarendon.

Cage, R. A. (1994). Infant mortality rates and housing: Twentieth century Glasgow. *Scottish Economic and Social History, 14*, 77–92.

Collins, B. (1983). The Edwardian city. In J. C. Beckett et al. (Eds.), *Belfast the making of the city, 1800–1914.* Belfast: Appletree Press.

Daunton, M. J. (1983). *House and home in the Victorian city: Working-class housing 1850–1914.* London: Edward Arnold.

Feeney, G. (1980). Estimating infant mortality trends from child survivorship data. *Population Studies, 34*, 109–128.

Fraser, M. (1996). *John Bull's other homes: State housing and British policy in Ireland 1883–1922.* Liverpool: Liverpool University Press.

Garrett, E., Reid, A., Schürer, K., & Szreter, S. (2001). *Changing family size in England and Wales: Place, class and demography, 1891–1911.* Cambridge: Cambridge University Press.

Garrett, E., Reid, A.,& Szreter, S. (2012). Fertility and child mortality in a household setting: Comparative perspectives from UK censuses, 1861–1921. *Popolazione e Storia*, 2010(2), 59–82.

Glasscock, R. (1967). The growth of the port. In J. Beckett & R. Glasscock (Eds.), *Belfast: The origin and growth of an industrial city*. London: BBC.

Goldstein, J. R., Gonzáles-Prieto, E., Gampe, J., & Peters, F. (2011). Missing children: Indirect estimation of child mortality from census microdata. Extended abstract of paper presented at PAA 2012. http://paa2012.princeton.edu/download.aspx?submissionId=121457. Accessed 16 May 2012.

Gray, F., & Boddy, M. (1979). The origins and use of theory in urban geography: Household mobility and filtering theory. *Geoforum, 10*, 117–127.

Gribbon, S. (1982). *Edwardian Belfast: A social profile.* Belfast: Appletree Press & Ulster Society for Irish Studies. (Picture Ulster Club, Castle Place).

Lee, R. (1991). Regional inequalities in infant mortality in Britain, 1861–1971: Patterns and hypotheses. *Population Studies, 45*, 55–65.

Luy, M. (2012). Estimating mortality differences in developed countries from survey information on maternal and paternal orphanhood. *Demography, 49*, 607–627.

Luy, M., Di Guilio, P., & Caselli, G. (2011). Differences in life expectancy by education and occupation in Italy, 1980–94: Indirect estimates from maternal and paternal orphanhood. *Population Studies, 65*, 137–155.

Lynch, J. (1998). *A tale of three cities: Comparative studies in working-class life*. Basingstoke: MacMillan.

McCracken, J. (1967). Early Victorian Belfast. In J. Beckett & R. Glasscock (Eds.), *Belfast: The origin and growth of an industrial city*. London: BBC.

Morgan, N. (1993). *Deadly dwellings*. Preston: Mullion Books.

Morgan, N. (2002). Infant mortality, flies and horses in later-nineteenth-century towns: A case study of Preston. *Continuity and Change, 17*, 97–132.

Pooley, C. (1979). Residential mobility in the Victorian city. *Transactions of the Institute of British Geographers New Series, 4*, 258–277.

Preston, S., & Haines, M. (1991). *Fatal years: Child mortality in late nineteenth century America*. Princeton: Princeton University Press.

Rodger, R. (1989). *Housing in urban Britain*. Cambridge: Cambridge University Press.

Rowntree, J. S. (1941). *Poverty and progress: A second social survey of York*. London: Longman, Green & Co.

Short, B. (1997). *Land and society in Edwardian British*. Cambridge: Cambridge University Press.

Sullivan, J. (1972). Models for the estimation of the probability of dying between birth and exact ages in early childhood. *Population Studies, 26*, 79–97.

Trussell, T. (1975). A re-estimation of the multiplying factors for the Brass technique for determining childhood survivorship rates. *Population Studies, 29*, 97–107.

United Nations. (1983). *Manual X: Indirect techniques of demographic estimation*. New York: The Department.

Watterson, P. (1986). Role of the environment in the decline of infant mortality: An analysis of the 1911 census of England and Wales. *Journal of Biosocial Science, 18*, 457–470.

Watterson, P. (1988). Infant mortality by father's occupation from the 1911 census of England and Wales. *Demography, 25*, 289–306.

Williams, N., & Galley, C. (1995). Urban-rural differentials in infant mortality in Victorian England. *Population Studies, 49*, 401–420.

Woods, R., & Shelton, N. (1997). *Atlas of Victorian mortality*. Liverpool: Liverpool University Press.

Woods, R., Watterson, P., & Woodward, J. H. (1988). The causes of rapid infant mortality decline in England and Wales, 1861–1921, Part 1. *Population Studies, 42*, 343–366.

Woods, R., Watterson, P., & Woodward, J. H. (1989). The causes of rapid infant mortality decline in England and Wales, 1861–1921, Part 2. *Population Studies, 43*, 113–132.

Chapter 5
Micro-Analysis of Mortality in Urban Areas. The Parish of Oliveira in Guimarães, in Northern Portugal Between the Eighteenth and Twentieth Centuries

Maria Norberta Amorim, Antero Ferreira, and Luís Meira-Machado

The systematic integration of all this information allows us to position adult individuals in their family and social life context, and to follow their life courses within a given adult community for a long period. The mortality register for individuals under the age of seven is not well maintained before 1860, according to the dispositions of the Diocese of Braga to which Guimarães belongs.

By extending the research up to 1910, we aim to systematically follow the adult population born between the late eighteenth century and the early nineteenth century, examining the risk of dying and relating it to the social environment. We also aim to examine infant-juvenile mortality from 1860 onwards by social status of the parents at birth.

The ultimate goal for demographic historians, even for those who chose the classical micro-analytical approach, is to explain the evolution of populations in light of the influence of demographic variables. This is difficult work, especially in urban settings, and is often pursued in stages but amply justified by the benefits of examining trends over a longer term time horizon. In historical demography, the methodological choices become crucial according to the nature of the sources; these

---

Research conducted within the Project "Espaços urbanos: dinâmicas demográficas e sociais (séculos XVII–XX)", with the reference FCT PTDC/HIS-HIS/099228/2008, co-funded by the budget of the COMPETE – Programa Operacional Factores de Competitividade in its ERDF component and the budget of the Fundação para a Ciência e a Tecnologia in its State Budget component.

M.N. Amorim (✉) • A. Ferreira
CITCEM – Transdisciplinary Culture, Space and Memory Research Centre, Universidade do Minho, Guimarães, Portugal
e-mail: mnsbamorim@gmail.com; anterof@gmail.com

L. Meira-Machado
Department of Mathematics for Science and Technology, Universidade do Minho, Guimarães, Portugal
e-mail: lmachado@math.uminho.pt

D. Ramiro Fariñas, M. Oris (eds.), *New Approaches to Death in Cities during the Health Transition*, International Studies in Population 12,
DOI 10.1007/978-3-319-43002-7_5

become more diverse in the long term, and particularly with reference to the key variables such as mobility and mortality. Thus, in the phase we are now pursuing – the analysis of mortality in the central parish of Guimarães,[1] the parish of Oliveira, between the eighteenth and twentieth centuries – we will present case-by-case explanations of the methods used and a brief description of the sources.

We start with a discussion of the main sources and databases, follow with a brief presentation of the study site, and explore the view of death in the city and how it was observed and explained by health professionals who lived in the transition between the nineteenth and twentieth centuries. A comparative approach highlights the specific characteristics of the Guimarães population during the period under study.

In a second phase, although limited by the characteristics of the sources, we address three types of approach to mortality from the eighteenth to the twentieth centuries, comparing the results, in the same chronology, with those extracted from the databases on the Azores Islands of Pico and Faial[2]:

(a) Life expectancy at age 30 for individuals born between 1750 and 1829 whose death was recorded.
(b) Life expectancy at birth for individuals born between 1835 and 1864 in stable families.[3]
(c) Life expectancy at birth for individuals born between 1881 and 1899.

The year 1884 will serve as a starting point for the analysis, for the parish of Oliveira, four rural parishes of the Island of Pico, and two urban parishes on the Island of Faial to detect any differences, in particular survival at older ages.

5.1 Data and Setting

Sources

Parish Records

When building the demographic-genealogical database for Oliveira on which our research is based, the basic sources used were the parish records for baptisms, marriages and deaths. Baptisms were considered for the period from 1590 to 1900, whilst marriage records were extended to include the first five decades of the twentieth century, and the death entries only ended in 1990.

---

[1] Research conducted within the Project "Espaços urbanos: dinâmicas demográficas e sociais (séculos XVII–XX)", with the reference FCT PTDC/HIS-HIS/099228/2008, co-funded by the budget of the COMPETE – Programa Operacional Factores de Competitividade in its ERDF component and the budget of the Fundação para a Ciência e a Tecnologia in its State Budget component.

[2] The databases referred to in this work were organized by Maria Norberta Amorim, with occasional support from experts.

[3] We assume stable families as those for which we were able to obtain data on the survival of all children up to the age of seven years.

The series are continuous, except for the disappearance of a marriage register book for the period 1728–1766 which does not significantly impact our work. Nevertheless, we did face the problem with of mortality records for children under 7, individuals to whom the Church had no obligation to provide comfort at the time of death. This situation is common to the large Archdiocese of Braga, and was generally overcome before the end of the 1850s, when civil legislation standardised procedures concerning the registering of all acts in the parishes. Despite the legal requirements, analysis of the sources reveals that only from 1881 were all deaths systematically and continuously recorded in Oliveira.

The róis de confessados (*status animarum*)

Other sources used were the *róis de confessados* (records of parishioners who confessed and took communion at Easter). The purpose of these documents was to monitor the religious Easter precepts, but they evolved throughout the nineteenth century into mechanisms for population censuses. They began to record all residents (and not only those aged over 7, as was the case formerly) by their name and age, grouped into households and houses and distributed by the streets and places in each parish. In relation to the head of the family, they contain information on the familial, professional or companionship relationships in each home. The same dwelling could include several family members of different generations or other individuals identified as "assistants" or "tenants", which, in the latter case, means the payment of a rent for the use of part of the property.

In the parish of Oliveira, we found *róis de confessados* from 1734 to 1944, but only from 1835 onwards did they tend to include all residents.[4]

These documents are difficult to process as each roll is the basis for drawing up the next roll, interspersed with new households and new individuals in each one of them, or households that have been totally crossed out because their members have left, or single members have been crossed out because they have left or died. The roll may or may not include an explanation as to why someone is absent or dead. All this information, both initial and that added later, is obviously important for our purposes, but when considering the resident population in a specific year, we count only those that were registered in the first instance. This difference is detectable by the placement of the data on the sheet, the ink colour and the handwriting.

Demographic-Genealogical Databases

Our work is based on the organisation of parish information on baptisms, marriages and deaths, through a methodology called *parish reconstitution* (Amorim 1991) using a computer application developed by Fernanda Faria (Faria and Henriques

[4] From the last years of the 19th century, not all *róis* include those under the age of 7.

2004), called SRP (acronym for *Sistema de Reconstituição de Paróquias*, i.e., Parish Reconstitution System) (Henriques 2001).

We followed the life courses of all individuals who were registered in the parish in defined time frame, in a genealogical sequence and according to matrimonial links, with open entries to references on their socio-professional and residence situations. Intersections were recorded between urban parishes and their urban locations, leading towards production of a *central database* (Henriques 2001).

Although the histories of a few dozen parishes have been reconstructed by a considerable number of authors in Portugal, for obvious reasons, there are few cases that draw on this methodology with regard to urban parishes in the long term, that is, until the nineteenth century. We have already completed this work for Oliveira, and, in part, for two parishes in the town of Horta, on the Azores island of Faial. In an ongoing project, we expect to have, in the near future, all 10 parish databases gathered into a single record applicable to the urban centre of Guimarães and surrounding parishes, as well as the urban centre of Horta with its rural surroundings, covering 17 parishes on the island of Pico and 13 parishes on the island of Faial. In the case of Guimarães, only the inter-parish intersections for the period before 1820 have been developed. Consequently, all we have is the analysis of the parish on which, in terms of time span, we conducted more extensive research: the parish of Oliveira.

Guimarães Between the Nineteenth and Twentieth Centuries

The town of Guimarães was, at the time, formed by three parishes: Oliveira do Castelo, S. Paio and S. Sebastião. Some of its streets expanded beyond these limits, extending to the neighbouring parishes of Azurém, Creixomil and Urgeses. Drawing on data from the first census carried out in Portugal, we present a table below showing the evolution of the town's population and its peripheral parishes between 1864 and 1900 (Table 5.1).

In 1853, Queen Maria II promoted Guimarães to the rank of a city, justifying this decision for historical reasons and, at the same time, its great development: "*uma das mais populosas da província do Minho, e a mais florescente em diversos ramos de industria, à qual são devidas a sua opulência e prosperidade, e as suas relações dentro e fora do país (…)*[5]" (Braga 1953).

The dynamism of the town became even more pronounced during the second half of the nineteenth century, culminating in 1884 with the inauguration of the rail link to Porto and the 1st Industrial Exhibition of Guimarães. This showcased the council's productive capacity and advertised the main products of the region, in particular textiles (linen, cotton), leather products, cutlery and jewellery, which were exported all over the country and abroad, especially to Brazil.

[5] "one of the most populated provinces of Minho, and the most flourishing in various branches of industry, to which it owes its opulence and prosperity, and its relations within and beyond the country".

Table 5.1 Population of the town of Guimarães (1864–1900)

	1864	1878	1890	1900
Oliveira (We have included inhabitants from the parish of S. Miguel do Castelo which, in the meantime, has been joined with the parish of Oliveira.)	3400	3626	3718	4006
S. Paio	1935	1956	2278	2467
S. Sebastião	2415	2535	2615	2631
Subtotal	**7750**	**8117**	**8611**	**9104**
Urgeses	648	752	812	940
Azurém	1029	1074	1107	1262
Creixomil	1579	1829	1963	2223
Total	**11,006**	**11,772**	**12,493**	**13,529**
Council	**45,015**	**45,744**	**49,695**	**54,723**

Source: Population Census of the Kingdom of Portugal (1864, 1878, 1890, 1900)

At the same time, a series of urban studies and initiatives were launched, clearly showing a major concern for health and sanitary conditions. We highlight the works carried out by the City Improvement Commission, chaired by Avelino da Silva Guimarães, where he proposes: "(...) *to build public washing facilities in Campo da Feira, near the creek; for the public slaughter house, select a plot of land on the upper side of Rua de Sta. Luzia, as clean water is available there; build latrines and public dumps; build bathrooms; forbid enclosed manure deposits; for every new street opened or improved, provide pipelines in proper sanitary and cleanliness conditions; (...) the gas lighting system; (...) remove firework workshops to a location far from the town; find the best way to improve the conditions of our tanneries located in the S. Francisco neighbourhood, not allowing the water running from the tannery sumps to contaminate the Caldeiroa creek, and the tanners' workshops (...) must be moved to outside the city; the prompt and immediate completion of the new market in the extinct S. Domingos Convent; (...).*" (Fernandes and Gonçalves 2005:224).

The mere listing of these proposals is sufficient to assess the health problems that the new city faced, especially in a period when it became one of the first cities in the country.

In a dissertation, João de Meira carried out a comprehensive study on the demography and diseases of Guimarães in the early twentieth century, a key requirement for the study of its population trends. Analysing the age-specific mortality rate between 1896 and 1905, he commented that its maximum value was found in the 0 to 4 age group (223 per thousand for male mortality and 199 per thousand for female mortality), although he believed that these rates were not very high compared with the values obtained for the city of Porto in the same period (respectively 307.2 per thousand and 219.4 per thousand). He further noted that, in 1904, 74 people who were strangers to the city had died in the hospital.

Table 5.2 Total mortality rate for the ten-year period 1895–1905 and rates per 1:000 deaths

Ages	Male	Female	Total	Rates per 1.000 deaths	
				Male	Female
0–4	2.481	2.213	4.694	223,25	199,13
05–09	267	234	501	24,02	21,05
10–14	98	88	186	8,81	7,91
15–19	120	151	271	10,79	13,58
20–24	151	152	303	13,58	13,67
25–29	107	135	242	9,62	12,14
30–34	95	114	209	8,54	10,25
35–39	89	123	212	8,00	11,06
40–44	116	130	246	10,43	11,69
45–49	124	129	253	11,15	11,60
50–54	173	178	351	15,56	16,01
55–59	172	208	380	15,47	18,71
60–64	269	312	581	24,20	28,07
65–69	246	264	510	22,13	23,75
70–74	333	418	751	29,96	37,61
75–79	247	346	593	22,22	31,13
80–84	234	299	533	21,05	26,90
85–89	92	98	190	8,27	8,81
90–94	32	36	68	2,87	3,23
95–99	10	11	21	0,89	0,98
100–	1	0	1	0,08	0,00
Unknown age	7	10	17	0,62	0,89
	5.464	5.649	11.113	491,51	508,17

Source: (Meira 1907:130)

Then he proceeded with the study of diseases and illnesses for the year 1904, based on the information collected at the Guimarães Hospital. He found that most of the patients admitted to this hospital lived in the town or in the council area, and few (less than 10 %) were from neighbouring councils. As for marital status, single women were the ones who most sought out the hospital, which can be related to the traditional imbalance in the sex ratio in this region and the high number of female servants (Table 5.2).

A very interesting observation compared the gender and age-specific number of patients treated at the hospital. He rightly noted that "*if we take into account that the earlier ages are always more maltreated through neglect by their families and seldom receive hospital care, this higher frequency of patients between the ages of 20 and 30 is in line with the data we presented earlier on the age-specific composition of the population*" (Meira, 1907: 135).

A brief analysis of the survey conducted by João de Meira on the professions of patients treated at the hospital allows us to immediately conclude that it is primarily the disadvantaged population that mostly used these services. The most common occupations for men were day labourers and servants (farming servants mostly). For women, they were mainly housewives, followed by servants and weavers.

Comparative Study of the Population of the Oliveira Parish in the Last Quarter of the Nineteenth Century

Appling the procedures mentioned with regard to the population survey conducted on the basis of the *róis de confessados*, the year 1884 was selected to compare the state of the population in Oliveira and in other communities for which we have studied the same type of documentation. These are the two urban parishes on the Island of Faial, Matriz and Angústias, and three rural communities on the Island of Pico, S. João, Santo Amaro and the rural setting of the town of Lajes.[6]

For 1884, we counted 3157 inhabitants[7] in the parish of Oliveira; the parishes of Matriz and Angústias in Horta, analysed together, had a population of 5465 inhabitants; in the rural parishes of S. João and Santo Amaro, and in the rural area of Lajes, in an aggregated manner, we counted 5379 people.

By simply comparing the profile of the pyramids (we used proportional values in each case), we note a marked difference between rural and urban populations with regard to distribution of people by age brackets. The numbers are larger in the 20–65 age group in cities, especially with regard to women.

In all parishes, both urban and rural, the sex ratio changes noticeably, indicating stronger differential mobility (Figs. 5.1, 5.2 and 5.3).

The comparison is easier to absorb in the following table, containing the percentage distribution by age and gender, in the parish of Oliveira and in the group of the said Azorean rural and urban communities.

We can see that in Oliveira, minors under 15 years of age constituted 36 % of the total for males and 25 % for females. In the urban communities of Faial, the percentages are 30 % and 24 %, respectively. In the rural communities of Pico, we find the percentage under age 15 to be 36 % for boys and 27 % for girls. Although interpretation is premature, we can assume that a higher fertility rate in the mainland parish affects the proportions, along with differential infant and child mortality rates in relation to urban or rural Azores parishes. We cannot, however, neglect that children abandoned in foundling wheels, and later left in the care of nannies in rural areas, are not represented in the *status animarum*.

For individuals aged 65 years and over, it is obvious that the rural parishes of Pico have more survivors, and 13 % of this age bracket is male and 11 % female. In the urban area of Faial, the percentages stand at 6 % and 7 %, respectively, whilst in Oliveira the weight of males in that age bracket does not rise above 4 %, although it reaches 7 % in the case of females.

[6] Faial and Pico are the two closest islands within the Archipelago of the Azores.

[7] We detected in this roll a relative lack of records for children in their first years of life. We corrected it, by approximation, considering, in the database, those born and died in the three years prior to 1884, admitting, for those years, the systematic use of the infant mortality registry. Following this, we rejected the observations collected in the roll on individuals in their 1st, 2nd and 3rd years of life.

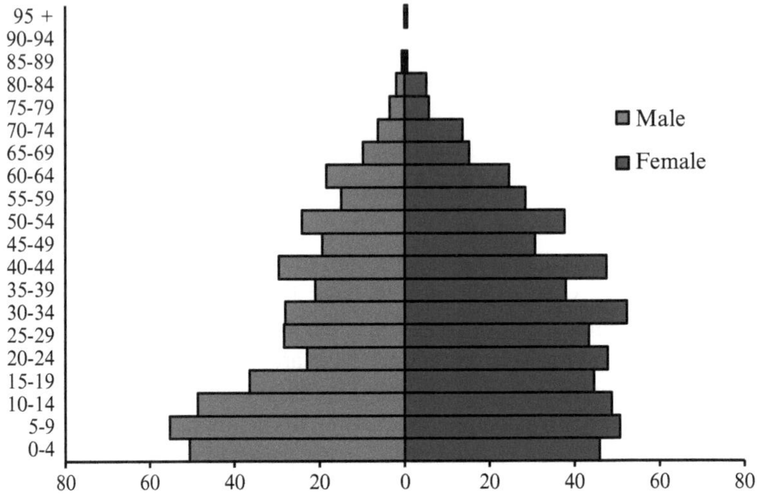

Fig. 5.1 Age pyramid in Oliveira (1884)

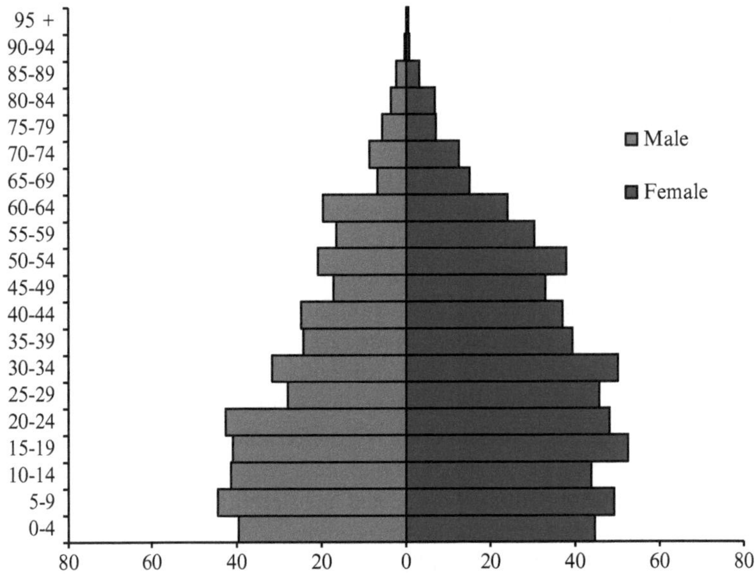

Fig. 5.2 Age pyramid in Matriz and Angústias (1884)

We began our analysis with the idea that, in the nineteenth century, life expectancy in the Pico rural communities would have been markedly more favourable in all age brackets, particularly in older ages, compared with the nearest urban area, or with the urban parish in the mainland (Table 5.3).

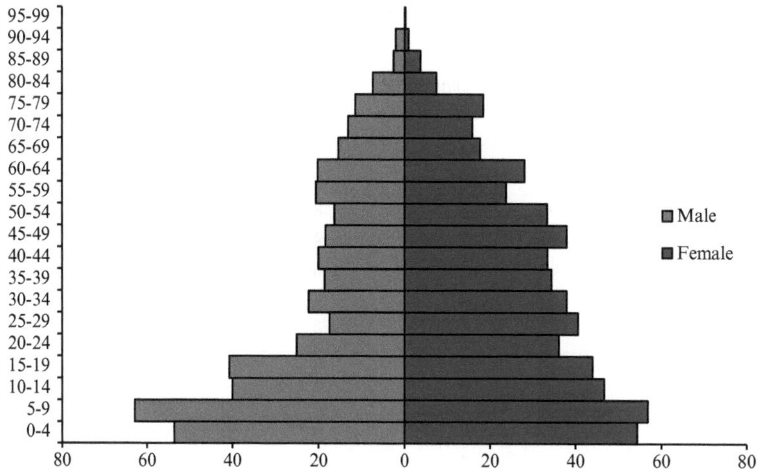

Fig. 5.3 Age pyramid in S. João, Santo Amaro and the rural area of Lajes (1884)

5.2 The Reconstruction of Life Expectancies in Guimarães

Life Expectancy at 30 of Individuals Born Between 1750 and 1829, Whose Death Was Recorded

In the parish of Oliveira, since the continuous, systematic recording of infant mortality only started in 1881, and the *róis de confessados* containing the entire resident population are only available from 1835 onwards, a valid approximation to the mortality patterns in previous periods is only possible, if solely middle aged adult individuals are considered in the analysis. In these circumstances, it is common practice to focus on married individuals over 25 years of age, considering them as the most stable sector of the population. In our case, we chose to consider 30 as the most stable age, given the relative frequency of mobility among younger couples in urban areas, and the fact that marriage took place at an older age in the Azorean rural parishes under study (Table 5.4).

Thus, our study took account of all the individuals identified at death by their birth date,[8] aged 30 years or over, in both the parish of Oliveira and the Matriz parish on the Faial island,[9] and in four aggregated rural parishes on the Pico island.[10] We

[8] We believe that the inclusion of single individuals did not affect the result.

[9] The parish of Angústias has a number of gaps in the death records between 1815 and 1843, compromising the analysis.

[10] The parishes of S. João and Ribeira, in the council of Lajes, and Santo Amaro and Prainha, in the council of S. Roque.

Table 5.3 Population (comparative analysis). Oliveira, urban parishes of Faial and rural areas of Pico (1884)%

Age brackets	Oliveira (1880) %		Urban parishes of Faial (1884) %		Rural areas of Pico (1884)%	
	M	F	M	F	M	F
0–4	12	8	9	8	12	9
5–9	12	9	11	8	15	10
10–14	12	8	10	8	9	8
15–19	9	8	10	9	9	8
20–24	6	8	10	8	6	6
25–29	7	7	7	8	4	7
30–34	7	9	7	9	5	7
35–39	5	6	6	7	4	6
40–44	7	8	6	6	5	6
45–49	5	5	4	6	4	7
50–54	6	6	5	7	4	6
55–59	4	5	4	5	5	4
60–64	4	4	5	4	5	5
65–69	2	3	2	3	4	3
70–74	1	2	2	2	3	3
75–79	1	1	1	1	3	3
80–84	0	1	1	1	2	1
85 e +	0	0	0	0	1	1
Total	**100**	**100**	**100**	**100**	**100**	**100**

Table 5.4 Life expectancy at 30 – Generations born between 1750 and 1829

Age	Oliveira (Guimarães)			Main parish/Faial			Rural parishes/Pico		
	M	F	MF	M	F	MF	M	F	MF
30	27.9	28.2	28.1	30.9	33.0	32.2	40.1	40.8	40.5
35	25.6	26.3	26.0	28.6	30.6	29.9	36.2	36.9	36.6
40	22.3	26.5	24.6	25.1	27.5	26.6	32.0	33.0	32.6
45	19.4	23.2	21.5	22.2	24.8	23.8	28.1	29.2	28.7
50	16.0	20.5	18.5	18.9	22.2	20.9	24.1	25.2	24.7
55	14.1	16.7	15.6	15.9	19.2	17.9	20.3	21.4	20.9
60	12.5	14.0	13.4	12.7	15.4	14.4	16.9	17.8	17.4
65	8.2	11.4	10.4	9.4	12.9	11.6	13.8	14.4	14.1
70	7.7	8.5	8.2	6.8	10.4	9.1	10.3	11.5	11.0
75	5.4	6.1	5.8	5.2	8.3	7.3	8.0	8.7	8.4
80	4.6	5.6	5.2	4.6	6.2	5.8	5.8	6.2	6.1
Obs.	**138**	**188**	**326**	**207**	**337**	**544**	**3397**	**3841**	**7238**

Comparison between Oliveira and the island communities

calculated the life expectancy between 30 and 80, and present the results in 5-year intervals.

Comparing the central parish of Guimarães with the central parish of Horta, on the island of Faial, with regard to life expectancy at 30 for individuals born between 1750 and 1829 identified as such at death, we find that, at this age, life expectancy was more higher in Horta by about 4 years, with less differences from the age of 40, but always more favourable in the island town, even in the older age brackets.

In the case of the four rural communities of Pico, life expectancy at the age of 30 was higher than in Oliveira by 12 years and higher than the Matriz parish of Horta by 8 years. In previous work, we had already called attention to Pico's striking survival rate in the eighteenth and nineteenth centuries (Amorim 2004b). It seems that the mild climate, its relative dryness, purity of water and a varied diet, with corn cake as a basic food, as well as potatoes, both the English variety and sweet potatoes, little meat but plenty of fish, milk and dairy products, some wine and fruit in abundance, may have influenced this result. Geographical factors, such as isolation, which prevented epidemics, cultural factors, related to prolonged breastfeeding, woman-mother and child protection, and even genetic factors, may also have been influential.

As we have a systematic record of infant mortality for the Pico island parishes, we can calculate with reasonable accuracy life expectancy at birth for generations born between 1750 and 1829. The results obtained for life expectancy at age 30 by tracking the life courses can then be compared with the results we presented earlier, covering only those individuals that were born and died in the communities in question.

For two of the Pico parishes (S. João and Santo Amaro), we intersected the demographic-genealogical databases with the *róis de confessados* to find the year in which those who did not die in their parishes no longer appeared on the records. As for Ribeiras and Prainha, without *róis de confessados* and no deaths in the parish, we had to resort to some conventions to mark the end of an observation, on a case-by-case basis. Thus, when a family moved, we assume the date of departure for each member of the household was taken to be the last known family date, generally at the time of the birth or death of a child. In the case of an isolated departure, the end of the observation was set conventionally at the 20th birthday, taking into account the main reasons for the absence. Emigration to Brazil or to the United States, or moving to Horta or Angra, took place in most cases at puberty, while at older ages people left (less frequently) as a result of marriage (Table 5.5).

As can be seen on the table above, observations that did not involve the case-by-case monitoring of life paths, reduce by about half a year the life expectancy at age 30 (which is understandable because, although more limited, there is still mobility of individuals at higher ages). The two curves then gradually draw closer together.[11]

[11] To compare statistically this fact, the chi-squared test was used as an adjustment test between the two independent samples. The test yielded a high corroboration value (close to 1), suggesting that there are no significant differences between the two groups.

Table 5.5 Life expectancy in the rural communities of Pico

	Monitoring of life paths			Stable individuals		
Age	M	F	MF	M	F	MF
0	52.9	55.8	54.3			
5	59.4	60.7	60.1			
10	56.2	57.4	56.8			
15	52.7	53.4	53.1			
20	48.6	49.4	49.1			
25	44.6	45.3	45.0			
30	40.7	41.3	41.0	40.1	40.8	40.5
35	36.6	37.3	37.0	36.2	36.9	36.6
40	32.4	33.3	32.9	32.0	33.0	32.6
45	28.4	29.4	29.0	28.1	29.2	28.7
50	24.3	25.4	24.9	24.1	25.2	24.7
55	20.5	21.6	21.1	20.3	21.4	20.9
60	17.0	18.0	17.5	16.9	17.8	17.4
65	13.8	14.5	14.2	13.8	14.4	14.1
70	10.4	11.6	11.1	10.3	11.5	11.0
75	8.0	8.8	8.4	8.0	8.7	8.4
80	5.8	6.3	6.1	5.8	6.2	6.1

Generations born between 1750 and 1829
Observation with the monitoring of life paths and stable individuals

Life Expectancy at Birth of Individuals Born Between 1835 and 1864 in Stable Families

As we have seen, from 1835 the Oliveira *róis de confessados* refer to all resident individuals, of any age. Since we have systematic records of births, which monitor stable families year after year, it is possible to calculate with reasonable accuracy the date on which children died without there being a death record. Then, we considered that missing entries in the roll for children from stable families after the age of eight stems from effects related to work or schooling, particularly in the case of future clergymen.

If we subtract half of those missing from the initial number at each age (Henry 1976:169), we are able to calculate the respective mortality ratios for each year, monitoring the generations until they become extinct.

Life expectancy at birth for generations born in the Horta parishes cannot be considered in this analysis due to two interruptions in the death records in Angústias in the first half of the nineteenth century, and also because the database for the Matriz parish has not yet been properly prepared for this complex study.[12] (Table 5.6).

[12] The monitoring of life paths, on a case-by-case basis, is a very delicate and lengthy work that has only been developed, in the case of Horta, for the parish of Angústias.

Table 5.6 Life expectancy at birth – generations born between 1835 and 1864

	Oliveira (Guimarães)			Rural communities/Pico		
Age	M	F	MF	M	F	MF
0	37.5	42.0	40.0	56.4	58.6	57.6
5	49.5	53.3	51.9	62.2	63.9	63.2
10	46.8	50.9	49.3	58.4	60.3	59.5
15	42.4	46.4	44.9	54.5	55.9	55.4
20	39.6	43.1	41.7	50.1	51.8	51.1
25	35.1	40.3	38.2	45.9	47.7	47.0
30	32.3	35.8	34.5	42.1	44.1	43.3
35	27.9	32.1	30.5	38.2	40.3	39.5
40	25.6	31.0	28.9	34.2	36.1	35.3
45	21.8	27.4	25.2	30.1	32.1	31.3
50	19.1	24.0	22.1	25.8	28.1	27.1
55	16.6	20.0	18.8	21.5	24.1	23.0
60	14.1	15.5	15.0	17.4	20.1	19.0
65	9.9	14.2	12.6	13.6	16.4	15.2
70	7.3	13.1	10.9	10.7	12.9	12.0
75	6.2	9.9	8.8	8.2	10.1	9.4
80	3.8	6.0	5.5	6.3	7.4	7.0
85	2.5	3.1	3.0	4.2	5.4	5.0

Comparison between Oliveira and the rural communities of Pico

Life expectancy at birth in Oliveira, for the generations born in stable families between 1835 and 1864, would have been around 40 years of age, whilst in the rural communities of Pico it was over 57. Gender differences, favouring females, are much sharper in Oliveira than in Pico.

According to Livi Bacci (del Panta et al. 1996:252), in the comparisons made between Italy and Europe, and considering the periods between 1750 and 1900,, we find that the Oliveira rates connote, for the same periods, with countries in which the mortality rate is more favourable. However, we have to bear in mind that we are analysing only the 'stable' families in Oliveira, excluding from the study children born out of wedlock, and especially, the abandoned children who were particularly vulnerable to an early death. If we were to include these risk groups in the analysis, life expectancy would certainly be lower.

Pico is a very special case which seems to show that prophylactic measures against disease, purity of air and water, a healthy diet, physical exercise and emotional balance, and the protection of mother and child, can improve survival to levels only possible in societies with advanced medical care.

The very methodical Governor of the Autonomous District of Horta, António José Vieira Santa Rita, in his 1861 Report, estimated that, for the four islands of his district (Pico, Faial, Flores and Corvo), there was one death in 55 inhabitants in 1859, the same proportion as in 1858. In the case of Pico, the proportion was one death in 67 residents, which means that, in the mid-nineteenth century, the crude

Table 5.7 Life expectancy in some western countries, 1750–1900

Countries	1750–1759	1800–1809	1850–1859	1880	1900
England	36.9	37.3	40	43.3	48.2
France	27.9	33.9	39.8	42.1	47.4
Sweden	37.3	36.5	43.3	48.5	54
Germany	–	–		37.9	44.4
Italy	–	–		35.4	42.8
The Netherlands	–	32.2	36.8	41.7	49.9
The Soviet Union	–	–		27.7	32.4
The United States (white population)	–	–	41.7	47.2	50.8
Australia	–	–		49	55
Japan	–	–		35.1	37.7

Source: (Livi-Bacci 1987: 252)

Table 5.8 Survivors at 35 years of age. Comparison between Oliveira, Angústias the Pico communities. Generations born between 1835 and 1864

Age	Oliveira	Angústias(a)	Comunidades do Pico						
	M	F	MF	M	F	MF	M	F	MF
1	811.8	849.7	830.4	816.6	853.5	834.3	881.4	898.1	889.7
5	678.4	713.2	695.5	733.6	764.8	748.6	836.3	848.0	842.0
10	648.3	679.1	663.5	721.2	739.3	729.9	820.2	829.8	824.9
15	639.3	672.2	655.5	715.0	728.5	721.5	804.0	820.3	812.2
20	605.8	647.7	627.3	710.0	716.4	713.1	795.7	807.6	801.5
25	597.2	613.9	604.3	699.8	708.1	703.8	781.2	792.0	786.5
30	560.0	605.8	583.9	690.7	702.5	696.3	760.5	769.3	764.6
35	547.9	583.2	565.9	685.4	698.1	691.5	740.0	746.3	742.7

Generations born between 1834 and 1864

death rate was below 15/1000. He himself notes that on Pico compared to other islands, although a population of 27,360 people, there was not *um único facultativo* [*a single doctor*] (Table 5.7).

If we now compare survivors per thousand births for 1 year, 5 years and then 5-year periods up to 35 for the Oliveria, Angústias and Pico communities, we see a greater similarity between the urban places than between the rural ones.

In the analysis of Oliveira, for generations born between 1835 and 1864, the mortality ratio in the first year of life per thousand births was 188, 150 and 170, for males, females and both genders, respectively. In Angústias, for generations born between 1834 and 1864 (there is a period missing before 1834), the corresponding results are 183, 146 and 166 in the Pico parishes, they are 119, 102 and 110, respectively (Tables 5.8 and 5.9).

Table 5.9 Survivors at 10 years of age. Comparison between Oliveira, Angústias and the Pico communities. Generations born between 1880 and 1899

	Oliveira (a)	Angústias	Pico communities						
	M	F	MF	M	F	MF	M	F	MF
1	799.0	828.8	813.3	806.9	816.2	811.3	886.7	904.1	895.3
5	653.2	664.1	658.4	718.2	763.1	739.3	849.7	867.9	858.7
10	632.7	641.0	636.6	707.0	752.3	728.4	839.2	859.4	849.2

Data for Oliveira goes from 1881 to 1889

Despite similarities between Oliveira and Angústias in survivorship beyond the first birthday, at age 566/1000 individuals survived in Oliveira, whilst in Angústias, the number was 691/1000.

Life Expectancy at Birth for Individuals Born Between 1881 and 1899

For the generations born in Oliveira between 1881 (the year in which the deaths of minors started to be recorded more systematically), and 1899, (including all the deceased in our analysis since the collection of death records goes up to 1990), we calculated life expectancy by monitoring the life courses on a case-by-case basis, following the procedure described in relation to the Pico parishes, without using the *róis de confessados*. For families that moved, we used the last known date for those families. For individuals that left separately, the date of marriage or the 20th birthday mark the end of the observation. It should be noted that the dates of death for the vast majority of individuals born between 1881 and 1899 but who left, are available from the 1930s from entries recorded on their baptism records. We did not consider deaths outside the parish as that would bias the analysis (Table 5.10).

Let's compare survival until 10 years of age, for Oliveira, Angústias and the Pico rural communities (analysis for Angústias only goes until 1911, when the Civil Registry is established in Portugal).

For the generations born in Oliveira in the last two decades of the nineteenth century, mortality in the first year of life is worse compared to those born between 1835 and 1864, with 201 deaths per thousand male births, 171 for females, and 187 for both genders. This decline is also found in Angústias, although less pronounced, with 193, 184 and 189, respectively. In the Pico parishes, infant mortality is even lower for the same period, with 113, 96 and 105, for males, females and both genders, respectively.

At 10 years of age, 636/1000 individuals had survived in Oliveira, 728/1000 in Angústias, and 849/1000 in the Pico parishes.

However, from the life expectancy table, we can see that death figures are slightly better for generations born in Oliveira in the last two decades of the nineteenth cen-

Table 5.10 Life expectancy at birth – Generations born between 1881 and 1899

	Oliveira (Guimarães)			Rural communities/Pico		
Age	M	F	MF	M	F	MF
0	39.0	44.7	41.7	59.2	60.4	59.8
5	54.0	61.6	57.7	64.5	64.5	64.5
10	50.7	58.8	54.6	60.3	60.1	60.2
15	46.3	54.1	50.1	55.9	55.5	55.7
20	42.0	49.4	45.6	51.9	51.6	51.7
25	38.0	45.3	41.5	47.3	47.9	47.6
30	33.9	41.9	37.7	43.4	43.7	43.5
35	31.7	37.7	34.7	38.8	39.5	39.1
40	28.8	34.0	31.5	34.3	35.8	35.1
45	24.6	30.0	27.4	29.9	31.9	30.9
50	20.6	25.9	23.4	25.4	27.3	26.4
55	16.4	21.9	19.2	21.3	23.1	22.2
60	14.1	18.3	16.4	17.3	19.0	18.2
65	11.2	14.2	12.9	13.7	15.2	14.5
70	8.2	10.3	9.5	10.5	11.9	11.2
75	5.5	7.3	6.7	8.7	9.5	9.1
80	5.1	4.9	5.0	6.0	6.9	6.5
85	3.6	3.8	3.7	4.3	5.1	4.8

Comparison between Oliveira and the rural communities of Pico

tury, in comparison to those born between 1835 and 1864. This improvement signals a major drop in adult mortality.

5.3 Final Notes

Over this three-century period, the basic sources for births, marriages and deaths changed and other serial sources emerged, particularly in the nineteenth century, thus shaping our methodological options.

Although we admit that the risk of death among children from these families was relatively low, the results obtained for the generations born in the two last decades of the nineteenth century do not discredit these values. This is an area of Portugal that in the first half of the nineteenth century was protected against epidemics that had a very strong impact on other parts of the country, as was the case of cholera, and then yellow fever. Nevertheless, the greater lack of sanitary conditions in urban areas and the concentration of foundling wheels in cities can cause a gap between urban and rural patterns with regard to death, as seems to be the case in the comparison with the Angústias parish, in the city of Horta.

In the course of the research, the results of the analysis of demographic behaviour from the eighteenth century seems be relatively sound, even those that were more difficult to examine, in relatively isolated rural communities, with systematic records of infant mortality and demographic-genealogical databases, prepared from the intersection of all events.

In urban communities, the volume of data and especially inter-parish mobility had a much more disturbing effect on the analysis of the more complex phenomenon of mortality, which suggested that intersecting urban centres with their surroundings could be useful.

We conclude with the conviction of the value of the monitoring life courses, from systematically organised demographic-genealogical databases, with the aim that they be successively enlarged, is the most reliable way to obtain a valid approach to the phenomenon of mortality in the long run.

References

Amorim, M. N. (1987). *Guimarães de 1580 a 1819. Estudo Demográfico*. Lisboa: I.N.I.C.

Amorim, M. N. (1991). Uma metodologia de reconstituição de paróquias desenvolvida sobre registos portugueses. *Boletin de la Asociación de Demografia Histórica, IX*(1), 7–25.

Amorim, M. N. (2004a). *O Pico. A abordagem de uma ilha. Vol.I – As Famílias. Tomo I – As famílias de S. João nos finais do século XIX*. Município das Lajes do Pico/NEPS.

Amorim, M. N. (2004b). O Pico (séculos XVIII a XX). A ilha açoriana mais poupada pela morte. *Boletin de la Asociación de Demografia Histórica, XXII*(II), 53–84.

Braga, A. V. (1953). *Administração Seiscentista do Município Vimaranense*. Câmara Municipal de Guimarães.

de Meira, J. (1907). *O Concelho de Guimarães*. Porto: Typografia a Vapor Da Empreza Guedes.

del Panta, L., Livi Bacci, M., & Sonnino, E. (1996). *La Populazione Italiana dal Medioevo a Oggi*. Roma: Editori Laterza.

Faria e Henriques. (2004). Sistemas Demográficos para a análise de dados demográficos. Guimarães: NEPS, Universidade do Minho.

Fernandes, M., & Gonçalves, M. (2005). *Urbanismo e Morfologia Urbana no Norte de Portugal: Viana do Castelo, Póvoa de Varzim, Guimarães, Vila Real, Chaves e Bragança entre 1852 e 1926*. Porto: Faculdade de Arquitectura da Universidade do Porto.

Henriques, P. (2001). Norberta Amorim, Antero Ferreira, Maribel Santos, and Fátima Rodrigues. "Reconstituição De Paróquias E Formação De Uma Base De Dados Central.". In *Congresso da Assosiação de Demografia Histórica: Actas* (pp. 57–66). Lisboa: ADEH.

Henry, L. (1976). *Demografía*. Barcelona: Labor.

Livi-Bacci, M. (1987). *Ensayo sobre la historia demográfica europea. Población y alimentación en Europa*. Barcelona: Ariel.

Part II
Urban Mortality in Transition

Chapter 6
Infant and Early Childhood Mortality in a Context of Transitional Fertility: Geneva 1800–1900

Reto Schumacher

6.1 Introduction

In the European past, infant and child deaths represented an important share of the total number of deaths and were mainly responsible for the low to very low figures in life expectancy at birth demographers have observed for pre-transitional Europe. In the mid-nineteenth century, when infant and early childhood mortality had already experienced their first decline in most parts of the continent, rates of infant mortality still reached levels of over 400 per thousand in Germany, over 350 per thousand in Switzerland and almost 300 per thousand in France. Early childhood mortality was clearly lower, but also reached levels higher than 150 per thousand (Van de Walle 1986; Knodel 1988; Perrenoud 1998).

Demographers and historians alike have intensively investigated the reasons for the large numbers of child deaths and for regional and social differences in child mortality in nineteenth century Europe. One could find in pre-transitional Europe comparatively low levels of economic development and standards of living, lack of medical knowledge and practices combined with difficult sanitary environments and pre-transitional patterns of reproductive behaviour that all contributed to high levels of infant and early childhood mortality. Spatial differences in reproductive behaviour, in nursing habits and in physical environments may explain regional and even local differentials in child mortality, whereas individual differences in economic and educational resources may explain why in many European regions socio-economic status and child mortality were inversely correlated.

R. Schumacher (✉)
Statistique Vaud, Lausanne, Switzerland

NCCR Lives, Lausanne, Switzerland
e-mail: Reto.Schumacher@vd.ch

D. Ramiro Fariñas, M. Oris (eds.), *New Approaches to Death in Cities during the Health Transition*, International Studies in Population 12,
DOI 10.1007/978-3-319-43002-7_6

Another characteristic of infant and child mortality in the past was its unequal distribution among families. An important part of all infant and child deaths occurred in a relatively small number of families, whereas many families did not experience any child deaths at all. In a study on a nineteenth century population in Northern Sweden, Brändström (1988) has shown that although infant mortality reached 400 per thousand, nearly 45 % of the families never experienced an infant death. Family-level heterogeneity in child mortality, that is the clustering of infant and child deaths in families, may be explained by genetic factors, but also by behavioural patterns such as childcare practice and breastfeeding. Residential conditions might also have played a role. However, given the scarce information one can extract from historical sources, it is difficult to assess the relative importance of the factors causing such family-level clustering of child deaths.

The aim of this chapter is to analyse family-level clustering in infant and early childhood mortality in the particular demographic context of nineteenth century Geneva. The city of Geneva experienced an early decline in fertility starting in the early eighteenth century among upper class families and then in the second half of the century among middle and lower class families (Perrenoud 1988). Throughout the nineteenth century, marital fertility remained at a moderate but clearly transitional level before pursuing its decline at the end of the nineteenth century (Schumacher 2010). Despite the generally low levels of fertility, multivariate analysis of family reconstitution data has shown considerable variation in marital fertility by socio-economic status and by migration history. Both infant and early childhood mortality started declining around the turn of the nineteenth century, with infant mortality lagging slightly behind. During the nineteenth century, infant and childhood mortality remained moderate, rose temporarily after the middle of the century and then definitely fell at the end of the century. Micro-level analysis has shown considerable clustering of infant and child mortality in families. In this exploratory contribution, I investigate the patterns of this clustering and aim to assess in particular whether it can be explained by variations in fertility behaviour.

6.2 Fertility and Child Mortality in the Past

The interdependent relationship at the family level between fertility and child mortality in past societies has been extensively studied in the demographic literature. As much of the historical-demographic literature has dealt with fertility and its decline in the nineteenth century, patterns of child mortality have mostly been considered an explaining factor of fertility behaviour rather than the result of reproductive patterns. In studies on pre-transitional fertility it has often been argued that the death of a breast-fed infant shortened the current birth interval by stopping the effect of post-partum infecundability (Knodel 1968; Preston 1978). While this lactation effect has been said to be purely biologic in nature and involuntary, the replacement effect found in transitional populations with moderate levels of child mortality has been seen as part of a deliberate family strategy (Knodel 1982, 1988; Legrand and

Sandberg 2006) when couples desiring a given number of children replaced a deceased child by a new birth. It has also been stated that in transitional populations with relatively high levels of child mortality, couples anticipated future child deaths by having more children than originally wanted in order to compensate for potential losses (Preston 1978).

The idea that fertility behaviour in the past may have had an effect on child mortality has first been put forward by Scrimshaw (1978) and Knodel (Knodel and van de Walle 1979; Knodel 1988). According to them, the high level of fertility in pre-transitional populations, or to put it differently, the couples' incapacity to efficiently reduce the family size explained why child mortality was so high. Child neglect and abusive childcare practices such as wet nursing and inappropriate feeding could have served as a way of limiting family size in high-fertility families, they have argued.

In the more recent literature, scholars have increasingly paid attention to reproductive patterns having an impact on child survival (Knodel and Hermalin 1984; Pebley and Stupp 1987; Nault et al. 1990; Lynch and Greehouse 1994). A U-shaped association has been found between maternal age at birth and child mortality, risks having appeared highest among very young and older mothers. The higher mortality among children of very young mothers may be due to insufficiently developed reproductive systems in very young women, whereas excess child mortality at older maternal ages may be related to decreasing efficacy of the reproductive system with age. The J-shaped association found between birth order and child mortality has been interpreted as the result of higher maternal age at higher birth orders (Pebley and Stupp 1987), but the effect of birth order often remains substantial in multivariate models controlling for maternal age. Nault et al. (1990) have hypothesized a selection effect due to generally higher child mortality in large families. In an analysis restricted to large families, they still found the J-shaped effect of birth order, which they interpreted as resulting from maternal age and short birth intervals in large families. Again, many studies have given evidence for an effect of birth order net of maternal age and degree of birth spacing, meaning that other things being equal, higher order children are frailer than lower order children. Reasons for this effect may lie in maternal depletion (Oris et al. 2004) affecting mothers' and their children's health and producing lower birth weights, or in the competition for resources among children (Knodel and Hermalin 1984).

The relationship between child spacing and child mortality has been demonstrated by many studies: children born after short birth intervals are subject to higher mortality risks than children born after longer intervals to preceding siblings. There are several reasons why the length of the previous birth interval can affect the index child's survival chances (Pebley and Stupp 1987). First, closely spaced births may lead to maternal depletion and affect thereby children's health. Second, the potential for resources competition among children increases when births are too closely spaced within a family. Finally, infectious diseases may spread more easily among siblings of similar age. Pebley and Stupp (1987) also warn against potential artefacts in the effect of the length of the previous birth interval. Especially if no data on breastfeeding are available, short birth intervals may also indicate short durations of breastfeeding, which might in turn explain why survival chances are low.

Several authors have identified the survival status of the previous sibling as the most powerful predictor of the index child's risk of dying (Nault et al. 1990; Lynch and Greenhouse 1994). In their paper on infant mortality in nineteenth century Sundsvall, Lynch and Greenhouse have demonstrated that the index child's risk of dying in infancy was higher not only if the previous child had died, but also if older siblings had died in infancy. This unambiguous demonstration of family-level clustering of child deaths can be found in many other studies on historical or contemporary populations (Das Gupta 1990; Guo 1993; Alter et al. 2001). Although most authors acknowledge the importance of parental (or maternal) behaviour in the explanation of child death clustering, only a few have tried to assess the contribution of family-level variables to clustering. In a study on family clustering of childhood mortality in North-east Brazil, Sastry (1997) has shown that birth order and the length of the preceding birth interval explain a substantial part of the variance of family-level frailty. Vandezande et al. (2010) have found similar results for nineteenth century Antwerp, where the death of the previous sibling captured a large part of the family-level frailty in infant mortality.

6.3 Data and Context

For the purpose of this study, I use data for nineteenth century Geneva. An independent city state since the middle of the sixteenth century, the city and its surroundings were annexed by Napoleon in 1798 and made capital of the French department du Léman. In 1814, Geneva entered the Swiss Confederation and the former Republic of Geneva became a Swiss canton. The city population rose from approximately 22,000 in 1800 to 59,000 in 1900. The overwhelming majority of this population growth was due to regional, national and international immigration. The proportion of the locally born population decreased from about two-thirds at the beginning of the century to less than 30 % at the turn of the twentieth century. The immigrant population originated from French-speaking Switzerland, Savoy (Kingdom of Sardinia until 1861, France afterwards) and the neighbouring French departments (Ain, Jura, Doubs), but also from German-speaking Switzerland, Southern Germany and Northern Italy. Since the eighteenth century, the local economy was dominated by the production of luxury goods such as watches, clocks and jewellery, and by the private banking sector. After the destruction of the medieval city walls in 1850, the construction sector was the main employer for immigrants, after the trade sector and domestic service. During the second half of the nineteenth century, light industry and services also gained considerable importance, for natives as well as for immigrants.

The demographic context of nineteenth century Geneva was characterized by transitional levels of fertility and child mortality. Throughout the nineteenth century, marital fertility remained at a moderate but clearly transitional level before

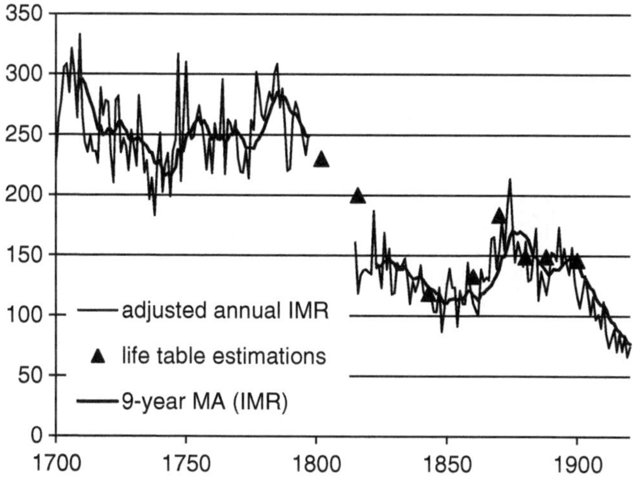

Fig. 6.1 The evolution of infant mortality, Geneva, 1700–1920 (Source: Schumacher 2010)

pursuing its decline at the end of the nineteenth century. Coale's index of marital fertility I_g declined from 0.515 in 1802 to 0.425 in 1843, before increasing again towards the middle of the century. In 1860, I_g reached a level of 0.490, fell to 0.380 a decade later and definitely declined after 1880 to reach post-transitional levels at the beginning of the twentieth century. Longitudinal analysis has shown that this temporary increase can be partly explained by a calendar effect in fertility, but it may also reflect a composition effect due to immigration (Schumacher 2010).

Figure 6.1 shows the long-term evolution of infant mortality between 1700 and 1920. Between 1780 and 1820 the infant mortality rate fell from levels higher than 200 per thousand to values oscillating between 100 and 150 per thousand. Between 1860 and 1875, infant mortality increased before falling below the 100 per thousand threshold towards the end of the century. This temporary increase in infant mortality in the second half of the nineteenth century has been observed in a variety of European contexts (Perrenoud 1998), but remains difficult to explain. Figure 6.2 shows the long-term evolution of early childhood mortality in the city of Geneva between 1700 and 1920. During the eighteenth century, child mortality was subject to periodic smallpox outbreaks, which can be seen in regular peaks occurring every 5–6 years (Perrenoud 1979). Although smallpox continued to outbreak irregularly until 1871, the diffusion of Jenner's vaccine during the first three decades of the nineteenth century (Schumacher 2010) contributed to reduce substantially levels of early childhood mortality. Between 1780 and 1870, the probability of dying between ages 1 and 4 (${}_4q_1$) oscillated around 110 per thousand. After the last outbreak of smallpox in 1871, early childhood mortality declined significantly to reach post-transitional values at the turn of the twentieth century.

To study the relationship between fertility behaviour and clustering in infant and early childhood mortality, I use family reconstitution data described in detail in

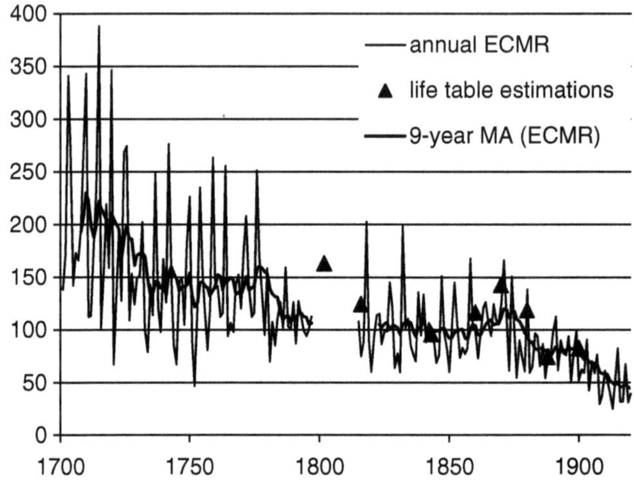

Fig. 6.2 The evolution of early childhood mortality (ECMR), Geneva, 1700–1920 (Source: Schumacher 2010)

Schumacher (2010). Based on an alphabetical sampling scheme, the database contains information on more than 2200 couples who got married in the city of Geneva between 1800 and 1880. Using civil registration records, censuses, immigration permits and nominative yearbooks, I reconstituted birth histories and determined the observed length of all family life courses. Birth histories include information on children's survival until the age of 5 years. For several reasons, the death records I used must be considered of high quality. First of all, registration of deaths had been carried out by the public authorities since the middle of the sixteenth century in registers covering the territory of the Republic of Geneva, including the rural areas. For the nineteenth century, decennial registers covering the canton of Geneva (elaborated by archival employees in the early twentieth century) allow one to follow families leaving the city to live either in one of the new neighbourhoods outside the city walls or in rural municipalities of the canton. The problem of wet-nursed children raised and deceased outside town, leading to potential under-registration of child deaths (cf. Rollet 1997), is insignificant in the case of Geneva: Perrenoud (1975) has reported on the widespread habit of repatriating bodies of wet-nursed children who died in neighbouring Upper Savoy, a catholic region where protestant children could not be buried. The present study uses data on 5147 children born in Geneva between 1800 and 1899, and stemming from 1749 families. A total of 1036 children died before the age of 5 years. These child deaths have been found clustered among 707 families, which means that for almost 60 % of the families, no child death could be observed.

6.4 Analytic Strategy

The aim of this study is to analyze the impact of fertility behaviour on child mortality in general, and on the clustering of child deaths in particular. As explained above, in a context of transitional demography the association between fertility and child mortality must be considered interdependent. When analyzing an interdependent relationship, one has always to bear in mind the problem of possible reverse causation. The strategy I have chosen to analyze the relationship between fertility behaviour and infant and early childhood mortality has been set up to minimize the problem of reverse causation, but cannot completely rule it out.

The present analysis comprises two steps. In the first step, I identify families of high and low child mortality risk respectively and study the characteristics of their birth histories. To identify the family-level risk of child mortality, I first run a multilevel piecewise-constant exponential hazard model of child survival, specified as a random-intercept Poisson model with an offset (Rabe-Hesketh and Skrondal 2008). In this null model, only the intercept and a categorical variable indicating the age band of the index child measuring the age schedule of mortality are included. The intercept is allowed to vary at both the individual and the family-level. This model can therefore be considered a nested frailty model (Mills 2011) with age spells s nested in children i who are nested in mothers j. Formally,

$$\lambda_{sij} = \ln\left(\frac{\mu_{sij}}{t_{sij}}\right) = \sum_{k} \beta_k d_{ksij} + \zeta_{ij} + u_j \qquad (6.1)$$

where λ_{sij} is the piecewise-constant incidence rate, μ_{sij} the number of deaths (0 or 1) in age band s of child i and mother j, t_{sij} is the exposure time child i of mother j spent in band s, d_{ksij} is a categorical variable indicating k different age bands, ζ_{ij} is a random intercept for child i of mother j and u_j a random intercept for mother j. The two random intercepts are assumed to be independent of each other and have a normal distribution with expectation 0 and variance ψ_1 and ψ_2 respectively. Based on the estimated coefficients of model 1, I then estimate the family-level random effects ($u_1, u_2, \ldots u_j$) as level-3 residuals to distinguish between high risk and low risk families. To compare the birth histories of high risk and low risk families, I apply a sequential data approach. Looking at the first 85 months since the first birth, I define 85 monthly states whose values correspond to numbers of achieved birth parities.

In a second step of the analysis, I run a series of models of the type of model 1 and look at the evolution of the family frailty term σ_{uj}^2 when individual and family-level variables are taken into account. Formally, these models can be written as

$$\lambda_{sij} = \ln\left(\frac{\mu_{sij}}{t_{sij}}\right) = \sum_{k} \beta_k d_{ksij} + \sum_{m} \beta_m X_{mij} + \sum_{p} \beta_p Z_{pj} + \zeta_{ij} + u_j \qquad (6.2)$$

where X is a vector of covariates characterizing index child i and Z is a vector of variables characterizing family j. The distinction between individual and family-level predictors is not always clear. The only true individual-level variable I include in X is the sex of the index child. All other variables in X are related to the child's family, but vary at the individual level: mother's age at birth, birth order, the length of the previous birth interval, the survival status of the previously born sibling at the conception of index child i, and the survival status of the previous sibling after index child i is born. In Z I include variables characterizing the families j: social status, migratory status of the mother and migratory status of the father.

An important aspect of my analytic strategy is to run the analyses separately for infant mortality and for early childhood mortality respectively. Oris et al. (2004) have convincingly shown for a series of different contexts that the determinants of infant and early childhood mortality differ from each other. Infants' survival chances have been shown dependent on their mothers' health, as reflected in maternal age and length of birth intervals, whereas children aged 1–5 have been shown responsive to the social status of the household and to economic stress.

6.5 Results

In this section I present and comment the results of the various analyses I have run for the purpose of this study.

Figure 6.3 shows the transversal monthly distribution of achieved birth parities among families of low infant mortality risk (1), families of lower to middle risk (2), families of middle to higher risk (3), and among high infant mortality risk families (4). The quartiles of the family-level intercepts have been used to define these four categories. The four graphs of Fig. 6.3 have been plotted by TraMineR, a package for sequence analysis in R (Gabadinho et al. 2011). The null model that allowed me to estimate the family-specific random intercepts (u_1, u_2, …, u_i) has been fitted in MLwiN using Markov Chain Monte Carlo estimation (Browne 2009). Both the null model and the sequence analysis have been restricted to 637 families who can be observed at least during 85 months after the first birth. An ANOVA-like discrepancy analysis (Studer et al. 2011) of the pair-wise dissimilarities (optimal matching distances) between individual sequences shows a statistically significant association between infant mortality risk and birth spacing. Lower to middle risk families in particular seem to have fewer births and tend to space them more than high risk families. However, there is no clear-cut difference between low risk and high risk families. In both groups, about 50 % of the families reach parity 4 before the end of the 85-month period, and about 20 % reach parity 5. In the group of low risk, parity 3 is even reached in higher proportions than in the high risk group; low risk families also seemed to space their births to a lesser extent. This first descriptive overview of the association between fertility behaviour and infant mortality illustrates that a high rhythm of childbearing may or may not increase the risk for infant mortality. In other words, there were families in which the high rhythm of childbearing may

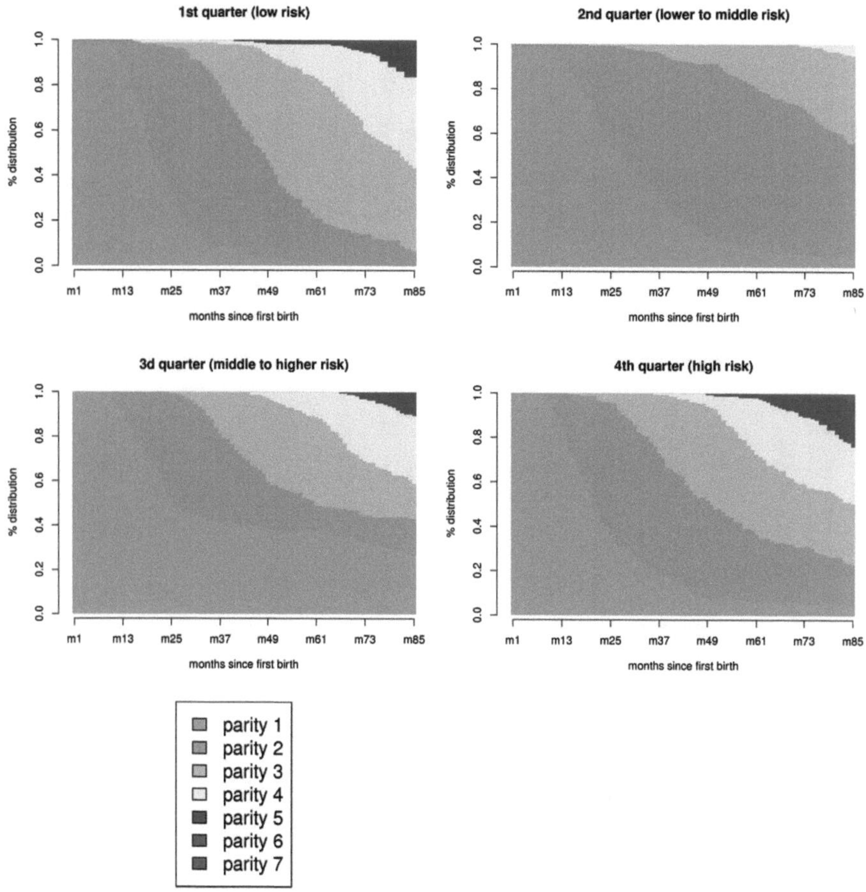

Fig. 6.3 Transversal distribution of birth parities, Geneva, 1800–1900, by level of infant mortality risk

have negatively affected the children's survival chances (or alternatively, in which the high level of infant mortality led the couples to rapidly replace the deceased children). At the same time there is evidence for families whose rhythm of child-bearing was high, but whose children were subject to very low risks of infant mortality. A logistic regression model predicting the probability for a given family *j* to be part of the high infant mortality risk group shows that upper class families were under-represented in this group, confirming the results of Edvinsson et al. (2005) for nineteenth century northern Sweden. Accordingly, upper class families were over-represented in the group of low infant mortality risk. The migratory status of the parents does not have any effect on the probabilities of belonging to either the high risk or the low risk group.

Figure 6.4 shows the transversal monthly distribution of achieved birth parities among families of different risk levels for early childhood mortality. As before, the

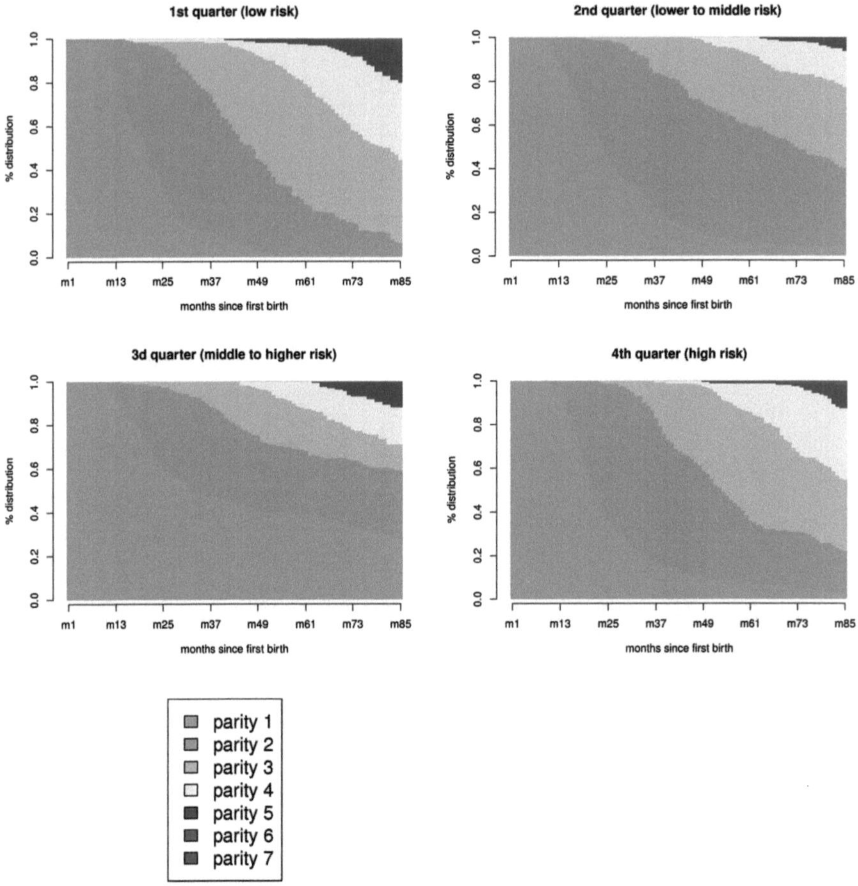

Fig. 6.4 Transversal distribution of birth parities, Geneva, 1800–1900, by level of early childhood mortality risk

four categories have been defined according to the quartiles of the family-level intercepts estimated in a piecewise-constant exponential hazard model without other covariates than the age bands d_{ksij}. The discrepancy analysis of the pair-wise optimal matching distances shows a significant association between the rhythm of childbearing and the risk of early childhood mortality. Families of lower to middle and middle to upper child mortality risk can be characterized by a lower rhythm of childbearing than low and high risk families. However, the birth histories of the latter hardly differ from each other. As in the case of infant mortality, a high rhythm of childbearing is associated with high risks of early childhood mortality for some families, but not for others. Logistic regression analysis highlights that upper class families are clearly underrepresented in the high risk group. The probability of belonging to the low risk group however does not differ between social classes.

Table 6.1 Comparison of models of infant mortality risk

Model	Variables	DIC	$\sigma_{\zeta ij}^2$	σ_{uj}^2	$\sigma_{uj,\xi j}$	$\sigma_{\xi j}^2$
m1.1	Base, age, age2, rank, sex	7025.5				
m1.2	m1.1+ζ_{ij}, u_j	6995.2	0.017	0.206		
m1.3	m1.2+length, previousdead, death	6951.9	0.013	0.465		
m1.4	m1.2+upper, momig, famig, bperiod	6964.4	0.005	0.312		
m1.5	m1.3+upper, momig, famig, bperiod	6932.7	0.001	0.465		
m1.6	m1.5+ξ_j	6918.0	0.002	0.409	−0.241	1.222
m1.7	m1.6+previousdead ·upper	6913.0	0.009	0.415	−0.283	1.371

While I have dealt with birth histories of various infant and child mortality risk groups in the first step of my analysis, I now look at individual and family-level risk factors for infant and early childhood mortality. Table 6.1 compares a series of survival models predicting the risk of infant mortality in nineteenth century Geneva. All models have been fitted using Markov Chain Monte Carlo estimation in MLwiN. Chains of 100'000 iterations have been run for all models. To compare models with each other, I use the deviance information criterion DIC.

Model 1.1 contains 5 individual-level variables. *Base* is a categorical variable distinguishing the 3 age bands'0 months','1–5 months' and'6–11 months'. *Age* and *age2* refer to the age at birth of index child's *i* mother *j*, whilst *rank* stands for birth order and *sex* for the child's sex. In model 1.2 two random intercepts at the individual level and at the family level are included. The decrease of the DIC shows that the inclusion of the two random effects is justified. However, only the family-level frailty term σ_{uj}^2 is substantial and statistically significant, whilst the individual-level frailty term $\sigma_{\zeta ij}^2$ is insignificant. In model 1.3 3 individual-level variables measuring the impact of birth spacing and previous child deaths on index child's *i* survival chances are further included. *Length* is a categorical variable distinguishing short, medium and long previous birth intervals, as well as first births. *Previousdead* is a dummy variable indicating whether the previous child was dead before the conception of index child *i* and *death* is a time-varying dummy variable indicating the death of the previous sibling after the index child's birth. The inclusion of these 3 variables clearly improves the preceding model, but leads to an increase of the family-level frailty, which might stem from variables that are differently associated with the outcome variable at the child level on the one hand and at the family level on the other hand. A closer inspection of model 1.3 has shown that the variable *previousdead* contributes most to this increase. Apart from the variables already included in model 1.2, model 1.4 further includes 4 family-level variables. *Upper* is a dummy variable indicating whether family *j* is part of the upper social class. The dummy variables *momig* and *famig* indicate whether the child's mother or father were immigrants, whilst *bperiod* is a categorical variable distinguishing the four periods of birth'1800–1829','1830–1859','1860–1879' and'1880–1899'. Strictly speaking, *bperiod* is an individual-level variable, but its value is constant within most families. The inclusion of these 4 variables also improves the fit of model 1.2, but not as much as the 3 individual-level models included in model 1.3. The family frailty term also increases in model 1.4 (when compared to model 1.2), but to a lesser extent than in model 1.3. Model 1.5 combines all individual-level and family-level variables. Its fit is clearly improved but its family frailty term remains high.

In a further step of this regression analysis, I have focused on the role played by the variable *previousdead*, the variable which led most to an increase in the family frailty term. In model 1.6, the coefficient of this variable is allowed to vary at the family level, which is reflected by the inclusion of the random coefficient ξ_j. The model fit is further improved and the family frailty decreases with this further complication. The variance of ξ_j is highly substantial and significant, which means that the effect of *previousdead* varied considerably between families. Finally, in model 1.7 a cross-level interaction between upper and *previousdead* is specified in order to test whether the variability of *previousdead* is related to social class. The interaction term leads to a decrease in the DIC, but the variance of the random coefficient does not decline.

Table 6.2 gives the regression estimates of models 1.5–1.7. With respect to individual-level variables it can be said that birth rank is clearly positively associated with infant mortality and that a short previous birth interval increases the risk of death. These two effects can be interpreted in terms of competition for resources or as the result of maternal depletion. The death of the preceding sibling within the index child's first year of life unambiguously lowers the latter's survival chances. The effect of the death of the previous child before the index child is conceived, however, is ambiguous. Its overall effect is negative, meaning that the index child's survival chances were on average higher when the previous sibling was dead before the birth of the index child, which points to the competition for resources hypothesis. The results of models 1.6 and 1.7 show, however, that the effect was negative in some families, and positive in others. It is shown in model 1.7 that among upper class families in particular the effect was positive, which is another illustration of infant death clustering, but also evidence for less resource competition in wealthy families.

Table 6.3 summarizes the results of a series of survival models for early childhood mortality in nineteenth century Geneva. Model 2.1 includes the same individual-level variables that have been specified in model 1.1 for infant mortality. In this series, *base* distinguishes the 3 age bands'12–23 months','24–35 months', and'36–59 months'. In model 2.2 the intercept is allowed to vary at the individual level and at the family level. The lower DIC in model 2.2 justifies the specification of these two random effects. However, as in the previous models for infant mortality, only the family-level frailty term is substantial and significant. Model 2.3 further includes 5 individual-level variables measuring the effects of the childbearing rhythm and of previous child deaths. *Length* and *previousdead* are defined as in the first model series. *Death* is again a time-varying dummy variable indicating the death of the previous sibling between age 1 and 4 of the index child. *Subseq1* and *subseq2* vary also with time and indicate the birth of subsequent siblings of the index child. As shown by the DIC statistic, the inclusion of these 5 variables does not improve model 2.2, but it leads to an insignificant family-level frailty. When the 5 variables are included one by one, it appears that the variable *death* contributes

Table 6.2 Piecewise-constant exponential hazard models of infant and mortality posterior means (p.m.) and empirical 95 % confidence intervals (C.I.)

	Model 1.5			Model 1.6			Model 1.7		
	p.m.	(C.I.)		p.m.	(C.I.)		p.m.	(C.I.)	
		(2.5	97.5)		(2.5	97.5)		(2.5	97.5)
Constant	−0.339	−2.75	1.58	−0.654	−2.22	1.14	−0.573	−2.69	1.16
Age band child									
0 months	Ref			Ref			Ref		
1–5 months	**−1.673**	−1.85	−1.50	**−1.667**	−1.85	−1.49	**−1.664**	−1.85	−1.48
6–11 months	**−2.111**	−2.31	−1.92	**−2.103**	−2.30	−1.91	**−2.098**	−2.30	−1.90
Age of mother									
Age	−0.107	−0.23	0.05	−0.083	−0.20	0.01	−0.096	−0.20	0.03
Age2	0.002	0.00	0.00	0.001	0.00	0.00	0.001	0.00	0.00
Birth rank	**0.090**	0.03	0.15	**0.085**	0.02	0.14	**0.085**	0.02	0.15
Sex									
Girl	Ref			Ref			Ref		
Boy	**0.243**	0.08	0.40	**0.233**	0.07	0.39	**0.232**	0.07	0.40
Previous birth interval									
Short	**0.320**	0.07	0.58	**0.330**	0.08	0.59	**0.333**	0.08	0.59
Medium	0.178	−0.07	0.43	0.170	−0.08	0.42	0.170	−0.08	0.42
Long	Ref			Ref			Ref		
First birth	0.093	−0.19	0.37	0.097	−0.18	0.38	0.093	−0.19	0.37
Previous child dead at conception of i	**−0.357**	−0.64	−0.08	**−0.532**	−1.00	−0.09	**0.251**	−0.71	1.11
Death of previous child after birth of i	**0.985**	0.21	1.65	**0.984**	0.22	1.66	**0.981**	0.23	1.64
Mother immigrant	−0.015	−0.22	0.19	−0.026	−0.22	0.17	−0.020	−0.22	0.18
Father immigrant	**0.207**	0.01	0.41	**0.203**	0.00	0.40	**0.200**	0.01	0.40
Upper class family	**−0.651**	−0.98	−0.35	**−0.658**	−0.98	−0.35	**−0.763**	−1.12	−0.44
Period of birth									
Born 1800–1829	Ref			Ref			Ref		
Born 1830–1859	0.112	−0.15	0.37	0.098	−0.16	0.37	0.109	−0.15	0.37
Born 1860–1879	0.204	−0.06	0.48	0.193	−0.07	0.46	0.199	−0.06	0.47
Born 1880–1899	0.142	−0.19	0.47	0.127	−0.20	0.46	0.134	−0.20	0.46
Previous dead · upper							0.861	−0.02	1.72

(continued)

Table 6.2 (continued)

	Model 1.5			Model 1.6			Model 1.7		
	p.m.	(C.I.)		p.m.	(C.I.)		p.m.	(C.I.)	
Random effects									
$\sigma_{\zeta ij}^2$	0.001	0.00	0.003	0.002	0.00	0.007	0.009	0.00	0.051
σ_{uj}^2	**0.465**	0.20	0.73	**0.409**	0.15	0.72	**0.415**	0.18	0.72
$\sigma_{uj,\xi j}$				−0.241	−0.68	0.10	−0.283	−0.74	0.09
$\sigma_{\xi j}^2$				**1.222**	0.52	2.32	**1.371**	0.53	2.65

Number of infants *i*: 5147
Number of families *j*: 1749
Number of person-years: 4679.7
Bold coefficients are significant at the 5 % level

Table 6.3 Comparison of models of early childhood mortality risk

Model	Variables	DIC	$\sigma_{\zeta ij}^2$	σ_{uj}^2
m2.1	Base, age, age2, rank, sex	4411.5		
m2.2	m2.1 + ζ_{ij}, u_j	4396.9	0.002	0.269
m2.3	m2.2 + length, previousdead, death, subseq1, subseq2	4416.9	0.004	0.042
m2.4	m2.2 + upper, momig, famig, bperiod	4396.5	0.002	0.225
m2.5	m2.3 + upper, momig, famig, bperiod	4411.7	0.006	0.061

most to the decline in σ_{uj}^2. Model 2.4 adds to model 2.2 the 4 family-level variables *upper*, *momig*, *famig*, and *bperiod*. It can be seen that none of these variables does substantially lower the family frailty. In model 2.5, all individual-level and family-level variables are included.

Table 6.4 finally shows the regression coefficients of models 2.2, 2.3 and 2.5. As in the previous models for infant mortality, birth rank is positively related to early childhood mortality. The length of the previous birth interval, the survival status of the previous child at the conception of index child *i*, as well as the birth of younger siblings, however, did not have any effect on child mortality in nineteenth century Geneva. The death of the previous child after the index child's 1st birthday tended to lower the survival chances of the latter (significant at the 10 % level). In the case of early childhood mortality, this correlation between the survival chances of two successive siblings captures almost completely the family-level clustering of child deaths. Finally, what has been highlighted by many other studies (see Oris et al. 2004) is confirmed by the present example: social status remains one of the most powerful predictors of early childhood mortality in transitional populations.

6.6 Discussion and Conclusion

The aim of this chapter was to shed new light on two old questions, namely whether reproductive patterns had an impact on the risk of infant and child mortality in transitional populations and whether the family-level clustering of child deaths can be

Table 6.4 Piecewise-constant exponential hazard models of child mortality posterior means (p.m.) and empirical 95 % confidence intervals (C.I.)

	Model 2.2			Model 2.3			Model 2.5		
	p.m.	(C.I.)		p.m.	(C.I.)		p.m.	(C.I.)	
		(2.5	97.5)		(2.5	97.5)		(2.5	97.5)
Constant	−1.625	−3.95	−0.11	−0.797	−3.27	1.57	−1.663	−3.41	0.09
age band child									
12–23 months	Ref			Ref			Ref		
24–35 months	**−0.410**	−0.65	−0.17	**−0.406**	−0.66	−0.16	**−0.400**	−0.65	−0.15
36–59 months	**−1.030**	−1.27	−0.79	**−1.028**	−1.30	−0.76	**−1.017**	−1.28	−0.75
Age of mother									
Age	−0.135	−0.23	0.01	**−0.186**	−0.34	−0.03	**−0.158**	−0.27	−0.05
Age2	0.002	0.00	0.004	0.003	0.00	0.01	0.002	0.00	0.00
Birth rank	**0.105**	0.04	0.17	**0.091**	0.02	0.16	**0.106**	0.04	0.17
Sex									
Girl	Ref			Ref			Ref		
Boy	0.010	−0.19	0.21	0.008	−0.20	0.21	0.023	−0.18	0.23
Previous birth interval									
Short				0.053	−0.27	0.36	0.039	−0.29	0.36
Medium				0.196	−0.10	0.49	0.181	−0.12	0.48
Long				ref			ref		
First birth				0.049	−0.30	0.39	0.027	−0.33	0.38
Previous child dead									
At conception of i				0.035	−0.27	0.33	0.009	−0.30	0.31
Death of previous child									
After birth of i				0.572	−0.02	1.10	0.540	−0.05	1.07
Subsequent birth 1				−0.088	−0.34	0.16	−0.095	−0.36	0.16
Subsequent birth 2				0.013	−0.54	0.53	0.003	−0.55	0.52
Mother immigrant							0.138	−0.09	0.37
Father immigrant							−0.058	−0.29	0.17
Upper class family							**−0.535**	−0.91	−0.18
Period of birth									
Born 1800–1829									
Born 1830–1859							−0.057	−0.35	0.24
Born 1860–1879							−0.060	−0.36	0.24
Born 1880–1899							−0.382	−0.79	0.02
Random effects									
$\sigma_{\zeta ij}^2$	0.002	0.00	0.01	0.004	0.00	0.02	0.006	0.00	0.02
σ_{uj}^2	**0.269**	0.03	0.57	0.042	0.00	0.10	0.061	0.00	0.25

Number of children *i*: 4493
Number of families *j*: 1701
Number of person-years: 16992.9
Bold coefficients are significant at the 5 % level

explained by differences in reproductive behaviour. To answer these questions, I used data on nineteenth century Geneva, a demographic context marked by an early decline in fertility and relatively moderate levels of infant and early childhood mortality. In such a context where overall levels of fertility were low but where individual heterogeneity was still important, the question whether child deaths were concentrated in high-fertility families suggests itself.

Given the interdependent relationship between fertility and child mortality, reverse causality is a major methodological challenge when studying the impact of fertility on children's mortality. The analytic strategy applied in this paper cannot completely rule out this problem. To avoid spurious conclusions I studied the association from two different perspectives and kept the interdependent nature of the relationship in mind when commenting the results of the analyses. An important ingredient of my analytic strategy was also to run separate analyses for infant mortality on the one hand and for early childhood mortality on the other hand, because previous studies have shown considerable differences in the determinants of mortality during the first year of life and during the period from age 1 to age 4 respectively.

In a first step I identified four groups of families differing in their risk for infant and childhood mortality and studied their rhythm of childbearing by means of sequence analysis. The analysis showed that high risk families and low risk families did not substantially differ from each other in their rhythm of childbearing. While lower-to-middle risk and middle-to-higher risk groups characterized themselves by low rhythms of childbearing, both high risk and low risk families were characterized on average by high rhythms of childbearing. While closely spaced births might have increased the risk for infant and child mortality in one group, the high rhythm of childbearing did not lower the children's survival chances in the other group. Bearing in mind that among high risk families, fertility could have been the consequence of child mortality rather than the other way around, I conclude from this first analysis that the heterogeneity in fertility behaviour in nineteenth century Geneva was *not* the reason for the clustering of infant and child deaths.

In a second step I ran a series of piecewise-constant exponential hazard models for the risks of infant and child mortality. The models showed substantial degrees of family-level clustering in infant mortality. Although reproductive behaviour clearly had an impact on the level of infant mortality, it cannot explain the clustering of infant deaths. As expected, the risk for infant mortality grew with birth order and was higher when the previous birth interval was short. The models for infant mortality revealed an interesting source of between-family heterogeneity: the death of the previous child before the conception of the index child had a positive impact on the index child's survival chances in some families, but a negative influence in others. There must be an association between infant death clustering and this variable, since its inclusion in the models increased the family-level frailty term.

The family-level clustering in child mortality was less important than in infant mortality. Family-level frailty in child mortality is definitely not explained by reproductive behaviour. Although the risk for child mortality grew with birth order, there was no association between child mortality on the one hand and the length of the previous birth interval and the occurrence of subsequent births on the other hand. The death of the previous child before the conception of the index child had no effect on children's survival chances. However, the death of the previous child after the index child's first birthday tended to increase the mortality risk of the latter. The inclusion of this last variable almost completely captures the clustering of child deaths. The death of the previous child is of course no explanation for clustering, or at least only a tautological explanation. After all this result is another illustration of the moderate level of child death clustering. Contrary to infant mortality, the phenomenon of family-level clustering in child mortality can be reduced to the correlation between the mortality risks of two consecutive siblings.

The main result of this study is that in nineteenth century Geneva, death clustering in infant and child mortality was not related to the between-family heterogeneity in reproductive behaviour. This conclusion remains of course context-specific. In the transitional context of nineteenth century Geneva, family limitation was achieved by a combination of birth stopping, birth spacing and high ages at marriage. Families who did not stop having children after achieving the desired family size were likely to practice birth spacing. The answer to the question whether fertility behaviour contributed to the clustering of infant and child deaths in transitional populations requires therefore further analyses in contexts where fertility was subject to important between-family heterogeneity and where birth spacing was less practiced. The secondary result of this study is the evidence for between-family heterogeneity in the way the death of the previous sibling (and the timing of this death) affected the survival chances of the index child. This result has two implications. First, the non-consideration of this heterogeneity in a hazard model can lead to biased estimations of family-level frailty in infant mortality. Second, this result asks for further analysis since the investigation of this variable may lead to better understanding of the unequal distribution of child deaths among families.

References

Alter, G., Oris, M., & Broström, G. (2001). The family and mortality: A case study from rural Belgium. *Annales de démographie historique, 1*, 11–31.

Brändström, A. (1988). The impact of female labour conditions on infant mortality: A case study of the parishes of Nedertornea and Jokkmokk, 1800–96. *Social History of Medicine, 1*, 329–358.

Browne, W. J. (2009). *MCMC estimation in MLwiN*. Bristol: Centre for Multilevel Modelling.

Das Gupta, M. (1990). Death clustering, mothers' education and the determinants of child mortality in rural Punjab, India. *Population Studies, 44*, 489–505.

Edvinsson, S., Brändström, A., Rogers, J., & Broström, G. (2005). High-risk families: The unequal distribution of infant mortality in nineteenth-century Sweden. *Population Studies, 59*, 321–337.

Gabadinho, A., Ritschard, G., Müller, N. S., & Studer, M. (2011). Analyzing and visualizing state sequences in R with TraMineR. *Journal of Statistical Software, 40*, 1–37.

Guo, G. (1993). Use of sibling data to estimate family mortality effects in Guatemala. *Demography, 30*, 15–31.

Knodel, J. (1968). Infant mortality and fertility in three Bavarian villages: An analysis of family histories from the 19th century. *Population Studies, 22*, 297–318.
Knodel, J. (1982). Child mortality and reproductive behaviour in German village populations in the past: A micro-level analysis of the replacement effect. *Population Studies, 36*, 177–200.
Knodel, J. (1988). *Demographic behavior in the past. A study of fourteen German village populations in the eighteenth and nineteenth centuries*. Cambridge: Cambridge University Press.
Knodel, J., & Hermalin, A. I. (1984). Effects of birth rank, maternal age, birth interval and sibship size on infant and child mortality: Evidence from 18th and 19th century reproductive histories. *American Journal of Public Health, 74*, 1098–1106.
Knodel, J., & van de Walle, E. (1979). Lessons from the past: Policy implications of historical fertility studies. *Population and Development Review, 5*, 217–245.
Legrand, T., & Sandberg, J. (2006). Effects of child mortality on fertility: Theoretical complexities and measurement difficulties. In *Entre nature et culture: Quelle(s) démographie(s)? Chaire Quetelet 2002* (pp. 181–205). Louvain-la-Neuve: Academia-Bruylant.
Lynch, K. A., & Greenhouse, J. B. (1994). Risk factors for infant mortality in nineteenth-century Sweden. *Population Studies, 48*, 117–133.
Mills, M. (2011). *Introducing survival and event history analysis*. London: Sage.
Nault, F., Desjardins, B., & Légaré, J. (1990). Effects of reproductive behaviour on infant mortality of French-Canadians during the seventeenth and eighteenth centuries. *Population Studies, 44*, 273–285.
Oris, M., Derosas, R., & Breschi, M. (2004). Infant and child mortality. In T. Bengtsson, C. Campbell, J. Lee, et al. (Eds.), *Life under pressure: Mortality and living standards in Europe and Asia, 1700–1900* (pp. 359–398). Cambridge, MA: MIT Press.
Pebley, A. R., & Stupp, P. W. (1987). Reproductive patterns and child mortality in Guatemala. *Demography, 24*, 43–60.
Perrenoud, A. (1975). L'inégalité sociale devant la mort à Genève au XVIIe siècle. *Population, 30*, 221–243.
Perrenoud, A. (1979). *La population de Genève du seizième au début du dix-neuvième siècle. Etude démographique*. Genève: Société d'histoire et d'archéologie de Genève.
Perrenoud, A. (1988). Espacement et arrêt dans le contrôle des naissances. *Annales de démographie historique, 1*, 59–78.
Perrenoud, A. (1998). Le recul de la mortalité ordinaire'. In J. P. Bardet & J. Dupâquier (Eds.), *Histoire des populations de l'Europe* (Vol. 2, pp. 57–82). Paris: Fayard.
Preston, S. H. (1978). Introduction. In S. H. Preston (Ed.), *The effects of infant and child mortality on fertility* (pp. 1–18). New York: Academic.
Rabe-Hesketh, S., & Skrondal, A. (2008). *Multilevel and longitudinal modeling using Stata*. College Station: Stata Press.
Rollet, C. (1997). Childhood mortality in high-risk groups: Some methodological reflections based on French experience. In C. A. Corsini & P. P. Viazzo (Eds.), *The decline of infant and child mortality: The european experience, 1750–1990* (pp. 213–225). The Hague: Kluwer.
Sastry, N. (1997). Family-level clustering of childhood mortality risk in Northeast Brazil. *Population Studies, 51*, 245–261.
Schumacher, R. (2010). *Structures et comportements en transition. La reproduction démographique à Genève au 19e siècle* (Population, famille et société, Vol. 12). Berne: Peter Lang.
Scrimshaw, S. C. M. (1978). Infant mortality and behavior in the regulation of family size. *Population and Development Review, 4*, 383–403.
Studer, M., Ritschard, G., Gabadinho, A., & Müller, N. S. (2011). Discrepancy analysis of state sequences. *Sociological Methods & Research, 40*, 471–510.
van de Walle, F. (1986). Infant mortality and the European demographic transition. In A. J. Coale & S. C. Watkins (Eds.), *The decline of fertility in Europe* (pp. 201–233). Princeton: Princeton University Press.
Vandezande, M., Moreels, S., & Matthijs, K. (2010). *Explaining death clustering. intergenerational patterns in infant mortality. Antwerp, 1846–1905*. Working paper 13 of the WOG Historical Demography.

Chapter 7
A Slow Transition. Infant and Child Mortality Decline in a Sardinian Community: Alghero (1866–1935)

Marco Breschi, Massimo Esposito, Stanislao Mazzoni, and Lucia Pozzi

7.1 Introduction

The decline in infant and child mortality in Italy is particularly discernible in the decades following national unification in 1861. On a national level, the probability of dying prior to the age of 5 fell from around 475 in 1861, to about 200 in 1931 (Del Panta 1997). However, the rates of decline were highly differentiated in Italy's large macro-areas, being faster in the northern and central regions and slower in the southern and island territories (Somogyi 1967; Del Panta 1997; Pozzi 2000; Breschi and Fornasin 2007).

These contrasts became even more pronounced from the end of the nineteenth century onwards, given that the northern and central towns experienced a socio-economic boom compared to the relative stagnation in southern urban areas. While the geographical patterns of this process are well documented, there has been little investigation into the reasons behind them. The generally accepted macro-level explanation hinges on the growing socio-economic north-south divide (Daniele and Malanima 2008). Similarly, the rapid decline in infant and child mortality experienced in north-central towns is commonly attributed to the benefits derived from the introduction of new health policies (Del Panta 1990).

To date, analysis of these dynamics is largely based on aggregate data and the scarce research conducted at the individual level rarely focuses on urban contexts.

The present study was carried out within the framework of the research project "Filling the gap: an Italian population microanalysis from the demographic ancient regime to the first transition", coordinated by Marco Breschi and funded by the Italian Ministry of University and Research. We would like to thank the staff of the Alghero Historical Municipal Archive, Baingio Tavera and Gianfranco Piras for their invaluable help and cooperation.

M. Breschi (✉) • M. Esposito • S. Mazzoni • L. Pozzi
Department of Economic and Business, University of Sassari, Sassari, Italy
e-mail: breschi@uniss.it; mesposito@uniss.it; smazzoni@uniss.it; lpozzi@uniss.it

D. Ramiro Fariñas, M. Oris (eds.), *New Approaches to Death in Cities during the Health Transition*, International Studies in Population 12,
DOI 10.1007/978-3-319-43002-7_7

The originality of this study lies in its use of individual, micro-level data in reference to a medium-sized urban community—the municipality of Alghero—in Sardinia. For the first time in the context of Italy, we are able to trace the first 5 years of life for cohorts born between 1866 and 1930 at the individual level, and, at the same time, examine the decline in mortality from an environmental perspective. Not only can we distinguish between people who lived in the original old town and those who lived in the countryside, but also a third "expansion area", created and designed in line with newly introduced standards of civic urban construction, following a radical redevelopment of the town towards the end of the nineteenth century. We therefore have the chance to compare infant-child mortality in three distinct populations from 1900.

The aim of this paper is threefold: (a) to analyse the role of socio-economic determinants affecting infant and child mortality; (b) to measure the differentials associated with the place of residence, in particular rural/urban localities; (c) to verify, albeit in a speculative way, the effects of sanitary and public health measures in the new urbanized area.

7.2 The Study Area

Alghero is a coastal town in northwest Sardinia that, before national unification, constituted, along with the regions of Piedmont and Liguria, the Kingdom of Sardinia. According to the first Italian Census (1861) Alghero was the island's fourth-largest municipality, with 8831 inhabitants. The territory includes the Nurra plain to the north, the region's only 'true scattered habitat area' (Le Lannou 2006). The presence of 100 hectares of stagnant, brackish wetlands favoured the spread of malaria, which greatly affected the health of local population, especially those living outside the old town, up until the 1920–1930s.

Around the time of unification, the Sardinian economy was essentially based on agriculture (engaging over half of the male labour force), sheep-farming, and mining. Farming was not intensive and traditionally limited to olives, vines, fruits, cereals and legumes. Cultivation and production techniques were extremely rudimentary, resulting in poor yields and unprofitable products and land use was still organised according to a long-standing semi-feudal land tenure system (Coda 1977). Farmers had low standards of living and were often obliged to supplement their meagre earnings with additional activities such as handicrafts (Coda 1977). Being a coastal town, there was also a significant presence of fishermen, sailors, and coral fishers, as well as artisans and traders. The male occupations nominated in marriage records for the years 1866–1925[1] indicate that farmers and the above-mentioned composite socio-professional group were comparable in number, jointly amounting to 45 % of

[1] Information on brides' occupations was not used since the female categories were deemed inaccurate and inadequate; in the overwhelming majority of cases the expression used is "housewife".

the total labour force. The socio-economic structure also included a small (3 %) but significant minority group of affluent individuals predominantly made up of professionals, executives, and the small number of local members of the nobility. As in the rest of Sardinia, over 75 % of the population was almost completely illiterate.

Hygienic conditions in the town were dire, as attested by a number of national surveys and a variety of documents kept in the historical municipal archive (petitions, requests and protestations). The population was dense and the sewer system particularly poor, especially in the harbour area, where water lacked in both quantity and quality. These problems were partially resolved towards the end of the nineteenth century, and further addressed in the first half of the twentieth century.

Although Alghero was better served with medical facilities than the island's interior municipalities, these were nonetheless largely defective and inadequate (Gatti 1999; Putzolu 1993). The national survey on hygiene in Italian municipalities carried out by the General Directorate of Statistics in 1885 (Maic 1886) records the town as having six medical doctors, three pharmacists and three registered midwives.[2] A contract existed between the municipal authorities and the local hospital, administered by the Congregazione della Carità, for the treatment of indigent citizens, who, according to the municipal historical archive, accounted for around 40 % of families.

During the period under analysis the town's old structure was radically modified (Principe 1983; Sari 1988, 1998). Following national unification, and particularly after 1867, when the Ministry of War ceased to consider Alghero a military stronghold (Sari 1988, 1998), an animated debate unfurled on whether to demolish the old walls that had long protected the town. As for many other Italian and European towns at the time, this dilemma was largely prompted by the necessity to modernize outdated structures and meet the needs of a growing population (Varni 2005). Eventually, the demolition was provided for in the "Plan of expansion" dated June 1881, and work began 5 years later.

Although this same process occurred in many other Italian and European towns, some of the underlying reasons in Alghero were specific to this particular context. First and foremost, the local authorities considered the walls an obstacle to the modernization and expansion of the town. Following French urban models, the local authorities wanted to widen the streets and remove the old districts to make way for large squares, boulevards, and gardens to provide the necessary space for a growing population. Secondly, there was also a pressing need to provide employment for a large number of masons and unskilled workers who were jobless due to the prevailing economic situation. Lastly, there were also concerns related to public health (Sari 1998). The walls were thought to prevent ventilation and account for the most frequent diseases that afflicted the town; their demolition would therefore have ensured better sanitary conditions in the town centre.

This widely held view is confirmed in all the council's official acts and documents regarding applications for funding to purchase and demolish the walls. The key figures involved in this process included not only progressives from local

[2] This does not necessarily mean they had adequate professional training.

authorities but also many real estate speculators, whereas the majority of ordinary citizens would have been excluded. In the space of a few years, the walls were demolished and recovered spaces put to new use. For example, the town's new marketplace was created where the Montalbano bastion had stood (Sari 1999).

With some modification, the rest of the "expansion plan" was subsequently carried out, resulting in a new and spacious urban area which greatly contrasted with the old and over populated town.[3] This included the partial construction of a modern sewer system, the supply of drinking water to every house, and the designation of many buildings, particularly on Via Nazionale, to the growing middle class.

A good snapshot of the new population distribution is provided by the original sheets from the 1921 census, stored in the local Municipal Historical Archive. The census records a lower number of inhabitants (11,900 individuals, see Table 7.1) than the 12,555 in the official statistics, but after adding the 474 prison inmates and 31 religious figures living in the seminary, this discrepancy is negligible (little more than 1 %) and probably attributable to the loss of documents. The detailed information available from this source allows us to identify 2711 households by residence (see Table 7.1). The vast majority of the population (around 88 %) lived in the old town centre; 8 % resided in the new urban expansion area; and the remaining 4 % was dotted around the countryside.

The number of inhabitants per room was lower in the new urban area (1.87) than both the town centre (2.32), evidence of its persistently high population density, and the countryside (2.36) which reflects the prevalence of rudimentary rural dwellings (the so-called "pinnette" and "cuili" – Baldacci 1952; Mossa 1957). The Hisco classification system (Van Leeuwen et al. 2002) allows us to see the differences in the socio-professional profile of households in the three areas. Reflecting the island's rural economy, the largest group was farmers (30 %), and not surprisingly, their presence increased with distance from the old town, reaching 50.5 % in open countryside. Another striking characteristic of the rural area is the low percentage of "housewives and retired"[4] compared to both urban areas. There are also some clear contrasts between the old and new urban contexts. Whereas the presence of the higher social strata (skilled and elite) was well attested in the new expansion area, constituting 30.9 % of the total 220 household heads, in contrast, 30.7 % of the total 2386 household heads in the old town centre belonged to the unskilled and low skilled categories.

[3] This plan included a plant in echelon formation with the national road towards Sassari—now Via Vittorio Emanuele—serving as a pintle. The present-day Via Mazzini and Via XX Settembre were aligned to this street, which then intersected with the road corresponding to the Via IV Novembre before widening into an open square. There were also four parallel streets to the left and right of Via Nazionale, intersected by eight side streets. The plan also included the urbanisation of the area recovered by the transfer of the cemetery elsewhere and the creation of a large public park (now Giuseppe Manno Park).

[4] Information available in the 1921 Census on the socio-professional status of female heads of family is imprecise and inadequate; in most cases the category used is "housewife". For this reason and considering their advanced ages, we have grouped female family heads with retired heads ("Housewives and retired").

Table 7.1 Population distribution in the municipal territory of Alghero according to the census of 1921

Areas	Inhabitants	Rooms	Individuals per room	Households	Professional status of the head of the household (HISCO)%						
					Unskilled	Low skilled	Farmers	Skilled	Elite	Housewives and retired	Total
Old town centre	10,428	4502	2.32	2386	13.7	17.0	28.7	9.3	9.4	21.9	100
New expansion area	956	510	1.87	220	5.0	12.7	33.6	10.0	20.9	17.8	100
Rural area	516	219	2.36	105	7.6	15.2	50.5	2.9	18.1	5.7	100
Total	11,900	5231	2.27	2711	12.8	16.6	29.9	9.1	10.7	20.9	100

7.3 Infant and Child Mortality: Source Materials and Results

Individual life-histories were reconstructed almost exclusively on the basis of civil and religious records of birth, marriage and death, although some information was drawn from additional sources such as military lists, population registers, and the censuses of 1852 and 1921, to control partially and indirectly for the migration and movement of individuals.[5]

The combined use of civil and religious documentation[6] was necessary for an accurate and comprehensive reconstruction of individual life histories due to the national law introduced in 1866, which meant the new Kingdom of Italy no longer recognised marriages celebrated in a church alone. This loss of basic civil rights remained in vigour until 1929. Most couples, following long-standing tradition, continued to marry in church, often postponing civic regularization until the arrival of their firstborn or later (Benini 1911; Livi Bacci 1977). In the absence of civic legalisation for marriage, not only did the Italian State not recognise spouses or offspring as legitimate heirs, but recorded children in civil registers as illegitimate, greatly biasing official statistics on illegitimacy (Benini 1911; De Vergottini 1965).[7] As elsewhere in Italy, the proportion of illegitimate births in Sardinia shot up after 1866, from 2 % to an average of 10 % for almost 30 years. The same trend progressed in Alghero, where illegitimacy reached 10 % in the mid-1870s and 20 % a decade later (Breschi et al. 2009), before returning to "original" levels in the years leading up to World War I (Fig. 7.1). Since much of Alghero's population refused to comply with this law, it was indispensable to use both civil and religious sources to reconstruct the sequence and timing of marriages and identify "genuine" illegitimate births (Breschi et al. 2009).

Religious sources could also help clarify questions regarding civil records of the stillbirth rate, which remained strikingly high until the early twentieth century. However, careful examination of both civil and parish records for Alghero[8] would appear to confirm that measuring the true stillbirth rate in Italy for this period is

[5] Reconstruction of the individual life-histories of Alghero's population proved to be quite complex, given that no *Stati Animarum* were available—a common situation in almost every Sardinian parish (Anatra and Puggioni 1983)—and only small fragments of population registers were found in the municipal archive.

[6] The borders of the municipality and parish coincided perfectly at the time, meaning the population of reference was essentially the same for both registration systems.

[7] The national proportion of illegitimate births increased from about 5 % (1862–1865) to 6.2 % in the 3-year period after the introduction of the law, to over 7.5 % in the mid-1880s. Not surprisingly, this increase was particularly pronounced in the ex-territories of the Church state, where roughly 1 child in 5 was recorded as illegitimate. This phenomenon was partly counterpoised through natural legitimizations after civil marriage and a specific decree, leading to about half of illegitimate births eventually becoming legitimated (Benini 1911).

[8] This issue is complex, controversial and little explored at the national level. See the specific paper dedicated to this subject based on the empirical evidence derived from this case study (Breschi et al. 2012).

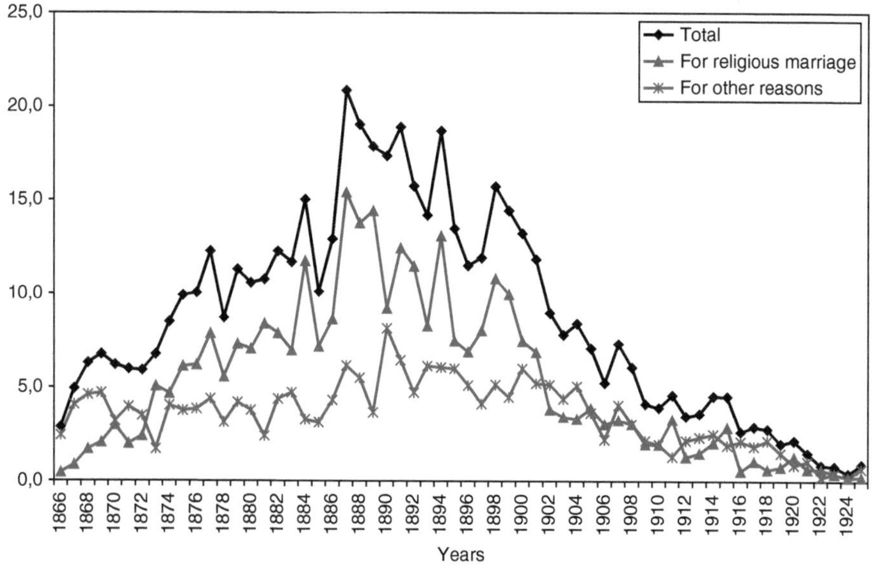

Fig. 7.1 Percentage of illegitimate births, Alghero 1866–1925

likely to remain an enigma. In this case study, at least one-third of official "still-born" babies probably correspond to "false still-born", in other words, babies who died some hours or days after birth but were not granted their due place in the "neonatal" category. Given that this study's main aim is to measure social and environmental differences in mortality, and in the light of empirical testing using a micro-analytical approach on individual and family biographies, we included all births (live and still) listed in the civil records.[9]

Before discussing the results of the micro-level analysis, it is worth considering the general characteristics of early-life mortality in the cohorts 1866–1930.[10] In Alghero, as elsewhere on the island, both infant and child mortality fell significantly (Fig. 7.2); the former by 40 % (from around 250 per thousand to 150 per thousand) and the latter by 60 % (from around 290 per thousand to 110 per thousand).

This trend is representative of Sardinia and also bears similarities to that in the south of Italy, where the decline in infant-child mortality encountered even more

[9] In the micro-level analysis of neonatal mortality, we adopted two models: one including the total number of births (live and still); and the second using only live births.

[10] Having adopted a cohort approach, we used the number of births for the years 1866–1930 and deaths for 1866–1935. We used two sets: the first covering all babies born to couples living in Alghero; the second including babies born to couples whose demographic history from marriage (civil or religious) can be reconstructed and whose presence in Alghero can be measured (until the fifth birthday of the last born). This was an attempt to capture the effects of migration on the measurement of infant-child mortality. The differences prove insubstantial, which is an indirect sign of the small incidence of migration, which was most often limited to single, predominantly male adults and not evident in Alghero until the twentieth century.

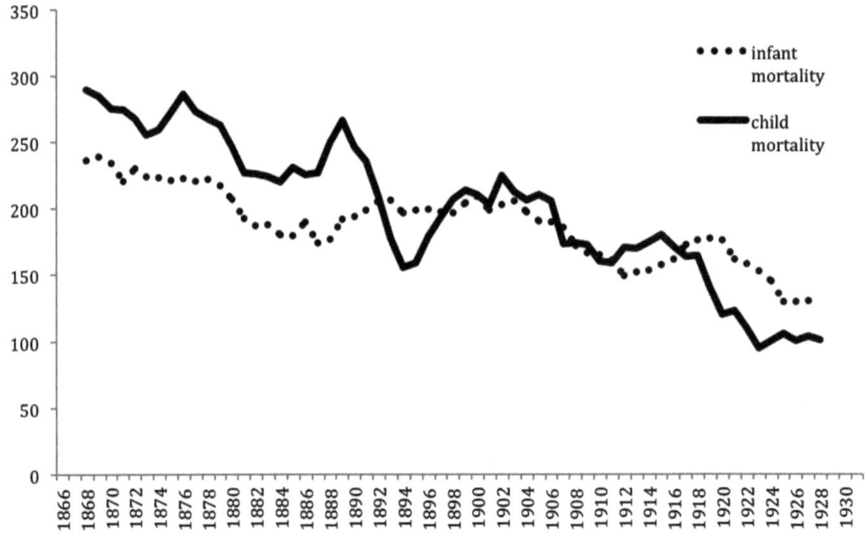

Fig. 7.2 Infant and child mortality rates (5-year moving averages), Alghero (1868–1927)

obstacles. Another feature seen here which is typical of the Mediterranean pattern is the "crossing-over" of the two rates. Whereas the mortality rate for infants is lower than that for children for cohorts born between 1866 and 1890, they subsequently intersect for the following thirty cohorts[11], and then invert their former positions after World War I. In relation to the general Mediterranean model, the most peculiar trait of the Sardinian pattern is the "moderate" level of infant mortality, at least for the period before the effective mortality decline.[12]

While explanations for the peculiarities of Sardinian mortality remain subject of debate (Pozzi 2000; Gatti 2002; Breschi et al. 2007), Colletti's hypothesis (1908) regarding the protective effects of prolonged breastfeeding is widely accepted. The benefits of late weaning contributed to keeping levels of infant mortality relatively low, or at least delaying death until childhood, balancing infant and child mortality levels (Goldman 1993; Hanson 1999).

[11] At the end of the nineteenth century, the probability of dying in the first year of life as opposed to in later childhood was more than double in France and Belgium, whereas in Italy the ratio was 1.2 and in Spain it was almost equal. There are strong regional differences within the Italian Kingdom, particularly in the south where this structural "Mediterranean" component was even more pronounced (Pozzi 2000).

[12] The infant mortality rate (Fig. 7.1) calculated on the basis of the total number of births, regardless of the official statement on viability, is over-estimated.

7.4 Individual-Level Analysis of Infant and Child Mortality

Although the decline in infant and child mortality regards all the cohorts examined, a difference emerges between urban and rural residence. A comparison using Kaplan Meier curves shows that children living in an urban setting had a higher survival rate than those in the countryside, and that this margin of difference was greater over the first 2 years (see Fig. 7.3).

Living in the town appears to have advantaged newborns, particularly in the first, delicate phases of life, with this effect tending to lose some of its impact in later childhood. A possible explanation for these differences is related to the presence of malaria, especially in remote areas. Sardinia was widely recognised as a high malaria-risk area at the time. Luigi Torelli, who conducted a well-known survey on malaria, including a detailed spatial distribution map of the disease in Italy, remarked that the island was almost entirely badly infested with malaria (Torelli 1883; Tognotti 1992).[13] The annual relative frequencies of malaria deaths in Sardinia were much higher than in the rest of Italy.[14]

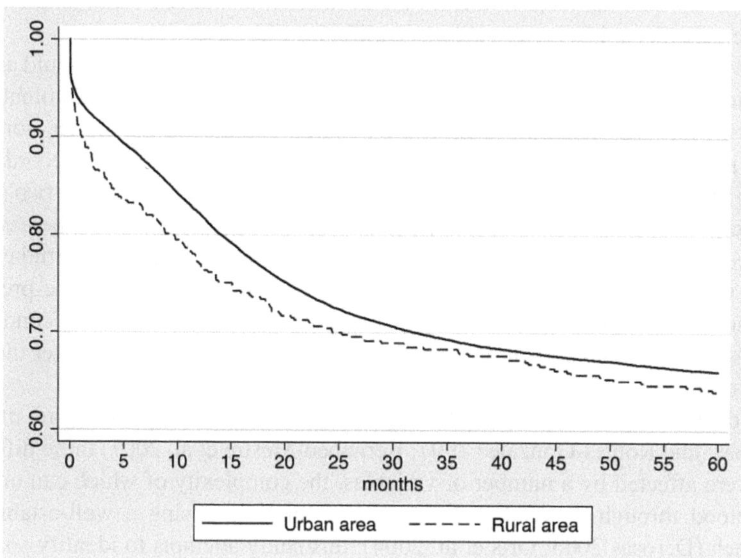

Fig. 7.3 Survival estimates by urban and rural area, Alghero (cohorts of birth 1866–1930)

[13] On Luigi Torelli and his work, see Eugenia Tognotti (1992) and Franco Della Peruta (1987).

[14] For a reconstruction of the role of malaria in Sardinia as well as a detailed analysis of the causes of the virulent resurgence of malaria after Italian unification, see Eugenia Tognotti (1996). Despite the gravity of the situation, significant countermeasures were not adopted until the mid-20th century, with a program funded by the Rockefeller Foundation that aimed to eradicate the vectors of disease (Donelli and Serinaldi 2003; Tognotti 2009).

The detrimental effects of malaria, particularly on the health of infants and pregnant women, were also well known. Not only did it increase the likelihood of premature birth, but in children it also caused swollen abdomens, damage to the liver, spleen and nervous system and delayed teething and walking. The full impact of malaria on infant health is now well understood from more recent research in developing countries (Guyatt and Snow 2004; Crawly et al. 2010).

Malaria infection during pregnancy is recognised as one of the major determinants of neonatal mortality, not only by provoking maternal anaemia (Gilles et al. 1969; Shulman et al. 1996; Cot et al. 1998), but primarily by causing low birth weight (LBW) (Brabin 1983, 1991; McGregor et al. 1983; Sullivan et al. 1999). Pre-term and full-term LBW and maternal fever close to delivery have been associated not only with neonatal mortality (in the first month of life) but also in the first trimester (Eisele et al. 2012). Any maternal infection capable of reducing the quantity or quality of breast milk can directly affect a new-born's health and chances of survival.

Despite a lack of precise information on the causes of child death in this context, it is reasonable to assume that differentials between urban and rural families can be partially linked to environmental factors. The town centre, while overcrowded, was further away than the rural area from the northern marshlands, where malaria vectors (female mosquitoes) were able to proliferate with ease.

The significant socio-economic differences between the two areas should also be taken into account. As mentioned (Table 7.1), the vast rural area was dominated by farmers, while the social fabric of the old and new urban areas was much more varied. It is well accepted that mortality selection is highly differentiated according to family SES. Analysis of the survival curves for children belonging to the two socio-economic extremes of the Alghero population (Fig. 7.4) reveals that whereas one-in-three children born to unskilled fathers failed to reach their fifth birthday, this figure was close to one-in-four in the case of elite families. Unlike the previous rural/urban analysis, this gap increases with age, suggesting that sanitary conditions and resources available for infant care became a more decisive factor after the cessation of the protective effect of breastfeeding.

As documented by conceptual frameworks on the determinants of infant mortality (Pozzi and Robles-Gonzalez 1997; Bernabeu-Mestre et al. 2007) these differentials were affected by a number of variables, the complexity of which can only be understood through detailed, individual-level analysis. Using a well-established approach (Derosas 2003; Oris et al. 2004), this study attempts to identify some of these determinants from a socio-ecological perspective using individual biographies for cohorts born between 1866 and 1930.

The variables included in our models largely depend on the characteristics and quality of data at our disposal. Although gestation, birth type and newborn immediate health status are widely recognised as having great importance in conceptual frameworks on the proximate determinants of mortality in early life (Cramer 1987; Shah et al. 2000; Misra et al. 2003; Oris et al. 2004; Titaley et al. 2008; Vandresse 2008), there are unfortunately no official records of this information in the period

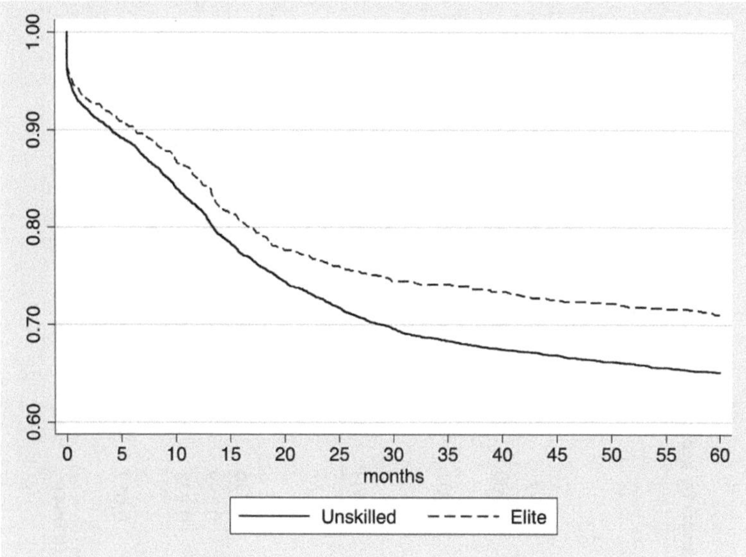

Fig. 7.4 Survival estimates by SES (unskilled and elite), Alghero (cohorts of birth, 1866–1930)

analysed (Istat 1957).[15] Despite these limitations, we devised four models, each relating to crucial phases in paediatric health over the first 5 years of life, in an attempt to measure the roles of changing relationship between biological, epidemiological, environmental, familiar, socio-economic and cultural determinants of infant-child mortality.

Given the risks associated with pregnancy, the predominance of bio-demographic factors and data limits regarding stillbirths, the first model relates to neonatal deaths (first month of life). Due to the largely insurmountable problem of data limits in civil records regards all Italy (Woods 2009), we used two versions of the first model to minimize possible effects: one including stillbirths and one without. We also made use of a previous study on Alghero that examines this issue in more detail (Breschi et al. 2012). The second model relates to the 1–7 month period and represents the breastfeeding phase. The third model spans the 8–15 month interval, and from literature of the time and examination of monthly mortality risks can be identified as the weaning period. The last model refers to the post-weaning period leading up to the fifth birthday ("child" mortality). The results are summarised in Table 7.2.

The gradual process of decline in mortality is captured by the covariate relative to the year of birth that in all models indicates a reduction of 1–2 % from one cohort

[15] In Italy, childbirth certificates were introduced in the late nineteenth century, but only for hospital births. At that time, very few women chose a hospital birth, and most of those who did were unmarried mothers. It is essential to take account of each mother's entire reproductive history to understand the risk factors for the health of an individual baby. See a recent study carried out at Udine hospital (Driul et al. 2010).

Table 7.2 Determinants of mortality. Alghero, cohorts 1866–1930: odds ratios and significance levels by age group

Determinants of mortality		Neonatal (0 month) with stillborn		Age (months) Neonatal (0 month) without stillborn		1–7		8–15		16–59		0–59		% 0–59
		Odds	P>z	Odds	P>z	Odds	P>z	Odds	P>z	Odds	P>z	Odds	P>z	
Year of birth	(Mean)	**0.988**	0.000	0.989	0.704	**0.990**	0.000	**0.993**	0.000	**0.979**	0.000	**0.983**	0.000	1902
Mother's age	(Mean)	**1.013**	0.013	1.006	0.387	1.008	0.121	**1.014**	0.001	**1.014**	0.000	**1.156**	0.000	29.2
Sex	(Male r.)	1.000		1.000		1.000		1.000		1.000		1.000		51.7
	Female	**0.818**	0.001	**0.813**	0.010	**0.880**	0.038	**0.854**	0.003	0.971	0.512	**0.885**	0.000	48.3
SES	(Un/lower-skilled r.)	1.000		1.000		1.000		1.000		1.000		1.000		38.9
	Farmers	0.965	0.673	1.005	0.963	1.119	0.127	0.930	0.236	**1.165**	0.003	1.076	0.059	44.7
	Skilled	0.935	0.621	0.894	0.495	1.127	0.299	0.950	0.599	1.065	0.447	1.027	0.667	10.4
	Elite	0.791	0.164	**0.644**	0.045	0.748	0.069	0.862	0.228	**0.712**	0.002	**0.739**	0.000	6.0
Zone	(Urban area.)	1.000		1.000		1.000		1.000		1.000		1.000		97.5
	Rural area	**1.538**	0.030	**1.980**	0.002	1.357	0.107	0.919	0.657	0.906	0.535	1.164	0.329	2.5
Events		1338		741		1210		1617		2580		6745		
σ^2		1.654 (0.147)		1.344 (0.179)		0.551 (0.095)		0.244 (0.064)		0.204 (0.047)		0.269 (0.030)		

to another. Only in the neonatal model (excluding stillbirths) does this covariate produce not significant results. This could be because excluding (true and false) stillbirths artificially lowers neonatal mortality levels, especially for the early cohorts, which are more prone to bias. In other words, it is possible that mortality in the neonatal phase declined much less, if at all, compared to subsequent periods of childhood (Breschi et al. 2012).

The influence of bio-demographic factors, or at least of those taken into consideration, is clearly evident. Firstly, female newborns have a 12–15 % lower risk than males up to the post-weaning phase, which is in line with a large body of research that shows that the reduction of higher male mortality levels commonly occurred after the second birthday for cohorts born before 1920 (Pinnelli and Mancini 1997; Breschi and Fornasin 2007). Secondly, a child's risk of death increases in relation to maternal age (1–1.5 % with each additional year), which along with results regarding the order of birth and vitality of the previous child, confirms that children born to older mothers, with a large number of siblings, encountered higher risks. Notably, it is only during the breastfeeding phase that maternal age lacks a statistically significant effect.

Possibly the most notable result that emerges regard SES, measured by father's occupation classified according to HISCO (Van Leeuwen et al. 2002). Again, this effect appears to have relevance in the post-weaning phase alone, when in relation to the reference category children of the elite class had around a 20 % lower risk of death, and the children of farmers around 15 % higher. While the SES effect lacks statistical significance in the neonatal, breastfeeding and weaning phases, the overall relationship up to the fifth birthday is clearly evident in the case of the elite, with a lower risk of about 26 % (last column, Table 7.2).

In the neonatal period a significantly lower mortality risk also emerges for the elite group (about one-third of the reference category's) when stillbirths are excluded. As suggested, discarding stillbirths means also eliminating cases related to delivery traumas and complications in the first most delicate hours of life. The pervasive low medical birth-attendance at the time meant that even children from well-off families were vulnerable during this crucial phase. Although the combination of factors related to the superior environmental and hygienic conditions, a richer and more regular diet and better provision of care offered by the higher social strata clearly favoured child survival, the fact that the benefits deriving from these factors are less apparent around the time of birth suggests that the risk of neonatal death was closely related to maternal bio-demographic characteristics and the perils of childbirth. Likewise, the protective immunity granted by breastfeeding extended to all babies, reducing the role or rather delaying the effect of environmental and hygienic conditions until the stage of weaning.

Of equal interest is the result observed in the first model, based on individual data, for the covariate on place of residence (urban vs. rural), which shows that the highest risks were encountered by newborns (with and without stillbirths) in the rural area. This empirical evidence appears to reinforce the previously advanced hypothesis (referring to Fig. 7.3), which related the survival differentials between

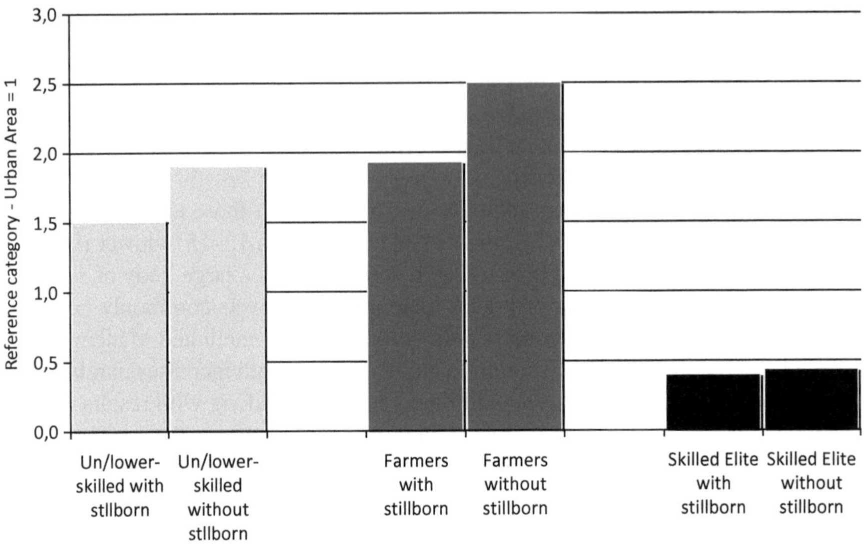

Fig. 7.5 Rural/urban odds ratios by SES, Alghero neonatal mortality, 1866–1930 cohorts

the town and countryside to the presence of malaria in the large and desolate rural municipal area.

This first model alone is however insufficient to determine the roles played by SES and place of residence, because: (a) the overall reduction in number of cases observed after SES and residence are taken into account suggests further simplifying the social classes; (b) besides the urban/rural contrast, significant variations also emerge between the old and new urban area; and (c) the population in the new urban area stabilized only after 1900. Three additional models were therefore applied that employ further simplified social classes (from a combination of the categories used in Table 7.2), newly delineated territorial areas, and different groups of cohorts.

First, we investigated any differential effects induced by place of residence (urban vs. rural) within the broadened social groups ("Un/lower Skilled", "Farmers", and "Skilled Elite"). The results from this analysis for neonatal mortality are summarised in Fig. 7.5 (dark patterning indicating the presence of statistical significance).[16]

Whereas the effect of place of residence on neonatal mortality lacks statistical significance at both extremes of the social scale, a significantly higher risk of death emerges for the newborns of farmers (with and without stillbirths) in the countryside, which would again appear to corroborate the hypothesis of a pathological effect of malaria on infant survival. The margin of difference is also larger in the absence of stillbirths, which, as established, implies the almost total elimination of

[16] The covariates are those included in the previous model (Tab. 7.2). Three different models were applied for each set of births using the social classes: Un/lower Skilled; Farmers; Skilled Elite.

deaths occurring soon after birth and largely affected by the bio-demographic conditions of the mother and inherent risks of childbirth.

Given the need to consider the effect of the differences between the old and new urban areas, it was also necessary to conduct an analysis limited to cohorts born after 1900. For the same reasons outlined above, the socio-economic structure was again simplified by combining the elite and skilled group into one higher class. The results of this analysis are detailed below (Table 7.3).

The rural area is absent from this model since the small number of higher class households provided insufficient events for analysis when restricted to cohorts 1900–1930, and moreover our interest here is to reveal any significant difference in mortality in relation to the two urban areas for children from the same social group.

As before, with the analyses covering all cohorts, statistically significant differences emerge only post-weaning. Children from the higher social class in the new urban area appear to have benefitted, at least partially, from a protective effect deriving from the far better living conditions. As mentioned, these advantages included fresher air, better sanitation, lower population density, and the availability of running water in wealthy homes along the axis coincident with the expansion zone (Via Vittorio Emanuele).

Further evidence of this environmental protective effect is also provided by the results of the empirical model referring to the most disadvantaged families (Table 7.4). This analysis included all three environmental contexts and revealed that children born to Un/Lower-skilled families living in the new urban area had a lower risk (about 60 %) during the weaning phase, even if the statistical significance is slight. It would appear that the better living conditions in the new urban area did improve infant survival.

However, as repeatedly stressed throughout this chapter, any hypothesis based on these results remains speculative, not least because the lack of information on cause of death in the civil status records does not allow for drawing irrefutable conclusions.

7.5 Final Remarks

This chapter examines the slow process of decline in infant and child mortality in a Sardinian community, which is in many ways representative of the broader Mediterranean context. The period analysed (1866–1930), roughly coincides with the first stage of demographic transition and partially with the first major improvements in hygiene and sanitary conditions, even if the true benefits of these, at least in the south of the country, were hardly perceptible until after World War II. Although this process has received much attention at the macro level, to date it remains largely unexplored at the individual level. Even if the period analysed coincides with the

Table 7.3 Determinants of mortality of skilled-elite children by place of residence, Alghero, cohorts 1900–1930

				Age (months)										
		Neonatal 0 month with Stillborn		Neonatal 0 month without stillborn		1–7		8–15		16–59		0–59		% 0–59
		Odds	P>z	Odds	P>z	Odds	P>z	Odds	P>z	Odds	P>z	Odds	P>z	
Zone	Town centre area	1.000		1.000		1.000		1.000		1.000		1.000		92.7
	New urbanization	1.148	0.580	2.526	0.062	0.809	0.690	1.164	0.694	**0.293**	0.021	0.741	0.289	7.3
Events		88		52		97		124		153		462		
σ^2		2.382 (0.847)		1.242 (0.572)		1.332 (0.547)		0.327 (0.298)		0.711 (0.327)		0.624 (0.167)		

Controlled for year of birth, sex, and mother's age

Table 7.4 Determinants of mortality of un/lower-skilled chidren by place of residence Alghero, cohorts 1900–1930

		Age (months)												%
		0 with stillborn		0 without stillborn		1–7		8–15		16–59		0–59		0–59
		Odds	P>z	Odds	P>z	Odds	P>z	Odds	P>z	Odds	P>z	Odds	P>z	
Zone	Town centre area	1.000		1.000		1.000		1.000		1.000		1.000		95.1
	New urbanization	1.311	0.535	1.406	0.463	1.108	0.794	**0.402**	0.047	1.008	0.980	0.898	0.609	3.2
	Rural area	0.597	0.421	0.202	0.149	0.899	0.845	1.496	0.271	0.717	0.428	0.963	0.885	1.7
Events		298		193		253		412		511		1474		
σ^2		2.360 (0.462)		1.923 (0.483)		0.501 (0.216)		0.330 (0.145)		0.174 (0.120)		0.221 (0.066)		

Controlled for year of birth, sex, and mother's age

beginnings of the great demographic transformation of the entire country, for a number of reasons it remains one of the least studied at the micro level.[17]

The life-history analysis carried out at the individual level with reference to the mentioned cohorts born in Alghero between 1866 and 1930 has allowed us to better understand the complex interactions between the bio-demographic, social, and environmental variables affecting the slow decline in infant and child mortality.

The weight of the bio-demographic variables (of mother and child) is clear throughout the period under examination. The role of the socio-economic component, measured albeit partially on the basis of father's profession, is also relevant. Micro-level analysis revealed that the higher socio-economic class was significantly advantaged and able to ensure the highest levels of child survival from birth through to the weaning phase and beyond.

We also saw that breastfeeding, which was widespread and prolonged in Sardinia, not only contributed to levelling out differences in SES, but also to maintaining relatively low levels of infant mortality. All socially related differentials become more apparent with the onset of weaning.

Analysis of place of residence also allowed for a better understanding of the role of environmental conditions. Despite certain insurmountable limitations in national documentation—most conspicuously on the cause of death—this study found that the children of farmers and shepherds living in the country experienced considerably higher risks compared to those of the same social group living in the town. We concluded that the action of malaria was much more relevant in the rural context, reflected by the modest direct and indirect effects of the disease on the health of mothers, unborn babies and infants living in the town.

We also ascertained a significant reduction in the risks of mortality (particularly after weaning) for children of the elite and skilled group who had the privilege of living in the new urban area, designed according to modern sanitary and hygienic principles. This result is particularly important in being the first empirical evidence, at least in the Italian context, of the benefits induced by the combination of two "conditions": being relatively "well-off"; and living in housing that was newly constructed, adequately ventilated, and equipped with running water.

This study allows us to affirm that the causal relationships outlined in the general theoretical frameworks find statistical support in the individual analyses carried out with reference to a real population during the process of demographic transition. We were able to discern the decisive contribution of social and environmental variables at a time of great transformation for the entire population but which, at least initially, mostly affected just a small minority of beneficiaries, which in the case of

[17] In Italy, the cut-off point between historical and contemporary demography is taken as coinciding with national unification (1861). Only from that time do we have a uniform statistical documentation for the whole country at our disposal. However, whereas studies on historical demography based on individual data rarely venture beyond 1860–1880, those on contemporary demography based on individual data essentially refer to the 1970s and later. The period 1880–1960 has become a sort of "no-man's land" for demographic studies based on individual data. For this reason, the process of demographic transition, at least in Italy, remains largely unexplored from a micro-analytic perspective.

Alghero were the higher social class living in the new urban area. It was precisely this combination—social advantage plus better housing—which underpinned the decline in child mortality observed in most of the urban populations of northern and central Italy from the late nineteenth century, and later in the south.[18]

We can note that in the case of Alghero, the already privileged social classes benefitted from the advantages derived from the new urban planning models promoted by the municipality and supported by government and private finance. To establish whether the characteristics of Alghero are typical of other such communities requires the study of other similar cases. In other words, the fundamental question remaining is whether the major urban transformations witnessed in all Italian towns in the late nineteenth and early twentieth century had a broad effect on the health of the general population or, as in the case of Alghero, was mainly limited to the higher social groups.

References

Anatra, B., & Puggioni, G. (1983). *Fonti ecclesiastiche per lo studio della popolazione della Sardegna centro-meridionale*. Roma: Cisp.

Baldacci, O. (1952). *La casa rurale in Sardegna*. Firenze: Centro di studi per la geografia etnologica.

Benini, R. (1911). *La demografia italiana nell'ultimo cinquantennio, in Cinquanta anni di storia italiana*. Milano: U. Hoepli.

Bernabeu-Mestre, J., Perdiguero, E., & Barona, J. (2007). Determinanti della mortalità infantile e transizione sanitaria. Una riflessione a partire dall'esperienza spagnola. In M. Breschi & L. Pozzi (Eds.), *Salute, malattia e sopravvivenza in Italia fra '800 e '900* (pp. 171–189). Udine: Forum.

Brabin, B. J. (1983). An analysis of malaria in pregnancy in Africa. *Bulletin of the World Health Organization, 61*, 1005–1016.

Brabin, B. J. (1991). *The risks and severity of malaria in pregnant women* (Applied field research in malaria reports, Vol. 1). Geneva: World Health Organization.

Breschi, M., & Fornasin, A. (2007). La mortalità per genere nei primi cinque anni di vita, Italia 1864–1959. In M. Breschi & L. Pozzi (Eds.), *Salute, malattia e sopravvivenza in Italia fra '800 e '900* (pp. 243–272). Udine: Forum.

Breschi, M., Mazzoni, S., Melis, P. M., & Pozzi, L. (2007). Nuove indagini per l'analisi della mortalità nei primi anni di vita in Sardegna. In M. Breschi & L. Pozzi (Eds.), *Salute, malattia e sopravvivenza in Italia fra '800 e '900* (pp. 195–220). Udine: Forum.

Breschi, M., Manfredini, M., Mazzoni, S., & Pozzi, L. (2009). Fertility and socio-cultural determinants at the beginning of demographic transition. Sardinia, nineteenth and twentieth centuries. In A. Fornasin & M. Manfredini (Eds.), *Fertility in Italy at the turn of the twentieth century* (pp. 63–78). Udine: Forum.

Breschi, M., Esposito, M., Mazzoni, S., & Pozzi, L. (2012). The Sardinian experience of the lowest Italian infant mortality rates at the turn of the twentieth century. True or false empirical evidence? *Annales de Démographie Historique*, 123, 63–94.

Coda, L. (1977). *La Sardegna nella crisi di fine secolo. Aspetti dell'economia e della società sarda nell'ultimo ventennio dell'Ottocento*. Sassari: Dessì.

[18]Much research is available at the macro level (e.g., Grottanelli 1980; Faccini 1984; Pogliano 1984; Piccinato 1989; Giovannini 1996).

Coletti, F. (1908). *La mortalità nei primi anni di età e la vita sociale della Sardegna*. Torino: Fratelli Bocca.

Cot, M., Le-Hesran, J. Y., Miailhes, P., Roisin, A., Fievet, N., Barro, D., et al. (1998). Effect of chloroquine prophylaxis during pregnancy on maternal hae-matocrit. *Annals of Tropical Medicine and Parasitology, 92*, 37–43.

Cramer, J. C. (1987). Social factors and infant mortality: Identifying high-risk groups and proximate causes. *Demography, 24*(3), 299–322.

Crawly, J., Chu, C., Mtove, G., & Nosten, F. (2010). Malaria in children. *The Lancet, 375*, 1468–1481.

Daniele, V., & Malanima, P. (2008). Divari di sviluppo e crescita nel Mediterraneo 1950–2005. *Rivista Italiana di Economia Demografia e statistica, 62*, 53–76.

Del Panta, L. (1990). Fattori e condizioni della mortalità tra 1800 e 1930: Igiene, salute e ambiente. La situazione in Italia. In *Popolazione, società e ambiente. Temi di demografia storica italiana (secc. XVII–XIX)* (pp. 245–273). Bologna: Clueb.

Del Panta, L. (1997). Infant and child mortality in Italy, eighteenth to twentieth century: Long-term trends and territorial differences. In A. Bideau, B. Desjardins, & H. P. Brignoli (Eds.), *Infant and child mortality in the past* (pp. 7–21). Oxford: Claredon Press Oxford.

Della Peruta, F. (1987). Luigi Torelli e la lotta contro la malaria. In C. Valenti (Ed.), *Aspetti storici e sociali delle infezioni malariche in Sicilia e in Italia. Atti del II seminario di studi (Palermo, 27–29 novembre 1986)* (pp. 183–188). Centro Italiano di Storia Sanitaria e Ospitaliera: Palermo.

Derosas, R. (2003). La mortalità infantile fatta a pezzi: Il caso di Venezia a metà '800. In M. Breschi, R. Derosas, & P. P. Viazzo (Eds.), *Piccolo è bello. Approcci microanalitici alla ricerca storico-demografica* (pp. 105–136). Udine: Forum.

De-Vergottini, M. (1965). Natalità e fecondità. *Annali di Statistica, 8*(17), 399–440.

Donelli, G., & Serinaldi, E. (2003). *Dalla lotta alla malaria alla nascita dell'Istituto di sanità pubblica. Il ruolo della Rockefeller Foundation in Italia: 1922–1934*. Roma - Bari: Laterza.

Driul, L., Londero, A. P., Bertozzi, S., Presessini, L., Vanin, M., D'Aietti, V., Fruscalzo, A., Biasioli, A., Salvador, S., Furlan, R., Petrovec, M. M., & Marchesoni, D (2010, June). Pregnancy outcome and neonatal health by mothers aged 40 years and over. *Journal of Medicine and Medical Sciences, 1*(5):148–155.

Eisele, T. P., Larsen, D. A., Anglewicz, P. A., Keating, J., Yukich, J., Bennett, A., Hutchinson, P., & Steketee, R. W. (2012). Malaria prevention in pregnancy, birthweight, and neonatal mortality: A meta-analysis of 32 national cross-sectional datasets in Africa. *Lancet Infectious Diseases, 12*(12), 942–949.

Faccini, L. (1984). Tifo, pensiero medico e infrastrutture igienico-sanitarie. In F. Della-Peruta (Ed.), *Storia d'Italia, Annali 7, Malattia e medicina* (pp. 705–737). Torino: Einaudi.

Gatti, A. M. (1999). Nascita dell'ostetricia e mortalità materna in Sardegna (XVII–XIX secolo). *Bollettino di Demografia Storica, 30/31*, 79–94.

Gatti, A. M. (2002). *La mortalità infantile tra Ottocento e Novecento. La Sardegna nel panorama italiano, Quaderni del Dipartimento di Ricerche Economiche e Sociali dell'Università di Cagliari. Sezione di Statistica*. Cagliari: Università di Cagliari.

Gilles, H. M., Lawson, J. B., Sibelos, M., Voller, A., & Allan, N. (1969). Malaria, anaemia, and pregnancy. *Annals of Tropical Medicine and Parasitology, 63*, 245–263.

Giovannini, C. (1996). *Risanare la città. L'utopia igienista di fine Ottocento*. Milano: Franco Angeli.

Goldman, A. S. (1993). The immune system of human milk: Antimicrobial, anti-inflammatory and immunomodulating properties [review]. *Pediatric Infectious Diseases Journal, 12*, 664–672.

Grottanelli, E. (1980). La politica dell'amministrazione comunale di Milano intorno ad alcuni problemi igienico-sanitari e della sicurezza collettiva. *Storia Urbana, 12*, 91–112.

Guyatt, H. L., & Snow, R. W. (2004, October). The impact of malaria during pregnancy on low birth weight in sub-Saharan Africa. *Clinical Microbiological Reviews, 17*(4):760–9.

Hanson, L. A. (1999). Human milk and host defense: Immediate and long-term effects [review]. *Acta Paeditrica Suppement, 88*, 42–46.

Istat. (1957). Le rilevazioni statistiche in Italia dal 1861 al 1956. Statistiche demografiche e sociali. *Annali di Statistica*, Serie VIII, Vol. 6.

Le-Lannou, M. (2006). *Pastori e contadini di Sardegna.* IV Italian Edition. Brigaglia M. (Ed.). Cagliari: Edizioni Della Torre.

Livi-Bacci, M. (1977). *A history of Italian fertility during the last two centuries.* Princeton: Princeton University Press.

McGregor, I. A., Wilson, M. E., & Billewicz, W. Z. (1983). Malaria infection of the placenta in The Gambia, West Africa: Its incidence and relationship to stillbirth, birth weight, and placental weight. *Transactions of the Royal Society of Tropical Medicine and Hygiene, 77*, 232–244.

Ministero di Agricoltura, Industria e Commercio (MAIC), Direzione Generale della Statistica. (1886). *Risultati dell'Inchiesta sulle condizioni igieniche e sanitarie nei comuni del Regno. Parte seconda: Notizie date per ciascun comune.* Roma: Tipografia dell'Ospizio di San Michele.

Misra, D. P., Guye, B., & Allston, A. (2003). Integrated perinatal health framework: A multiple determinants model with a life span approach. *American Journal of Preventive Medicine, 25*(1), 65–75.

Mossa, V. (1957). *Architettura domestica in Sardegna: Contributo per una storia della casa mediterranea.* Cagliari: Edizioni La Zattera.

Oris, M., Derosas, R., & Breschi, M. (2004). Infant and child mortality. In T. Bengtsson, C. Campbell, J. Z. Lee, et al. (Eds.), *Life under pressure. Mortality and living standards in Europe and Asia, 1700–1900* (pp. 359–398). Cambridge, MA: The Mit Press.

Piccinato, G. (1989). Igiene e urbanistica in Italia nella seconda metà del XIX secolo. *Storia Urbana, 27*, 47–66.

Pinelli, A., & Mancini, P. (1997). Gender mortality differences from birth to puberty in Italy, 1887–1940. In C. A. Corsini & P. P. Viazzo (Eds.), *The decline of infant and child mortality. The European experience: 1750–1990* (pp. 73–93). The Hague: Martinus Nijhoff Publishers.

Pogliano, C. (1984). L'utopia igienista (1870–1920). In F. Della-Peruta (Ed.), *Storia d'Italia, Annali 7, Malattia e medicina* (pp. 589–631).

Pozzi, L. (2000). *La lotta per la vita. Evoluzione e geografia della sopravvivenza in Italia fra '800 e '900.* Udine: Forum.

Pozzi, L., & Robles-González, E. (1997). L'analisi della mortalità infantile negli anni della transizione: Una riflessione sull'esperienza italiana e spagnola. In *Studi di Popolazione. Temi di ricerca nuova* (pp. 147–171). Roma: Dipartimento di Scienze Demografiche.

Principe, I. (1983). *Le città nella storia d'Italia. Sassari, Alghero.* Bari: Laterza.

Putzolu, F. (1993). Prime tappe dell'ostetricia in Sardegna. In L. Orrù & F. Putzolu (Eds.), *Il parto e la nascita in Sardegna. Tradizione Medicalizzazione Ospedalizzazione* (pp. 25–66). Cagliari: CUEC.

Sari, G. (1988). *La piazza fortificata di Alghero: analisi storico-artistica.* Alghero: Edizione del Sole.

Sari, A. (1998). Alghero nel XIX secolo. I piani d'ingrandimento. *Revista de l'Alguer, 9*(9), 69–87.

Sari, A. (1999). Alghero fuori le mura. I primi interventi urbanistici. *Revista de l'Alguer, 10*(10), 85–102.

Shah, N. M., Shah, M. A., Khalaf, A. A., Mustafa, M. M., & Al-Sayed, A. (2000). Searching for socioeconomic risk factors in perinatal mortality in Kuwait: A case-control study. *Social Science & Medicine, 51*(4), 539–550.

Shulman, C. E., Graham, W. J., Jilo, H., Lowe, B. S., New, L., Obiero, J., et al. (1996). Malaria is an important cause of anaemia in primigravidae: Evidence from a district hospital in coastal Kenya. *Transactions of the Royal Society of Tropical Medicine and Hygiene, 90*, 535–539.

Somogyi, S. (1967). *La mortalità nei primi cinque anni di età in Italia, 1863–1962.* Palermo: Università di Palermo, Istituto di Scienze demografiche.

Sullivan, A. D., Nyirenda, T., Cullinan, T., Taylor, T., Harlow, S. D., James, S. A., & Meshnick, S. R. (1999). Malaria infection during pregnancy: Intrauterine growth retardation and pre-term delivery in Malawi. *The Journal of Infectious Disease, 179*, 1580–1583.

Titaley, C. R., Dibley, M. J., Agho, K., Roberts, C. L., & Hall, J. (2008). Determinants of neonatal mortality in Indonesia. *BMC Public Health, 8*, 232.

Tognotti, E. (1992). La carta della malaria d'Italia (1880–82). *Quaderni internazionali di storia della medicina e della sanità, 1*(2), 23–34.

Tognotti, E. (1996). *La malaria in Sardegna. Per una storia del paludismo nel Mezzogiorno (1880–1950)*. Milano: Franco Angeli.

Tognotti, E. (2009). Program to eradicate malaria in Sardinia, 1946–1950. *Emerging Infectious Diseases, 15*(9), 1460–1466.

Torelli, L. (1883). *La malaria d'Italia*. Roma: Stabilimento Tipografico Italiano.

Vandresse, M. (2008). Estimation of a structural model of the determinants of neonatal mortality in Hungary, 1984–88 and 1994–98. *Population Studies, 62*(1), 85–111.

Van-Leeuwen, M. H. D., Maas, I., & Miles, A. (2002). *HISCO. Historical International Standard Classification of Occupations*. Leuven: Leuven University Press.

Varni, F. (2005). *I confini perduti. Le cinte murarie cittadine europee tra storia e conservazione*. Bologna: Editrice Compositori.

Woods, R. (2009). *Death before birth: Fetal health and mortality in historical perspective*. Oxford/New York: Oxford University Press.

Chapter 8
The Democratization of Longevity: How the Poor Became Old in Paris, 1880–1913

Lionel Kesztenbaum and Jean-Laurent Rosenthal

> "Mais comme il y a deux sortes de richesse, la richesse qui ne produit rien, et la richesse qui produit, que l'industrie sait partager pour l'accroître, j'ai été curieux de savoir si elles ont une influence également heureuse sur la durée de vie."[1]
>
> Louis-René Villermé, « De la mortalité dans les divers quartiers de la ville de Paris », *Annales d'hygiène publique et de médecine légale*, 1830

8.1 Introduction

In the 1860s, Parisians had a life expectancy at age five that was 4 or 5 years less than other French people. The gap did not begin to narrow until the 1880s and it did not close until the 1930s. Even in the 1890s, there were huge differences within Paris: the denizens of those neighbourhoods where life was long enjoyed an additional 14 years above what those in the worst neighbourhoods could expect (a difference that was almost twice as large as that between the best and worst departments within France). Those differences based on residence are also observable in differences in age a death between the bottom and the top part of the wealth distribution.

[1] "As there are two different forms of affluence, the one that don't produces anything, and the one that produces, and as industry knows how to share that one in order to increase it, I wanted to understand if they both positively influence the length of life."

L. Kesztenbaum (✉)
INED (Institut National d'Etudes Démographiques) and PSE (Paris School of Economics), 133, boulevard Davout, 75980 Paris Cedex 20, France
e-mail: lionel.kesztenbaum@ined.fr

J.-L. Rosenthal
Division of the Humanities and Social Sciences, Caltech (California Institute of Technology), Pasadena, CA 91125, USA
e-mail: rosentha@caltech.edu

D. Ramiro Fariñas, M. Oris (eds.), *New Approaches to Death in Cities during the Health Transition*, International Studies in Population 12,
DOI 10.1007/978-3-319-43002-7_8

In nineteenth century Paris, life was both brutally short and massively unequal, yet each year the city attracted hordes of migrants and, over the century after 1850, completely overhauled its sanitary infrastructure. While differences remain based on wealth, or neighbourhood, their relative importance has massively diminished.

This synopsis of the Paris experience poses two questions, one about the sources of differential mortality, the other about how it changes over time. Scholars have identified two opposed forces that drove life expectancy before World War II: first, the negative impact of having an ever increasing proportion of the population living in crowded and adverse urban environments (among others, Preston and Van de Walle 1978 or Cain and Hong 2009); second, increases in income and knowledge that in the long run offset the negative effects of urban living (see for instance Floud et al. 2011). In their pure form, income and knowledge are quite distinct. Higher income allowed individuals to purchase goods and services that prolonged life (e.g. better nutrition, clothing, and housing) that they consumed privately. Save for possible epidemiological effects, the better housing of one family has little effect on the life expectancy of another. At the other extreme we can place pure knowledge effects (like home cleanliness or boiling milk), once the survival value of such techniques are known they can be adopted by everyone because their costs are low. Here we focus on the correlation between mortality and income because the results are very striking in a city as unequal as Paris.

Paris turns out to be a very good laboratory to study differential mortality because the municipal statistical office was dominated by individuals who were obsessed with collecting and publishing detailed demographic data. Beyond the contrast between Paris and France that we can estimate for two centuries, we can track the evolution of mortality on a smaller scale (in each of Paris's 20 districts (*arrondissements*)) from 1880 to 1940 and, between 1880 and 1913, for each of the 80 neighbourhoods (*quartiers*) of the city. The municipal statistical office produced these disaggregated reports to spur public action to reduce both mortality and morbidity in the city. Yet during this period (unlike the interwar period) their efforts did not lead to major changes in policy. Additionally, the treasury collected (even though it did not publish) information on direct taxation for the same 80 neighbourhoods, which were also the units for the census of housings. Finally individual data sets on wealth at death enable us to produce estimates of average wealth levels for the same neighbourhoods. As we will show, there is extraordinary stability in the ranking of these neighbourhoods in terms of their real estate stock, their average wealth levels and in their relative life expectancy.

This chapter documents the long term evolution of life expectancy in Paris and its extraordinarily marked spatial variation. It is no great surprise that the poorest neighbourhoods were the deadliest, but the extent of the mortality differential between rich and poor is striking. Second, convergence to the low mortality regime was slow: although over time the variation in life expectancy within Paris fell, it has not disappeared.

Data

Paris has many advantages for studying differential mortality; the most straightforward of these is that the within Paris variances in incomes, wealth, and life expectancy were extremely large. There are some serious complications, however, the most obvious of these being that the individuals who were living in Paris at a point in time were not a randomly drawn sample. Thus, the choice of focusing on one large city rather than France as a whole as would be more conventional needs some defence.

The whole set of French localities would be an attractive laboratory for studying differential mortality because among the countries on both sides of the North Atlantic, France is the one with lowest levels of migration (either inward or outward). Hence, if one were to estimate differential mortality rates in a cross-section, one would not need to worry about the extent to which the individuals observed were selected, something that comes up if one deals with other countries that have high rate of emigration or immigration. However, scholars have long established that mortality rates varied by location (e.g. urban vs. rural) and we know that location was correlated with income. Hence in cross section it is difficult to separate income effects from other effects. Using time to help sort out these correlations reintroduces the thorny problem of endogeneity because even if French people did not often fall victim to the siren calls of North America, they moved around within their country quite a bit, and in particular cities were growing steadily since the beginning of the nineteenth century and the largest ones (Paris among them) fastest of them all (Guérin-Pace 1993). However, Paris also offers some important advantages to study mortality differentials.

Paris is obviously interesting in and of itself, but it presents a remarkable contrast with the country as a whole. In 1880, Parisians could expect to live 4 years (or nearly 10 %) less than French people as a whole (Fig. 8.1). Over the next three and a half decades, life expectancy in France increases by 4 years but that of Paris by nearly 7 years leading to a convergence that would turn into Paris' advantage in the interwar period. Thus, the patterns of spatial differential demography went through a great reversal. Yet at the same time the pattern of spatial differential demography changed very little before World War I.

As noted above and as we discuss below the difference between the worst and best decile of neighbourhoods is nearly 15 years in life expectancy, which is enormous. The distribution within the city highlights the large variations between neighbourhoods, even adjacent ones (Fig. 8.2). Furthermore, the spatial variation is stable over time and is measured after the city had provided broad access to clean water: building could connect to the water system to provide running water to each dwelling, a faucet at every floor or simply one on the ground floor, and there were also local fountains (Bocquet et al. 2008). It was in fact the other side of the water question: wastewater disposal that was going to occupy Parisians and mobilize investment in the half century following 1880. But the diffusion process favoured rich neighbourhoods over poor ones and thus actually further the spatial inequality within the city.

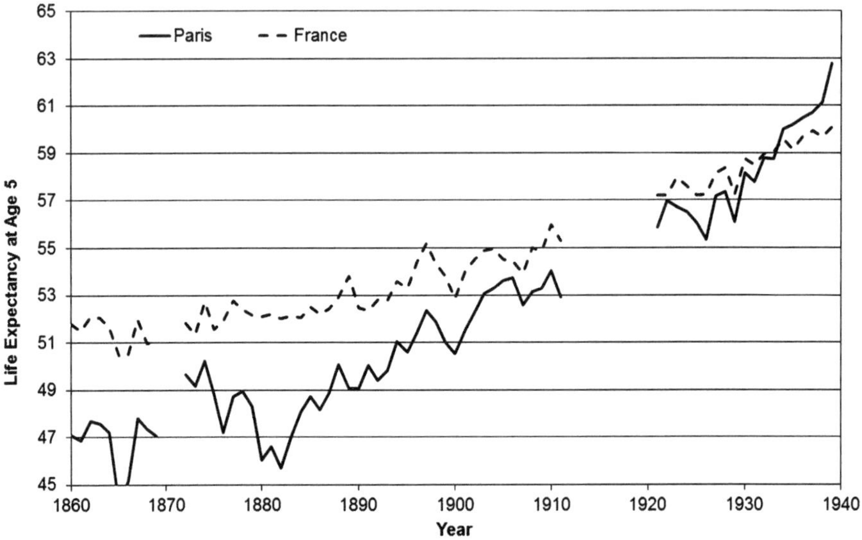

Fig. 8.1 Life expectancy at age 5, Paris and France, 1860–1939

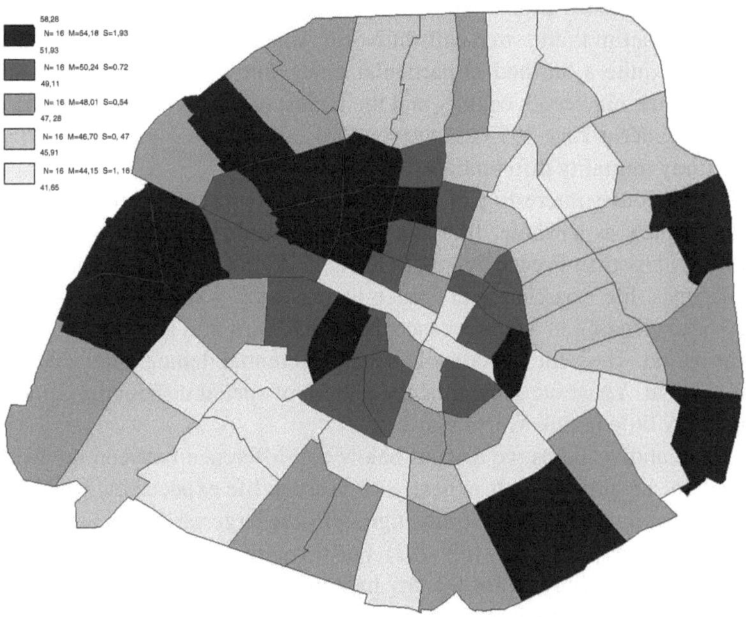

Fig. 8.2 Life expectancy at age 5 in Paris by neighborhood, 1881

The main reason for focusing on Paris is that we can carry out our analysis at three level of aggregation over long periods of time: the city (1820–1939), its 20 districts (1880–1939), and its 80 neighbourhoods (1880–1913). We can do so because the statistical department of the Paris municipality under the lead of Louis-Adolphe and Jacques Bertillon produced a regular flow of statistics about mortality. Jacques Bertillon himself was concerned with reducing the impact of communicable diseases in the city and with establishing the causes behind the dramatic differences in life expectancy. In fact, Paris was the birth place of studies of the relationship between mortality and wealth, with the work of Louis-René Villermé at the beginning of the nineteenth century (Villermé 1823, 1830). Indeed, Villermé was certainly one the first – if not the first – to explore the link between affluence and life expectancy, breaking a long established belief that mortality risk was the same for all (Villermé 1828; Lécuyer and Brian 2000).

Since Villermé, many studies have explored the income gradient in mortality and its evolution over time – not to mention a wide range of works that focus on this gradient nowadays (Williams 1990; Hummers et al. 1998; Cambois et al. 2001). Some look at this relationship from a macro perspective in order to explain "the mortality transition" (Kingsley 1956; Preston 1975; McKeown 1976), others – probably most – look at specific times and places. Both macro and micro level studies, however, try to learn what produce a socio-economic gradient in mortality, whether it is better nutrition (Harris 2004), better housing, better hygiene, or better access to medical resources, among others. They try also to establish what may be called the historical origins of health inequality. Some think that the social gradient has always existed and stays more or less the same over time while others propose a divergence-convergence pattern with the gradient rising – for instance during the industrial revolution – and then declining (Haines and Ferrie 2011). According to the first hypothesis, the mechanisms that link a fundamental cause (wealth) and mortality may change over time (for instance lack of sanitation and bad housing in the nineteenth century, smoking and bad habits in the twentieth century) but the association stays the same. The second hypotheses postulates that mortality inequalities were small before the industrial revolution as both income inequalities and medical knowledge were limited. Then it rises with income inequalities and access to better quality medicine for the wealthiest before diminishing again as public infrastructure were developed on a large scale, therefore beneficiating disproportionately to the poorest part of the society.

In fact it is now clear that the income gradient in mortality did not appear with the industrial revolution and nor did it disappear with the diffusion of health infrastructure. This leads to rich and insightful debates but also tends to somehow reduce the importance of the socio-economic gradient in mortality analyses. Environmental effects were put forward: first with a simple rural-urban opposition, hence the "urban disamenity" effect (Szreter and Mooney 1998; Woods 2003; Cain and Hong 2009), second in relation with a more detailed account of living conditions (Brown 1989; Cain and Rotella 2001; Ferrie and Troesken 2008). As a result, most studies conclude that there was a much weaker link between mortality and wealth than was assumed before, in favour of a strong environmental effect on mortality. In fact, some recent works are challenging the very existence of any causal relationship between income and mortality (Bengtsson and van Poppel 2011).

Our hypothesis lies somewhere between these two extremes. Indeed while money per se has no effect on either morbidity or mortality, it does influence consumption. More income affords people the option to live in better apartments, eat fresher food, wash themselves and their possessions more often, get better health care and so on and so forth. In the case of Paris the extraordinary variance in housing conditions lays bare these relationship which might not be so easy to pin down in small settlements where food and housing are cheap.

From the Data to Life Expectancy

Starting in 1817, the city began to publish death by age totals for each gender by 5 year age intervals. Then from 1880 to 1913, the *Annuaire statistique de la ville de Paris* reports death totals for each sex broken down into six age categories for each neighbourhood. The statistical office also published a series of detailed abstracts for the city drawn from the national censuses from 1881 forward that give us the age distribution of the living by neighbourhood.[2] Taking these two datasets together allows us to compute life expectancy at the *quartier* level.[3]

Indeed, the ideal way to measure differential mortality is to break down life expectancy by class or place of residence. One might want to compute life expectancy at birth. For Paris, at least, this would, however, present insurmountable problems because of severe under counts of both infant deaths and infant population. To begin, there was a massive recourse to wet nurses who lived a distance from the capital until very late in the century (Rollet-Echalier 1982). Such wet nursing was associated with very severe mortality, but the deaths were not recorded in the capital, thus any computation of life expectancy in early years would suffer from massive undercounting. Moreover, still birth registration remains a problem until late with some newborns being reported as still born even though they may have lived for a very short moment after birth, and vice versa.

Thus, we prefer life expectancy at age 5 and for comparability with the estate tax data (that are censored to age 20 or higher), we also compute life expectancy at 20. Even then, both because the age categories reports at the *quartier* level are not stable over time and do not necessarily accord between the *Annuaires* and the Censuses, we have to make some corrections. We proceed in three steps.

First, we adjust both mortality and population reports in order to obtain the number of deaths and the number of living for the same six age intervals: before age one; between one and 4 years; between 5 and 19 years; between 20 and 39 years; between 40 and 59 years; and over 60 years old. In all cases, we have very detailed reports at

[2] Since the French Revolution, population censuses were performed every 5 years; they have been kept in the archives from 1831 on in most cases. Here we use data on censuses from 1881, 1886, 1891 and so on.

[3] The *quartiers* have a population of at least 10,000 and with these six age categories the number of empty cells is essentially zero.

the Paris level (reports every 5-year) so we take advantage of them to correct the report at the *quartier* level. Take for instance the death reports before 1893: instead of reporting deaths for 5–19; 20–39 and 40–59, they use the age intervals 5–14; 15–34; 35–59. So we estimate, from data pertained to Paris as a whole, the share of the deceased aged 15–19 among those aged 15–34. We apply this share to the groups defined at the *quartier* level and we get, for each *quartier*, the number of deaths between 15 and 19 years old. We add this number to the total number of deaths in the age group 5–14 and extract from it from the number of deaths in the age group 15–34. We proceed in the same way for the age groups 15–34 and 35–59.

Second, we estimate inter-census populations for every year. It is standard to do so by combining the effect of aging and net migration. If the population were closed, then a cohort-based analysis will do (a new cohort is born each year, all other cohorts age by 1 year and loose some members due to mortality). If the population is open and migration rates just depend on age, then one has to add that factor back in. In other words two elements influence the growth rate of the population between censuses: deaths and migrations within each age group. When the first are the most important one can follow the evolution of each 5 year cohort from one census to the next. Then, the number of individuals of age (a) in year t depends on the number of individuals of age (a-5) in year (t-5) and one must then simply allocate the variation between the two values to the intervening years. However, when migration is significant, then the size of the age group (a) in year t depends less on the size of the age group (a-5) at (t-5) than on migration. For Paris where migration was very large, we estimate the size of an age group between census years from the variation between census years at age (a). In other words the size of the population of age (a) in year t is an interpolation of the size of that group in the two adjoining censuses.

Third, we compute a life table for each year and neighbourhood: to do so we calculate the age-specific mortality rate ($_nm_x$) for each age group by dividing the number of death in the age group by the number of individuals living in that age group for each year and neighbourhood. We can then produce death probabilities ($_nq_x$) where $q = n*m/(1 + (n - a)*m)$ where n is the length of the age group and a is the time lived by those who died within this age group. This last value is taken from Keyfitz and Flieger (1968:491) for individuals older than 5 and Coale and Demeny (1983) for ages 0–5 (but we focus here on life expectancy after 5 years old). Given death probabilities, we can immediately calculate mortality tables and life expectancy at each age (Preston et al. 2001: 42–50).

The assumptions we make in these computations do affect the results. In particular, the person-years lived by those who die in the oldest age group comes out at just under 8 years which is perhaps slightly optimistic. More importantly, it is quite realistic to think that this number is likely to have varied across neighbourhoods: it seems sensible to assume that mortality is more severe in the poorest parts of the city than in the richest parts. In this case the mortality differential would be even larger since mortality in the poorer neighbourhood is underestimated. Yet it seem logical, at least as a start, to make the same assumptions for all the neighbourhoods and avoid producing differential mortality by construction. It is also probably not true that migration affects all ages and neighbourhoods in the same way. It is more likely that migration is more intense in the poor neighbourhood –this would increase the population of rich neighbourhoods and thus reduce their mortality. Because our computations probably understate mortality differences across neighbourhoods this approach only strengthens our findings. After all the life expectancies we compute for the census years (when we have the exact population) are very similar to those for inter-census years. Varying the average life span per interval or the maximal age in the life table change very little on the between neighbourhoods differences in Paris.

Beyond these published data we have access to a series of cross sections drawn from estate tax records that provide wealth, gender, and age for the entire population of decedents roughly once every 5 years from 1807 to 1937. To match the life expectancy by neighbourhood one would want to have life expectancy by wealth percentiles. We cannot, however compute such measures. Indeed we do not have an age distribution for the living that are in a given wealth percentiles. In particular at the top end of the wealth distribution, one has to worry about endogeneity. Indeed, we need to purge from the empirical age-wealth at death relationship the part that runs from age to wealth. To be sure, it is likely that wealth helps prolong life (thus distribution of ages for the top percentiles is likely to be to the left of the age distribution of lower percentiles), that is the phenomenon we would like to capture. It is also true that at high levels of wealth, the older an individual lives, the larger the estate that person will leave behind, first because of unrealized capital gains and because the likelihood that he or she will inherit from collateral lines increases with age. Because of the latter channel we cannot compute life expectancy by wealth percentiles without some joint distribution of wealth and age among the living. Thus here we will simply present age at death by percentile.

Finally, there exist four real estate censuses (1878, 1890. 1900, and 1910) that provide number of housing units as well breakdowns of these units by their fiscal assessment. The data are reported by household (*ménage*) and break down rents into up to nearly two dozen categories including one that are below the threshold at which one would be liable for the *taxe mobilière* (a direct tax assessed on the basis of the occupation of the household head and of the rental value of the household's dwelling). The largest category in 1890 included those 521 dwellings assessed at more than 16,000 francs in rent. We define three categories of households, the poor are those who pay less than 300 francs a year in rent, then comes the middle class which pays between 300 and 1000 francs (per capital income in the 1880s for France), the rich pay more than a 1000 francs.

The halcyon days of the statistical office ended abruptly in 1913. Afterwards, and despite a massive increase in the city involvement in sanitation and other life preserving activities, its expenditures on publishing the life outcomes of its inhabitants declined massively. After WWI, the demographic data are only given by arrondissement and there were no real estate censuses published. Now we focus on the period for which the most detailed data are available: 1881–1913.

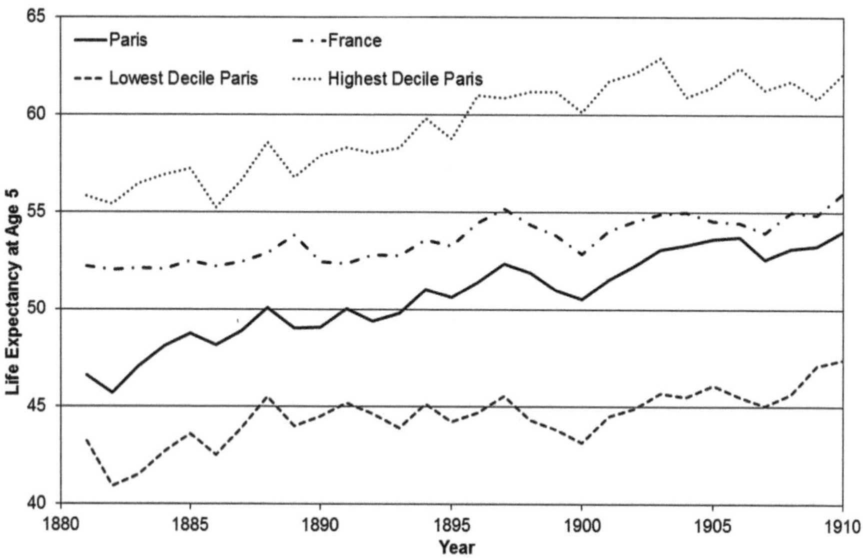

Fig. 8.3 Life expectancy at age 5 within Paris, compared to France

Inequalities in Time and Space

Figure 8.3 above presents mortality patterns across neighbourhoods within Paris compared with the average life expectancy for Paris (the plain line) and for France (dotted line). The figure also shows the life expectancy for the best eight (circle dotted line) and worst eight neighbourhoods (square dotted line) in Paris. In this scale the difference between the average life expectancy in Paris and France do not seem so large any more. In fact, the worst neighbourhoods in Paris have a life expectancy that is always about 8 years less than the average in the city and 10–12 years less than all France. At the other end of the spectrum, in the early 1880s the best neighbourhoods in Paris had a 7-year advantage over the rest of the city and a 4-year advantage over the rest of France. Over the next three decades, life expectancy rose quickly and neared 62 years; over that time these neighbourhoods saw their differences with all other benchmarks increase. Economic growth did not translate into a reduction of life expectancy inequality.

The inequality in life expectancy within Paris is particularly striking because it was in fact much larger than the difference observed across departments.[4] As Fig. 8.4 shows, the gap between the nine departments with the highest and lowest life expectancy was about 12 years in the 1880s; by 1910 it had shrunk to seven years. Most of the gain came from the worst departments where inhabitants experienced large (six years) gains in life expectancy while those in the best departments only eked out a gain of about one year. This pattern of rough stability at the top and big gains at the bottom is the reverse of Paris, where the bottom managed at best a

[4] Life expectancy by *départements* are taken from (Bonneuil 1997).

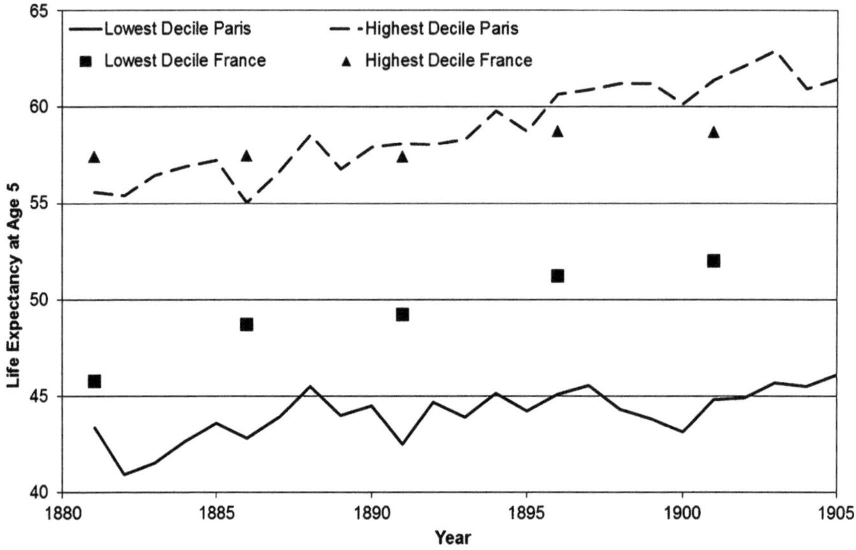

Fig. 8.4 Life expectancy at age 5 within Paris and within France

3-year gain in life expectancy when the top gained six years. As a result the worst departments, which started out with higher life expectancy than the worst neighbourhoods in Paris pulled away with a difference that jumped from about two years to almost seven. At the top the capital's neighbourhoods with the lowest mortality experienced enough gains to become the healthiest areas of France.

This is not simply an effect of picking tiny populations with unusual life circumstances. Even as early as the 1870s, the rich neighbourhoods had, each, populations of about 20,000 and the largest of the poor neighbourhoods had a population above 35,000. The primary reason for these differences comes from deep difference in the material circumstances of the residents of these neighbourhoods.

Mortality and Wealth

Looking at 1878, the city's income inequality becomes instantly obvious (Fig. 8.5). The share of rich (defined as paying at least 1000 francs in rents) was less than 10 %, and the poor (paying less than 300 francs in rent) made up 68 % of households. These different classes lived in different places. Twelve neighbourhoods (principally in the eastern edge of the city) had more than 90 % of their households paying less than 300 francs in rent, and in these neighbourhoods less than 0.7 % of households were rich. In contrast in five neighbourhoods more than 40 % of households could be classified as rich (all in the northwest), and in most of those the share of poor was less than half that of the city. Average rents reflect these contrasts and had been noted at the time. Rents in the Champs Elysées neighbourhood averaged 3400

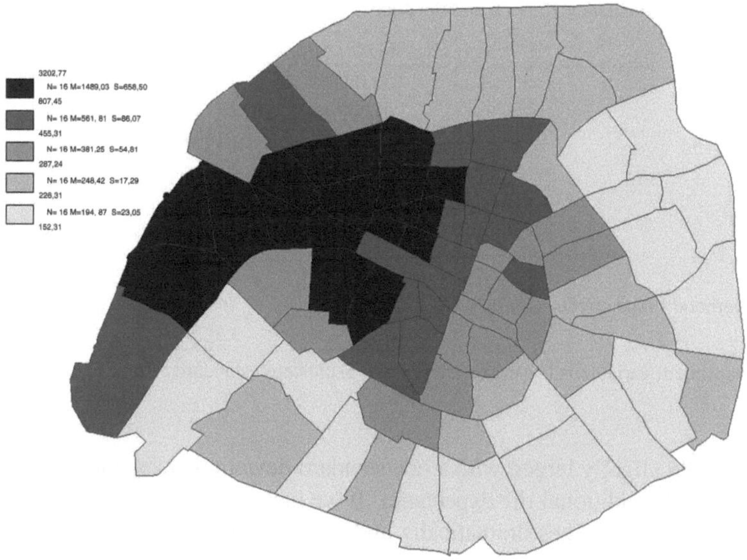

Fig. 8.5 Average rents by quartiers in Paris, 1878

francs while in the Charonne neighbourhoods they were 179 francs; in our twelve poor neighbourhoods rents average 186 francs while in the five rich ones they average 2204 francs. This higher than ten to one difference in rents in part reflects the massive differences in the size of apartments (the census provides the distribution of apartments by number of rooms), in amenities like running water, toilets within the apartment rather than in the hallway or on the ground floor, in air quality (prevailing winds being from the west, the east end of Paris was more polluted than the west) but it is also clear that there were location rents, indeed the high rent districts are clustered around the financial centre (the Bourse) and its political counterpart (the Élysée).

To evaluate the role of wealth or income we proceed in two steps. First we explore the links between mortality and wealth within neighbourhood. To do so we use a panel regression with four observations that link housing census with its nearest mortality year (1878 with 1880, 1890 with 1890 mortality and so on). Because we only have four housing surveys our panel has four cross sections for a total of 320 observations (Table 8.1). The advantage of this approach is that it allows us to include fixed effects that absorb any constant characteristics of the neighbourhood (hence the estimates are based on the within neighbourhood change over time). Those regressions show that increases in a neighbourhood share of poor were strongly associated with mortality: an increase of one standard deviation of the share of poor reduces life expectancy in the neighbourhood of three years.[5] Increases in the share of rich were conversely good for life expectancy and the implied elastic-

[5] Both the share of poor and the share of rich are standardized and thus the coefficients can be directly expressed as variations in life expectancy, the constant measuring the life expectancy at the average value of the share of poor/rich.

Table 8.1 Life expectancy, the rich and the poor

	(1)	(2)	(3)
Share of poor	−3.08***		−2.95***
	(0.29)		(0.34)
Share of rich		4.12***	0.67
		(1.16)	(1.12)
Constant	51.55***	51.91***	51.36***
	(0.19)	(0.49)	(0.40)
R^2	0.81	0.72	0.81
Neighborhood Fixed effects	Yes	Yes	Yes
N	320	320	320

Note: Dependent variable is life expectancy at age 5, clustered standard errors in brackets

ity is actually slightly larger, with a one standard deviation change leading to more than 4 years of additional life expectancy. If we include both variables the effect of the share of rich declines dramatically and becomes statistically insignificant, but the coefficient on share of poor is essentially unchanged.

An alternative approach is to focus on the cross sectional variation and estimate the impact of the share of poor across neighbourhoods at each census date. Figure 8.6 shows the fitted values for regressions we do not report. The first set for 1881 shows a negative association between life expectancy and the share of poor, then with each decade the relationship steepens, in part because of increased in life expectancy in richer (fewer poor) neighbourhood and because the fraction of poor tended to decline over time even though their mortality patterns did not change much. The line for 1911 is in fact the steepest, consistent with an increase in differential mortality as was suggested by Fig. 8.3.

To net out the effect of a decline in the share poor we re-ran the regressions from Fig. 8.6 but instead of using the contemporaneous survey, we used only the first census as an explanatory variable (Fig. 8.7). Again the 1881 predicted mortality ranges from 45 to 54, then 1891 show both an increase in life expectancy everywhere and a steeper slope suggesting that part of the increase in life expectancy in 1891 was associated with a decline in the share of poor. The 1901 data is even steeper suggesting that while things continued to improve in the richer neighbourhoods, they had improved little in the poorer ones. 1911 is then flatter and higher with the richest neighbourhoods (as defined in 1876) having gained almost seven years in life span since 1881 while the poorest ones had a gain of about three years or less than half. The timing of both increases is very different though: the wealthiest neighbourhoods gain a lot between 1881 and 1891 and again between 1891 and 1901 and then nothing up to 1911 whereas the poorest ones gain almost nothing before 1901 and then get better in the last period.

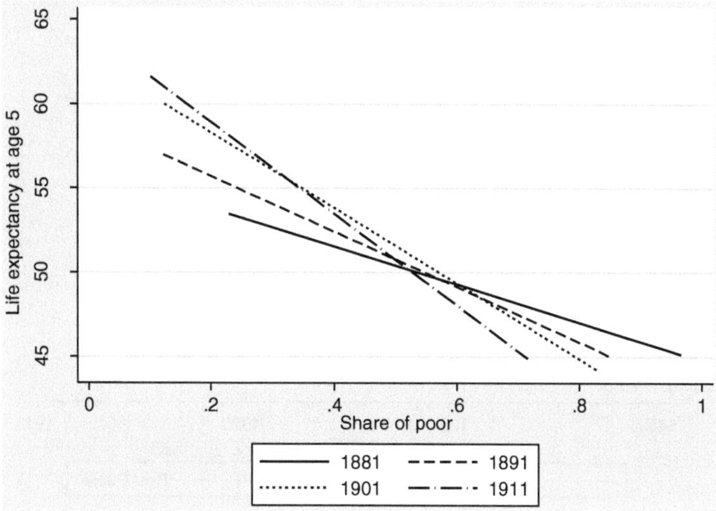

Fig. 8.6 Life expectancy and the share of poor households

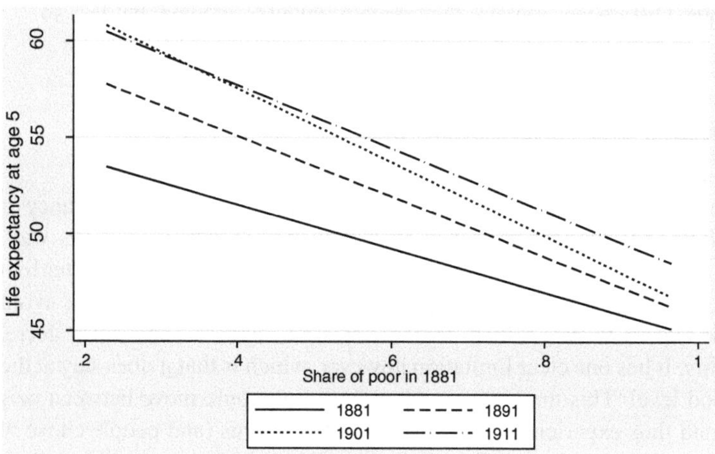

Fig. 8.7 Life expectancy and the share of poor in 1876

Finally, we can turn to the analysis at the district (arrondissement) level in order to get a broader picture. At that level, we can extend the analysis up until WWII (Fig. 8.8). The interwar period saw a relative convergence between the best and the worst neighbourhoods in Paris, although it is far from complete. Interestingly, the effect of income remains: the share of poors in 1878 still affects negatively life expectancy in 1939. Overall, though, the importance of rents fell by half: on average in the 1880s one additional standard deviation of poor means 2.5 less life expectancy at age 5; in the 1930s it's down to 1.3. Since life expectancy also increased in that period, the

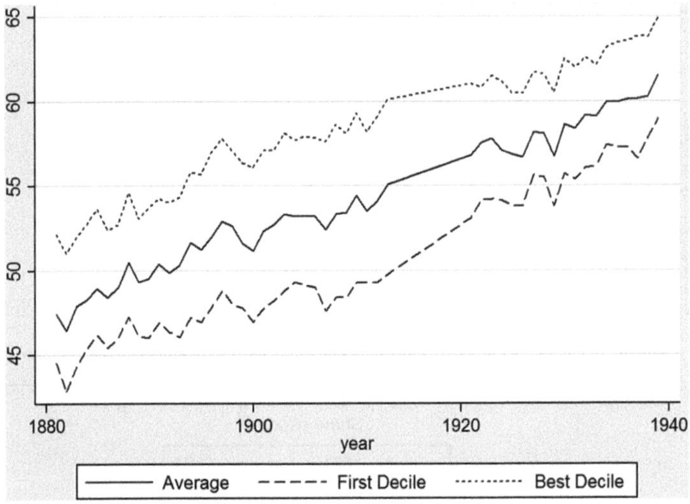

Fig. 8.8 Life expectancy by district, 1880–1940

relative gain is even stronger: from 5 % less life expectancy in the 1880s to 2 % in the 1930s. Differences remain, they remain linked to income, but less so.

Individuals and Neighbourhoods

The analysis so far highlights the huge differences in life expectancy between neighbourhoods within Paris. It is clear that life expectancy in Paris was closely related to income, because income is what allows people to afford better living conditions including better housing. It also gives some clues about the evolution of mortality up to W.W. I which demonstrates an increase –and not a decrease– of inequality. It has one clear limitation however, which is that it does stay at the neighbourhood level. This may be a problem because people move between neighbourhoods and thus experience different mortality patterns (and people chose where to stay at least in part because of the living conditions in a given neighbourhood). And at the same time it does not link directly the wealth of the individual with their mortality.

A way to overcome this limitation is to use individual data. We can rely on an alternative dataset assembled to study wealth inequality in the city from 1807 to 1937 (Piketty et al. 2006; 2014). These data culled from estate tax records provide age, marital status, and wealth for all wealthy Parisian decedents once every 5 years. Using the decedents' addresses we can measure the share of wealthy individuals that live in each *arrondissement*. Because of small numbers problem we aggregate all the relevant data across the period 1872–1912 (6 cross sections). Not surprisingly, the residential patterns of the wealthiest Parisians are very similar to the resi-

Table 8.2 Place of residence according to wealth (1872–1912)

	Wealth>4 million	4 M>Wealth>1 million	1 million wealth>500 K	500 K> wealth>250 K	250 K> wealth>125 K
N	97	850	1040	1455	2091
Richesse	8 702 609	2 562 100	698 441	350 078	178 848
	Fraction that reside in what arrondissement				
1	3.1	2.8	4.3	2.7	2.8
2	0.0	3.2	1.8	1.7	2.2
3	0.0	0.9	1.7	1.9	2.3
4	0.0	2.8	3.3	4.1	4.7
5	0.0	1.8	2.5	4.9	4.6
6	0.0	4.0	7.9	7.0	6.6
7	13.5	11.3	8.6	6.8	7.2
8	52.1	36.5	22.7	19.3	12.5
9	12.5	13.4	15.6	14.7	12.3
10	0.0	3.2	5.8	6.7	6.1
11	1.0	1.9	3.2	5.5	6.4
12	0.0	0.9	0.8	1.7	3.2
13	1.0	0.6	0.6	0.9	1.1
14	0.0	0.2	0.7	1.4	2.5
15	0.0	0.5	1.4	1.3	2.6
16	13.5	11.9	11.1	10.3	9.6
17	2.1	2.6	5.2	5.1	6.2
18	1.0	1.0	1.4	2.0	2.4
19	0.0	0.4	0.5	1.2	2.5
20	0.0	0.1	0.7	0.9	2.2

dential patterns given by the tax record (Table 8.2). And it reveals concentration indeed: of those who died with a half million francs or more with between a quarter and half of the wealthiest living in the 8th arrondissement alone. More surprisingly, even among the wealthiest, geographic concentration diminishes greatly as wealth declines, as people less wealthy are forced to live in adjacent neighbourhoods.

The same data allow us to study mortality at the individual level. Unfortunately no source would give the same data for the living and, as a result, we have to stay with the information on deceased only. As we noted previously, we cannot compute life expectancy by wealth percentile without additional data, which we do not have. Thus here we will simply present age at death by wealth percentile (Table 8.3). This indicator is without doubt biased because we observe wealth only at death; it nonetheless go in the same direction as the results we have seen in the previous section, age at death being inversely related to wealth. And again the effects are incredibly strong. The differences in age at death between the wealthiest (the top 2 % among the deceased of a given year) and the poorest (the 86 % poorest among Parisians) come in at just under 17 years in 1872. And just as in the previous analysis, one

Table 8.3 Age at death according to wealth at death

	1872	1877	1882	1887	1902	1912
Top 2 %	65.0	66.2	66.1	67.3	67.3	68.4
Next 4 %	61.2	62.5	62.5	63.1	63.6	65.6
Next 8 %	56.4	57.1	55.3	58.0	58.0	58.3
Rest	48.0	49.8	47.9	49.6	52.0	52.9
Av age	49.5	51.2	49.5	51.2	53.2	54.2
Total deaths	24,348	28,777	36,790	34,410	36,366	36,681
N with age and wealth	15,576	18,597	24,831	20,860	26,624	29,323

Note: The estate tax sample are comprised of all the individuals who died in a given year (e.g. 1872) and filed a return within 30 months of January 1 of that year, not all individuals with tax data have an age, we accordingly trim the population of no wealth individuals by the same proportion

striking feature is the stability of this pattern over time, the difference being roughly the same 40 years later.

8.2 Concluding Remarks

Why was it that Paris was so exceptional? It was, at the turn of the twentieth century, one of the major cities of the North Atlantic. As a metropolis Paris was a magnet for the rich. In fact, in this period, more than a quarter of the total French wealth was concentrated in Paris even if only 5 % of the French population lived in the City (Piketty et al. 2004). At the same time, the city attracted large numbers of people who came to the capital to provide their labor and lived in very low quality housing. The result was extremely brutal: strong and persistent mortality inequalities, the wealthiest living on average almost a quarter longer than the poor (even when excluding infant mortality). As we show in a companion paper, it was not until the end of the period that the diffusion of infrastructure began to reduce these inequalities (Kesztenbaum and Rosenthal 2014). In this chapter, we take advantage of these data in order to build the first step towards exploring in details this health-wealth nexus and the urban mortality transition. We provide a whole set of results –at the neighbourhood or individual level, based on demographic or taxation data, and so on– that demonstrate the extent of the mortality inequalities in Paris before WWI.

References

Bengtsson, T., & van Poppel, F. (2011). Socioeconomic inequalities in death from past to present: An introduction. *Explorations in Economic History, 48*(3), 343–356.

Bocquet, D., Chatzis, K., & Sander, A. (2008). From free good to commodity: Universalizing the provision of water in Paris (1830–1940). *Geoforum, 39*, 1821–1832.

Bonneuil, N. (1997). *Transformation of the French demographic landscape 1806–1906*. Oxford: Clarendon.
Brown, J. C. (1989). Reforming the urban environment: Sanitation, housing, and government intervention in Germany, 1870–1910. *Journal of Economic History, 49*, 450–472.
Cain, L., & Hong, S. C. (2009). Survival in 19th century cities: The larger the city, the smaller your chances. *Explorations in Economic History, 46*(4), 450–463.
Cain, L., & Rotella, E. (2001). Death and spending: Urban mortality and municipal expenditure on sanitation. *annales de démographie historique, 1*, 139–154.
Cambois, E., Robine, J.-M., & Hayward, M. D. (2001). Social inequalities in disability-free life expectancy in the French male population, 1980–1991. *Demography, 38*(4), 513–524.
Coale, A. J., & Demeny, P. (1983). *Regional model life tables and stable populations* (2nd ed.). New York: Academic.
Ferrie, J. P., & Troesken, W. (2008). Water and Chicago's mortality transition, 1850–1925. *Explorations in Economic History, 45*(1), 1–16.
Floud, R., Fogel, R. W., Harris, B., & Hong, C. S. (2011). *The changing body. Health, nutrition, and human development in the western world since 1700*. Cambridge: Cambridge University Press and NBER.
Guérin-Pace, F. (1993). *Deux siècles de croissance urbaine: la population des villes françaises de 1831 à 1990*. Paris: Anthropos.
Haines, M. R., & Ferrie, J. P. (2011). Socioeconomic inequalities in death from past to present: A postscript. *Explorations in Economic History, 48*(3), 441–443.
Harris, B. (2004). Public health, nutrition, and the decline of mortality: The McKeown thesis revisited. *Social History of Medicine, 17*(3), 379–407.
Hummers, R. A., Rogers, R. G., & Eberstein, I. W. (1998). Sociodemographic differentials in adult mortality: A review of analytic approaches. *Population and Development Review, 24*(3), 553–578.
Kesztenbaum, L., & Rosenthal, J.-L. (2014). *Income versus sanitation; mortality decline in Paris, 1880–1914* (PSE Working Paper n°26).
Keyfitz, N., & Flieger, W. (1968). *World population: An analysis of vital data*. Chicago: The University of Chicago Press.
Kingsley, D. (1956). The amazing decline of mortality in underdeveloped areas. *American Economic Review, 46*, 305–318.
Lécuyer, B.-P., & Brian, É. (2000). L'Argent, la vie, la mort: les recherches sociales de Louis-René Villermé sur la mortalité différentielle selon le revenu (1822–1830). *Mathématiques et sciences humaines, 149*, 31–60.
McKeown, T. (1976). *The modern rise of population*. London: Academic.
Piketty, T., Postel-Vinay, G., & Rosenthal, J.-L. (2004). *Wealth Concentration in a developing economy: Paris and France, 1807–1994* (CEPR Discussion Papers 4631, C.E.P.R. Discussion Papers).
Piketty, T., Postel-Vinay, G., & Rosenthal, J.-L. (2006). Wealth concentration in a developing economy: Paris and France, 1807–1994. *American Economic Review, 96*(1), 236–256.
Piketty, T., Postel-Vinay, G., & Rosenthal, J.-L. (2014). Inherited vs self-made wealth: Theory & evidence from a rentier society (Paris 1872–1927). *Explorations in Economic History, 51*(C), 21–40.
Preston, S. H. (1975). The changing relation between mortality and level of economic development. *Population Studies, 29*(2), 231–248.
Preston, S. H., & van de Walle, E. (1978). Urban French mortality in the nineteenth century. *Population Studies, 32*(2), 275–297.
Preston, S. H., Heuveline, P., & Guillot, M. (2001). *Demography: Measuring and modeling population processes*. Oxford: Blackwell Publishers.
Rollet-Echalier, C. (1982). Nourrices et Nourrissons Dans Le Département de La Seine et En France de 1880 À 1940. *Population, 3*, 573–606.

Szreter, S., & Mooney, G. (1998). Urbanization, mortality, and the standard of living debate: New estimates of the expectation of life at birth in nineteenth-century British cities. *Economic History Review, LI*(1), 84–112.

Villermé, L.-R. (1823). Note sur la population de Paris. *Archives générales de médecine, 3*, 468–471.

Villermé, L.-R. (1828). Mémoire sur la mortalité en France dans la classe aisée et dans la classe indigente. *Mémoires de l'Académie Royale de médecine, 1*, 51–98.

Villermé, L. R. (1830). De la mortalité dans les divers quartiers de la ville de Paris, et des causes qui la rendent très différente dans plusieurs d'entre eux, ainsi que dans les divers quartiers de beaucoup de grandes villes. *Annales d'hygiène publique de médecine légale, 3*(2), 294–341.

Williams, D. R. (1990). Socioeconomic differentials in health: A review and redirection. *Social Psychology Quarterly, 53*(2), 81–99.

Woods, R. (2003). Urban-rural mortality differentials: An unresolved debate. *Population and Development Review, 29*(1), 29–46.

Part III
Urban Mortality in the Developing World

Chapter 9
Estimating Area-Based Influences on Urban-Rural Inequalities in Health Outcomes: A Longitudinal Multilevel Epidemiological Investigation

Barthelemy Kuate Defo

9.1 Introduction

The majority of the world's population (51 %) now lives in urban areas. While cities offer prospects of often better social and economic opportunities and contribute to national development, rapid and often unplanned urban growth is often associated with poverty, environmental degradation and population demands that outstrip resources availability and service capacity, and place human health at risk (Woods 2003; Sverdlik 2011). By and large, urbanization is one of the most important demographic shifts worldwide during the past century and the global demographic shift now is the world's urban population exceeding the world's rural population (UN-Habitat 2011). Over the last 25 years or so, many middle and low income countries have experienced major shifts in the demographic and epidemiologic profiles of their populations, with salient ramifications on our understanding of health, disease and mortality patterns within and across those countries. The Demographic and Health Survey (DHS) programme has provided the international community and policy decision makers with some population and health information they need to plan, monitor, and evaluate population, health, and nutrition programmes, with a sense of continuity and history. There have been over 260 surveys in more than 90 developing countries since its inception in 1984. A number of potential problems and limitations in existing analyses of the urban environment in relation to urban

---

This work was supported in part by a grant from the International Relations Office of the University of Montreal, Canada. Supplemental support was provided by the International Union for the Scientific Study of Population (IUSSP).

B. Kuate Defo (✉)
Public Health Research Institute, Department of Demography & Department of Social and Preventive Medicine, School of Public Health, University of Montreal,
C.P. 6128 Succursale Centre-Ville, Montréal H3C 3J7, Quebec, Canada
e-mail: Barthelemy.Kuate.Defo@umontreal.ca

D. Ramiro Fariñas, M. Oris (eds.), *New Approaches to Death in Cities during the Health Transition*, International Studies in Population 12,
DOI 10.1007/978-3-319-43002-7_9

health hinge on changing contexts of individuals and families, confounding effects, the confusion between spaces and places that are notorious in cross-sectional analyses and snapshot studies using DHS-type data; these shortcomings can be addressed when new methodologies are developed to extend the use of these data beyond the confines of their cross-sectional nature for a country at one point in time. In fact, this largest sample survey programme in history involving several waves for the same countries provides unparalleled opportunities to address the dynamic relationships between urban environment and urban health during transitional periods characterizing the processes of urban transformation in those countries over time. This study considers the extent to which risk factors characteristic of the urban environment (in contrast to those characteristic of the rural environment) affect population health outcomes (World Health Organization 2002).

Three important trends characterize the urbanization process in this new urban era (UN-Habitat 2011). First, the biggest cities in the world are expected mainly in the developing world, with megacities of more than 20 million people now gaining ground in Asia, Latin America and Africa. Second, the majority of urban migrants are moving to small towns and cities of less than one million inhabitants. Natural population increase, rather than rural-to-urban migration, is becoming a more significant contributor to urban growth in many regions, as is reclassification of rural areas into urban areas. The scale of the environmental impact of megacities is likely to exacerbate urban health disparities due in part to the limited infrastructure such as roads, water supply and communication facilities in many small and intermediate-sized cities (Henderson 2010; United Nations 2011; Green 2012). This makes them less competitive locally, nationally and regionally, and leads to a lower quality of life for their citizens. Third, cities of the developing world are expected to absorb 95 % of urban growth in the next two decades, and will be home to 80 % of the world's urban population by 2030. After 2015, the world's rural population will begin to shrink as urban growth becomes more intense in cities of Asia and Africa, two continents where the world's largest urban populations in 2030 will reside. Urban poverty and inequality will characterize many cities in the developing world, and urban growth will become virtually synonymous with slum formation in some regions (Stephens 2011). Asia is already home to over 50 % of the world's slum population (581 million) followed by sub-Saharan Africa (199 million) and Latin America and the Caribbean (134 million). In the world, Sub-Saharan Africa has both the highest annual urban growth rate (4.58 %) and the highest slum growth rate (4.53 %), more than twice the world average. The continued threat of conflict in several African countries is a significant contributing factor in the proliferation of slums in the region's urban areas. These trends will most likely concern policymakers in the developing world as they confront the reality of growing inequality and poverty in their cities. There is overwhelming evidence suggesting that the wealth generated by cities does not automatically lead to poverty reduction but instead in many cities, fosters inequalities between the rich and the poor and mushrooming of the sizes and proportions of slum populations (UN-HABITAT 2007; Stephens 2011; Weeks et al. 2013). Although poverty remains a primarily rural phenomenon, urban poverty is becoming a severe and pervasive feature of urban life. UN-HABITAT

(2011) shows that the incidence of disease and mortality in some cases, such as HIV prevalence and other health indicators, is much higher in slums than in non-slum urban areas, and, is equal to or even higher than in rural areas.

Our research questions inherently ask about the changes over time and space in covariates of infant mortality in urban environments versus rural environments, while addressing issues of variability in exposure and outcome variables. Much of the published research on urban health has usually relied on cross-sectional information or on data measured at only one point of time in particular location. By ignoring the temporal dimension in research questions, such studies often confound the cause with the effect. Furthermore, they are especially vulnerable to distorted findings when the model excludes important measures that are also related to predictors. While studies have consistently identified clustering of poor health and mortality in urban areas, relatively little research has examined how stable space–time clustering are over an extended period of time. Our study proposes the integration of spatial and temporal analysis to explicitly model the possible patterns and changes in space–time clustering in health and survival in urban areas, in order to more fully inform policymakers and researchers about their dynamics.

9.2 Multilevel Framework of Urban-Rural Disparities in Health

Researchers have generally used one of three different approaches when considering the association between cities and health (Stephens 1995; Vlahov et al. 2007; Galea et al. 2005; Bilger and Carrieri 2013; Bocquier et al. 2011; Günther and Harttgen 2012; Konteh 2009; Xu et al. 2014). The first and most common approach, contrasts urban to non-urban (frequently rural) areas, in an effort to isolate living in urban areas as a primary determinant of interest and has often produced conflicting results (e.g., Paykel et al. 2002; Blazer et al. 1994; Yamamoto and Watanabe 2001). The second approach has focused on differences across cities in one or more countries. Using the city itself as the key determinant of interest, these studies compare different cities in order to reach conclusions about urban characteristics associated with health (e.g., Rodwin and Gusmano 2002). A third line of inquiry involves the study of intra-urban differences and how they are associated with variability in health within cities. This research is rooted in the observation that specific characteristics of small areas may be associated with health; most empirical work in this regard has focused on how characteristics of neighbourhoods of residence affect health (Ross 2000; Diez-Roux 2002). This research has shown associations, for example, between characteristics of the built environment and neighbourhood socio-economic status with sexually transmitted disease prevalence and cardiovascular disease mortality. Studies using these approaches to urban health have contributed to the understanding of the relation between city living and health. Much of this work has suggested that urban residents have worse health than rural residents, a disparity sometimes called the urban health penalty (Gould 1998). However, it is now evident that cities have positive as well as negative effects on health and well-being. This body of work suggests that a more nuanced appreciation of the complicated association between the urban/rural context and health is needed (Jedrychowski et al. 1997; Shima et al. 2002; Takano et al. 2002; Weeks et al. 2013; Bilger and Carrieri 2013; Bocquier et al. 2011; Günther and Harttgen 2012; Konteh 2009; Xu et al. 2014). Therefore, a fuller understanding of urban health will necessitate studies that include an appreciation of the dynamic nature of cities, the specificity of context, and a detailed consideration of the pathways by which changes in the urban context affect health. The dominant approaches used to study urban health to date have often focused on a single line of inquiry. Thus, the inter-city studies of urban health suggest that municipal-level factors (e.g., policies) may be important determinants of the health of city residents (Rondinelli 1986; Jerrett et al. 2003; Konteh 2009). Studies that have focused on differences within cities suggest that intra-urban factors (e.g. residential segregation) play a role in shaping health (Galea et al. 2005; Günther and Harttgen 2012). Ultimately however, it is the multiplicity of factors at different levels that shape the health of urban/rural residents. While this complex causal chain is not unique to urban health, it is particularly germane given the complexity of the urban context. Thus, a comprehensive model is needed that can incorporate and integrate the multiple levels of factors that affect health in cities and that considers features of cities that may either promote or harm health.

In this study, we propose a multilevel framework that captures these factors through national urban and rural populations of different size, density, diversity and complexity, and that recognizes that health in urban populations is a function of living conditions shaped by individual behaviours and attributes, municipal determinants, and national and global trends in contextual risk and protective factors of health. This framework will be used in all three dominant research strands highlighted above, that is, to study intra-urban differences in the health of populations, to compare the health of groups across cities, and to frame contrasts between urban and rural populations among countries across major regions of four continents of the world. We assess how the different levels of influences may contribute to health of 217 national populations in urban versus rural areas of 86 countries from four continents of the world.

Growing social and economic disparities in a country, region or continent, across urban and rural areas can intensify health inequalities already thought to exist. But studies that have attempted to quantify these inequalities over time are inexistent across middle and low income countries. Although an urban advantage has been reported, less frequently studied have been the mechanisms accounting for this advantage. It is conjectured that these mechanisms include the higher socio-economic status and consequent superior access to health service for people living in urban areas, and the fact that urban neighbourhoods are wealthier and consequently offer superior availability of health services. This implies that mechanisms operate at several levels —individual, household, community, country, regional and continental levels. This study considers the following research question: How great is the urban advantage, how has it changed over time, and to what extent is it accounted for by a series of multilevel characteristics? Differences in health by urban versus rural residence have been observed since the industrial revolution when urban living brought hazards owing to communicable diseases that were transferred easily across populations living in close proximity (Kearns 1988). An epidemiological shift, from communicable to degenerative disease, benefited urban dwellers, mostly due to public health, political factors and social dynamics. In the developing world, urban/rural health differences have received less attention (Kinsella 2001). Much of what is known was summarized by the National Research Council's Panel on Urban Population Dynamics (Montgomery et al. 2003) which indicated that on average, urban populations in modern-day periods live longer than do rural populations, and with the exception of HIV/AIDS, exhibit healthier levels across a range of indicators. Part of the advantage is thought to be a function of environmental factors, such as better equipped and a greater concentration of health facilities, and part a function of individual factors, such as characteristics among urban dwellers that relate to better health, like higher levels of income and education. Yet, the issue of health advantage in the developing world is far from settled. Importantly, there is wide intra-region variation. Urban areas tend to include sub-populations of slum living poor, who constitute a subset of extremely disadvantaged city dwellers (Montgomery and Hewett 2005). There is also some evidence suggesting that within-region inequalities may be widening, perhaps a result of economic globalization, concomitant market transformations, growing returns to education and weakening inequality-reducing infrastructure (Goesling 2001). While virtually no studies have compared urban versus rural poor, data indicate that the former are substantially worse off than the average in urban areas. Within-region inequalities in health are compounded by a number of related factors. The provision of public services and infrastructure, such as health care facilities, safe drinking water and sanitary waste disposal are often unequally distributed within regions, despite their increased availability on average in cities. This type of infrastructure is, in turn, exceptionally important in determining individual health risks (UN-Habitat 2011). In addition, across the developing world, urban health care systems tend to be characterized by increasing privatization and monetization, in part due to rising average incomes and costs of healthcare associated with increasing prevalence of non-communicable diseases such as diabetes and chronic infectious diseases such as HIV/AIDS.

Our conceptual framework for health disparities between rural and urban areas rests on the premise that multiple levels of influences shape population health. This framework is grounded in our understanding of the extant public health literature and builds on several other published conceptual frameworks that have considered the social and economic determinants of population health. Indeed, over the past 30 years or so, several conceptual frameworks have considered how multiple determinants of health may affect the health of particular populations (for reviews, see Evans and Stoddart 1990, 2003; Galea et al. 2005; Kuate Defo 2014). These frameworks have synthesized research about the contribution of nonmedical determinants to population health and offered refinements on how multiple determinants affected one another and ultimately affected the health of populations. These frameworks suggest that human activities and environmental conditions may be associated with factors such as economic development and social attitudes to shape population health in general and in the urban/rural context in particular where multiple factors interact to shape the health of populations. More specific to health in cities, there has been growing interest in the relations between the built environment and health and several frameworks have considered how features of the built physical environment may affect population health and how social and economic determinants shape the health of urban populations (Northridge et al. 2003; Frumkin 2002; Galea et al. 2005; Williams 2013). Thus, urban/rural environment in its broadest sense (physical, social, economic, and political) affect all strata of residents, either directly or indirectly. Our effort is to consider these influential factors directly (via the estimation of effects of measured factors) and indirectly (by accounting for unobserved variabilities at the multiple levels of influential factors), how they affect the health of rural/urban populations, and what are the mechanisms through which these variables may influence the conditions that are the primary determinants of the health of rural/urban populations.

9.3 Data Sources: The Demographic and Health Surveys (DHS)

This study carries out an examination of urban versus rural health outcomes in four continents using country-level and region-level time series data. These data come from successive waves of the Demographic and Health Surveys (DHS) in 86 countries from four continents, and involve 217 national populations which are the lowest units of analysis. The DHS are nationally representative household sample surveys that measure population, health, socio-economic and anthropometric indicators, emphasising maternal and child health. The DHS are an important data source for studying population health across low and middle income countries due to their extensive coverage, comparability and data quality. Urban/rural residence is a critical health determinant which has historically been found to distinguish health experiences across human populations. In this study, we assess driving forces behind urban advantage or disadvantage through a series of country-level summary indicators constructed from the DHS data.

Specific categorizations for rural and urban areas in most studies are complicated by a system of definitions that differ across agency and have changed over time. We use DHS data which have consistent definition of urban areas across DHS surveys for assessing changes over time through repeated cross-sectional DHS survey data spanning the period from 1985 through 2010 and involving multiple waves of follow-up surveys per country. We examined urban/rural variation in health by constructing the indicator variables for urban and rural areas. The aim in constructing these multilevel repeated cross-sectional survey data is to derive a set of variables for each cohort of countries under observation (same year of survey) – hence our country-year variable – that is comparable over time. The comparable methodology

Table 9.1 Hierarchical clustered distribution of 217 national populations studied by continent, region within continent, and countries within regions in the world: 1985–2010

Continent	Regions within continents	Countries within regions	Number of surveys
Africa	Western Africa	Benin, Burkina Faso, Cape Verde, Cote d'Ivoire, Ghana, Guinea, Liberia, Mali, Mauritania, Niger, Nigeria, Senegal, Serra Leone, Togo	39
	Middle Africa	Angola, Central African Republic (CAR), Cameroon, Chad, Congo, Congo DR, Gabon, Sao Tome and Principe	11
	Eastern Africa	Burundi, Comoros, Eritrea, Ethiopia, Kenya, Madagascar, Malawi, Mozambique, Rwanda, Tanzania, Uganda, Zambia, Zambia	42
	Southern Africa	Botswana, Lesotho, Namibia, South Africa, Swaziland	7
	Northern Africa	Egypt, Morocco, Sudan, Tunisia	10
Asia	Western Asia	Armenia, Azerbaijan, Georgia, Jordan, Turkey, Yemen	15
	South-Central Asia	Bangladesh, India, Kazakhstan, Kyrgyztan, Maldives, Nepal, Pakistan, Sri Lanka, Turkmenistan, Uzbekistan	21
	South-Eastern Asia	Cambodia, Indonesia, Philippines, Thailand, Timor-Leste, Vietnam	17
Latin America and the Caribbean	South America	Bolivia, Brazil, Colombia, Ecuador, Guyana, Paraguay, Peru	23
	Central America	El Salvador, Guatemala, Honduras, Mexico, Nicaragua	14
	Caribbean	Dominican Republic, Haiti, Jamaica, Trinidad and Tobago	11
Europe	Southern Europe	Albania	2
	Eastern Europe	Moldova, Romania, Ukraine	5
Total			217

of DHS surveys for calculating the indicators used under the same survey design and question wording ensure that there are no gaps in the time series because standardized questions were asked the same way in all survey years and coding of responses was consistent over time across countries. These multilevel distributions of these surveys by country, regions within continent and continents are presented in Table 9.1. About half (109) of these national surveys are conducted in Africa.

9.4 Summary Indicators and Outcome Variable

The dependent variable is the infant mortality rate, which is measured by 5-year periods preceding the survey (excluding month of interview from analysis). The exposure variables, which are time-dependent, include, in addition to time period: total fertility rate, median age at first marriage for age group 25–49 years, place of delivery (percent distribution of live births in the last 3 years preceding the survey, whose place of delivery was a health facility), vaccinations (percentage of children 12–23 months who had received all specific vaccines at any time before the survey and the percentage vaccinated by 12 months of age), median breastfeeding durations (exclusive breastfeeding), respondent level of education (proportion of respondents with the highest educational level, that is, secondary or higher), and housing characteristics (percent of households with electricity). These summary statistics from repeated cross-sectional survey data generate for each country, longitudinal data that can be used to infer behavioural relationships for the cohort of countries as a whole just as if panel data were available. Procedures for constructing such cohorts and for estimation using the resulting data are described below. Although the methods discussed here are primarily formulated as a response to the absence of panel data, it is not necessarily the case that they will give inferior results. The attrition problem that effectively curtails the useful length of much panel data is absent here. Because new samples are drawn at each DHS survey for a given country with multiple waves of DHS surveys, representativeness of the national population for a country is constantly maintained.

Following Baltagi (2008), the panel data in this study therefore consists of the pooling of these summary statistics (observations) related to urban environmental covariates of infant mortality on a cross-section of 86 countries over several waves of DHS surveys (time periods) from 1985 through 2009. Such Panel data allow controlling for variables that cannot be observed or measured like cultural factors or variables that change over time but not across entities including national policies and regulations, and international agreements. There are several benefits from using such constructed panel data for this study (for review, see Baltagi 2008). First, they allow controlling for individual heterogeneity. Panel data suggest that individuals, households, communities, countries, regions and continents are heterogeneous. Time series and cross-section studies not controlling for this heterogeneity run the risk of obtaining biased estimates. This may happen if some covariates vary with countries (or any other unit-level of observation within a country) and time while others may be country-invariant or time-invariant. In addition, some of these variables are difficult to measure or are not measurable; omission of these variables leads to bias in the resulting estimates. Panel data are able to control for these country- and time-invariant variables whereas a time series study or a cross-section study cannot. Second, panel data give more informative data, more variability, less collinearity among the variables, more degrees of freedom and more efficiency. Time series studies are plagued with multicollinearity; for example, there is high collinearity between exposure variables in the aggregate time series data. This is less likely with a panel across countries since the cross-section dimension adds a lot of variability, adding more informative data on exposure variables. In fact, the variation in the data can be decomposed into variation between countries of different sizes and characteristics, and variation within countries. The former variation is usually bigger, as our findings below substantiate. Third, panel data are better able to study the dynamics of adjustment. For example, in measuring exclusive breastfeeding in cities (or median duration of exclusive breastfeeding), cross-sectional data can estimate what proportion of children is exclusively breastfed at a point in time in a country.

Repeated cross-sections can show how this proportion changes over time, which has important policy implications for urban health. Fourth, such panel data are better able to identify and measure effects that are simply not detectable in pure cross-sections or pure time-series data. Fifth, panel data models allow us to construct and test more complicated behavioural models than purely cross-section or time-series data (Hsiao 1986).

9.5 Statistical Methods: Multilevel Log-Log Models of Repeated Cross-Sectional Data

Multilevel models are increasingly been used in analyzing survey data on participants from different geographical places such as countries or sub-regions. There are growing numbers of these datasets spanning multiple waves in low and middle income countries, and researchers are beginning to face the challenges of how to incorporate this longitudinal dimension into their studies. Implementing simultaneously comparative and longitudinal models to such repeated cross-sectional survey data should provide insightful understanding on the spatial effects that operate at different levels to influence health outcomes and social change. This study is an environmental and epidemiological investigation of such complex spatial processes. It uses multilevel modelling of area-based health data constructed from DHS surveys to disentangle these spatial effects that occur at different scales in a geographical hierarchy.

Our population at risk in each geographical area is made of national population of children less than 1 year of age, and their areal mortality is assessed within the exposure variables in their urban versus rural environments. The likely effects of influential areal variables on national infant mortality rate are separated into three distinct categories. The first category consists of the within-area effects, such as social characteristics of the national population at risk, using summary statistics (mean and proportion) for each area. We model unmeasured variables by allowing for variation in geographical hierarchy. The second category entails the hierarchical effects; these are due to the fact that small areas are grouped into larger areas. The third category involves the neighbourhood effects, since areas that are close to each other in geographical space (in the continent and sub-continent, across countries) may share common environmental or demographic factors which influence the outcome of interest. Such multilevel models are a powerful tool for analyzing and deriving inferences from these comparative survey data about the macro-level determinants of individual-level outcomes.

In this study, we incorporate multiple waves of comparative survey data from DHS in the formulation of the multilevel models considered in this study, and fit a three-level model, where individual units (*i*) are nested within country-years (*j*), nested in turn within countries (k). Our model also includes a vector of coefficient capturing the effect on the outcome variable of time period variable that varies both across countries and within countries over time. This time period variable is considered to be a characteristic of country-years, and is indexed t_k, because it is constant for respondents within a given country-year, and non-constant across both countries and the country-years nested within a given country. The multilevel model for the repeated cross-sectional data is formulated as follows:

$$y_{ijk} = \beta_{0ijk} + \beta_1 t_k + \beta_2 x_{ijk} + \delta z_{ijk}$$
$$\beta_{0jk} = \beta_0 + v_{0k} + u_{0jk} + e_{0ijk}$$

β_0 is the intercept, i is the level-1 units corresponding to national population, j is the level-2 units corresponding to the country-years (or number of national populations observed per country in its successive waves of cross-sectional survey), *k* is the level-3 units (country). In the models, x and z represent the exposure variables and possible interactions, respectively; v_{0k} is the random effect capturing between-country variability which is supposed to vary vis-à-vis the grand mean; u_{0jk} is the random effect at the country-years level, capturing within-country variability; and e_{ijk} is the random effect associated with variability across individual survey units. This approach investigates social change with all the available survey data which happen to have a longitudinal dimension through repeated cross-sectional data collection in multiple waves. Though the time period variable considered varies both over time and across countries, these two dimensions of its variability are treated singly in this study, which means that we are not trying to know whether just one dimension is driving any covariations found with the outcome variable, or even potentially whether the two effects have opposing signs. This approach effectively assumes that the cross-sectional and longitudinal associations between time period and the outcome variable are the same: a single coefficient β_1 linked to variable *tk* captures both effects. Further extensions of this model, which are beyond the scope of this paper, will allow clarifying the distinction (if any) between cross-sectional and longitudinal effects.

Before we discuss the structure of these spatial effects, we must first account for the fact that we have a non-linear (logarithmic) relationship between the outcome variable (infant mortality) and the predictors considered in this study. Since the cases in each area are sufficiently large (greater than 10), it is reasonable to model the logarithm of the relative risk directly (Clayton and Hills 1993), assuming these follow a Normal distribution. In this case, heterogeneity effects can be accommodated by weighting the random part of the model by some function of the population at risk in each area; we use the number of waves for each country in this respect. After careful review of the extant literature, two broad multilevel models were considered: the linear and log-linear multilevel models to be fitted to repeated cross-sectional data presented above.

Various methods for testing the linear model versus log-log model have been proposed (MacKinnon et al. 1983; Morris 1991; Rao and Wu 1989). Linear regression modelling, by definition, seeks to identify linear relationships between specified exposure and outcome variables. That is, relationships are assessed on the extent to which unit increases in X are constantly related to unit increases in Y; in social sciences and public health, no systematic (linear) relationship exists. It would perhaps be wise to consider the possibility, if not the probability, that within matrices of data on which we focus in this study, there are actually some non-linear relationships that are beyond and above some linear relationships. These relationships, where their curvilinear nature substantially violates assumptions of linearity, may go unrecognized or their magnitude underestimated when using linear methods. A common a priori assumption of non-linearity embedded in the economic theory is that of diminishing returns: the health production function, like all well-behaved production functions, is subject to diminishing returns. This behaviour is generally well captured by applying a log–log specification of predictors of mortality and longevity (Basu and Rathouz 2005). Our primary objective as researchers is to determine the extent to which reality or data generated by the underlying processes of our reality "behaves" according to the mathematical specification of our conceptual model of that process. We carried a series of graphical analyses of mortality patterns to determine that the log-log specification of model formulation was indeed capturing the behaviour of the data at hand which all have positive values since the log transformation is only applicable when all the observations in the data set are positive (although this condition can be guaranteed for any variable by using a transformation like $\log(X+k)$ where k is a positive scalar chosen to ensure positive values, although careful thoughts should be given to the interpretation of the parameter estimates in this special case). For a given data set there may be no particular reason to assume that one functional form is better than the other. Thus, we also compared the log-log specification with alternative specifications, but the latter poorly fitted the data. Henceforth, we used multilevel log-log models for assessing the relationships between changes in summary indicator variables considered and trends in infant mortality rates in urban populations versus rural population between 1985 and 2010 in 217 populations from 86 countries in Africa, Asia, Latin America and the Caribbean and Europe. The log-logistic distribution is a continuous probability distribution for a non-negative random variable used in survival analysis as a parametric model for events whose rate increases initially and decreases later, for example mortality from specific causes following health-related interventions (Collett 2003). The most common practice in empirical applications has been to transform the multiplicative model by taking natural logarithms and to estimate the log-linear model using ordinary least squares.

The multilevel model to repeated cross-sectional DHS survey data we have formulated here is therefore a multilevel log-log model since the dependent variables and all explanatory variables are logarithmically transformed into log-variables. Parameter estimation in models such as the ones we have formulated here can be performed using estimation methods based on a first-order or a second-order Taylor expansion of the link function. We estimated parameters using the MLwiN statistical software, given the stability of the algorithm, its statistical efficiency, the dataset at hand, and the complexity of the fitted models in this study. Parameter estimates were computed by the PQL estimation procedure with second-order Taylor expansion. This procedure is computationally more demanding, but results in more reliable parameter estimates than the MQL estimation procedure with first-order Taylor expansion that is used for model building. Flexible non-linear models of the type specified here are free of a priori assumptions of functional form, deriving equations from available data and selecting predictors that best serve the modelling objective which is prediction accuracy. Cross-sectional predictive and time series forecasting accuracy of flexible non-linear models similar to the ones we have specified has been validated in different fields, including the fields of medicine (Collett 2003). Time trend (the time periods 1985–1989, 1990–1994, 1995–1999, 2000–2004, 2005+) was included in the fitted models in order to account for changes over time and long-term trends resulting from changes in, for example, population structure, socio-economic conditions, enduring social structures and conditions, urban living conditions, and the provision of health care over time for instance. The period 1985–2010 under consideration witnessed major changes in all four continents and countries, caused partly by social and economic changes as well as changes in development, social and economic policies and programs, interventions and actions with influences on health and well-being of populations across these countries in the context of global and national demographic and epidemiologic shifts described above.

9.6 Findings

Table 9.2 presents the national populations with infant mortality rates in urban areas higher than infant mortality rates in rural areas from the DHS surveys, for the period 1987–2009: a total of 18 national populations from 16 countries, out of 214 countries for which data are available on infant mortality rates by geographical location of residence. Five African countries (six national populations) fall into this group: four from Eastern Africa – Tanzania (1991–1992 and 2010), Kenya (2008–2009), Eritrea (1995), and Namibia (1992) – and Mauritania (2000–2001) from Western Africa, suggesting an Eastern African regional pattern of urban disadvantage in these African populations, despite improvements in recent years for all these countries but Kenya where immunization coverage is lower in urban than rural settings (the proportion of children fully vaccinated is 62 % in urban areas compared with 69.9 % in rural areas) and the median duration of exclusive breastfeeding is lower

Table 9.2 National populations with infant mortality rates in urban areas higher than infant mortality rates in rural areas from the DHS surveys: 1987–2009

Continent	Region	Country (year)	Infant mortality rates (p. 1000)			Total fertility rate		Median age at first marriage: age group 25–49		Vaccinations: all		Median duration of exclusive breastfeeding		Electricity in the house		Delivery in a health facility	
			Urban	Rural	Diff.	Urban	Rural	Urban	Rural	Urban	Rural	Urban	Rural	Urban	Rural	Urban	Rural
LAC	South America	Colombia (1990)	28.9	23.4	−5.5	2.5	3.6	21.4	20.2	69.2	66.7	0.5	0.7	97.9	71	86.6	59.2
LAC	Caribbean	Dominican Republic (2007)	33.1	31.4	−1.7	2.3	2.8	19.2	18	56.5	60.8	0.5	0.5	98.6	89.3	98.3	96.5
LAC	Caribbean	Dominican Republic (1986)	71.9	67.9	−4			19	17.7	0.8		0.5	0.5				
LAC	Central America	El Salvador (2002)	29.6	28.6	−1	2.3	3.5	20.4	18.2	69.9	69.7	0.4	1			89.2	59.1
Africa	Eastern Africa	Eritrea (1995)	79.8	74.4	−5.4	4.2	7	18	16.3	79	30.6	3.6	3.3	80.6	2.1	58.4	6.3
LAC	South America	Guyana (2009)	45.1	31.7	−13.4	2.1	3	23.6	19.9	60.2	64.3	1.9	1.1	90.9	72.3	97.9	86.1
Asia	Western Asia	Jordan (2009)	26.8	20.6	−6.2	3.8	4	22.4	22.4					99.6	98.5		
Africa	Eastern Africa	Kenya (2008–09)	62.8	58.5	−4.3	2.9	5.2	22.2	19.4	62.9	69.9	0.6	1.1	65.6	8.1	75.2	36
Asia	South-Central Asia	Maldives (2009)	22.9	22.4	−0.5	2.1	2.8	20.4	18.5	91.4	93.5	2.2	2.3	99.9	99.8	98	96

(continued)

Table 9.2 (continued)

Continent	Region	Country (year)	Infant mortality rates (p. 1000)			Total fertility rate		Median age at first marriage: age group 25–49		Vaccinations: all		Median duration of exclusive breastfeeding		Electricity in the house		Delivery in a health facility	
			Urban	Rural	Diff.	Urban	Rural	Urban	Rural	Urban	Rural	Urban	Rural	Urban	Rural	Urban	Rural
Africa	Western Africa	Mauritania (2000–01)	74.2	61.6	−12.6	4.1	4.8	17.5	16.8	38	27.4	0.8	0.6	49.7	2.5	82.8	23.8
Africa	Southern Africa	Namibia (1992)	63.1	60.7	−2.4	4	6.3		24	59.6	57	0.5	0.5	66	4.2	86.9	58.4
LAC	South America	Paraguay (2008)	26.4	22.4	−4	2.2	3			76.8	74.1					94.7	77.2
Europe	Eastern Europe	Romania (1999)	32.2	26.1	−6.1	1	1.8									99.6	97.5
Asia	South-Central Asia	Sri Lanka (1987)	34.4	32.2	−2.2	2.1	2.8	24.3	22	59.8	65.1	0.5	0.5				
Africa	Eastern Africa	Tanzania (2010)	62.8	59.5	−3.3	3.7	6.1	19.8	18.5	85.6	72.6	1.9	2.5	46.2	3.7	81.8	41.9
Africa	Eastern Africa	Tanzania (1991–92)	108.3	97.1	−11.2	5.1	6.6	18.3	17.8	83.8	67.8	0.6	0.7	23.9	1.3	85.3	43.4
LAC	Caribbean	Trinidad and Tobago (1987)	34.2	27.9	−6.3	3	3.1	19.9	19.4			0.5	0.5				
Europe	Eastern Europe	Ukraine (1999)	13.7	6	−7.7	1.7	1.3									95.4	91.3

Note: Author's calculations based on DHS data

Table 9.3 Summary statistics on variables utilized in analyses of 217 national populations from 86 countries

	Urban environment			Rural environment		
	Min	Max	Average	Min	Max	Average
Infant mortality rate (p. 1000)	12.1	140.4	55.7	6.0	160.7	74.0
Total fertility rate	1	6.4	3.4	1.3	8.2	5.0
Unmet need of family planning (%)	3.6	41.6	19.3	5.1	46.2	23.0
Median age at first marriage (in years)	14.8	24.8	19.8	13.8	24.0	18.4
Median age at first sex (in years)	15.4	23.6	18.6	15.1	21.8	17.6
All vaccinations taken (%)	0.8	97.1	60.2	0.8	93.9	49.5
Median duration of exclusive breastfeeding (in months)	0.3	4.9	1.1	0.4	5.8	1.5
Has secondary education or more (%)	4.3	99.9	50.1	0.3	99.8	23.8
House has electricity (%)	3.5	100	71.5	0.1	100	32.6
Delivery at a health facility (%)	19.9	100	75.0	1.7	99.7	43.9

among urban children (0.6 month) than rural children (1.1 months). The highest urban disadvantage in all national populations is found in Guyana (gap of 13.4 points) in 2009; here, the proportion of children fully immunized in urban areas (60.2 %) is inferior to that of their counterparts in rural areas (64.3 %) while all the other summary statistics show lower estimates for rural than urban areas in Guyana. Thus, other contextual factors may be in operation; hence the multivariate analyses conducted below.

Table 9.3 shows the summary statistics on selected variables for analyses, based on the multilevel framework described above and within the limits of the international data at hand. These statistics highlight important variations in measures across national populations and countries. For instance, infant mortality rates vary from 12.1 per 1000 live births to 140.1 per 1000 live births in urban areas, and from 6.0 per 1000 live births to 160.7 per 1000 live births in rural areas. Similarly, the total fertility rate varies from 1 birth to 6.4 births per woman in urban environments and from 1.3 births to 8.2 births per woman in rural settings. For all environmentally measured risk and protective factors, the estimated figures indicate that the median duration of exclusive breastfeeding is lower in urban than rural areas.

Tables 9.4 and 9.5 present the findings from the most completed multilevel models fitted to the longitudinal (repeated cross-sectional) data constructed and analyzed.

Table 9.4 shows no significant variation across continent in the influences of urban or rural environments on infant mortality rates at the national level. When the analyses are refined by sub-regions within continents in Table 9.5, significant regional differences in national estimates of infant mortality rates separately for urban dwellers and for rural dwellers, allowing independent assessment of the effects of urban environments in these regions on population health outcomes, as well as differences in mechanisms in operation for the manifestation of these effects. National populations from South-Eastern Asia, Southern Europe and to some extent from Central

Table 9.4 Multilevel estimates of area-based aggregate risk factors of infant mortality rates across continents

Variables	Urban environment		Rural environment	
	Coefficient	Standard	Coefficient	Standard error
Fixed part				
Intercept	8.057***	1.572	8.150***	1.644
Continent				
Africa (Reference)				
Asia	–0.107	0.075	–0.040	0.081
Latin America and Caribbean	–0.024	0.080	0.015	0.089
Europe	–0.083	0.149	0.027	0.155
Time period				
1985–1989 (Reference)				
1990–1994	0.006	0.061	0.053	0.057
1995–1999	–0.001	0.059	0.084	0.056
2000–2004	–0.022	0.064	0.061	0.060
2005+	0.061	0.058	0.111**	0.054
Aggregate risk and protective factors				
Total fertility rate	0.070*	0.039	0.095**	0.041
Unmet need of family planning	0.207**	0.073	–0.043	0.078
Median age at first marriage	–0.540	0.543	–0.116	0.586
Median age at first sex	–0.429	0.510	–0.241	0.533
All vaccinations taken	–0.060	0.070	–0.030	0.068
Median duration of exclusive	–0.054*	0.031	–0.014	0.031
Has secondary education or more	–0.070	0.088	–0.213**	0.090
House has electricity	–0.117*	0.067	–0.137**	0.073
Delivery at a health facility	–0.302***	0.103	–0.303**	0.109
Random part				
Between-country variance	0.040***	0.010	0.062***	0.014
Between-survey variance	0.024***	0.004	0.020***	0.004
–2 Log Likelihood	26.248		22.006	
Number of surveys utilized in analyses	214 (three national populations had no infant mortality data)			
Number of countries	86			
Number of regions across continents	13			
Number of continents	4			

*p<0.10; **p<0.05; ***p<0.01.

America, have significantly lower levels of infant mortality rates than national populations from Western Africa (the reference region); similar findings emerge as regards the rural environment. Growing social and economic disparities in a country, region and continent across urban and rural areas seem to intensify health inequalities already thought to exist across middle and low income countries.

Table 9.5 Multilevel estimates of international area-based aggregate risk factors of infant mortality rates across regions

Variables	Urban environment		Rural environment	
	Coefficient	Standard Error	Coefficient	Standard Error
Fixed part				
Intercept	6.442***	1.388	7.687***	1.601
Sub-continental regions				
Western Africa (Reference)				
Middle Africa	–0.074	0.101	–0.191	0.128
Eastern Africa	0.086	0.077	0.015	0.100
Southern Africa	–0.011	0.192	0.104	0.229
Northern Africa	0.001	0.001	0.001	0.001
Western Asia	0.144	0.191	0.083	0.230
South-Central Asia	0.084	0.125	–0.043	0.152
South-Eastern Asia	–0.365**	0.141	–0.264*	0.175
South America	0.020	0.117	–0.138	0.149
Central America	–0.254*	0.144	–0.418**	0.190
Caribbean	–0.161	0.136	–0.276	0.185
Southern Europe	–0.913***	0.248	–0.711***	0.298
Eastern Europe	0.001	0.001	0.001	0.001
Time period				
1985 – 1989 (Reference)				
1990–1994	0.015	0.059	0.048	0.056
1995–1999	–0.002	0.055	0.078	0.053
2000–2004	–0.002	0.061	0.072	0.059
2005+	0.084	0.054	0.120	0.053
Aggregate risk and protective factors				
Total fertility rate	0.072**	0.036	0.112**	0.040
Unmet need of family planning	0.164**	0.065	–0.096	0.075
Median age at first marriage	–0.209	0.533	–0.033	0.625
Median age at first sex	0.004	0.545	–0.065	0.603
All vaccinations taken	–0.102*	0.064	–0.038	0.065
Median duration of exclusive breastfeeding	–0.058**	0.028	–0.018	0.030
Has secondary education or more	–0.157**	0.078	–0.220**	0.088
House has electricity	–0.080	0.057	–0.093	0.068
Delivery at a health facility	–0.348***	0.093	–0.350***	0.109
Random part				
Between-country variance	0.018***	0.006	0.044***	0.011
Between-survey variance	0.024***	0.004	0.020***	0.003
–2 Log Likelihood	–57.621		38.513	

(continued)

Table 9.5 (continued)

Variables	Urban environment		Rural environment	
	Coefficient	Standard Error	Coefficient	Standard Error
Number of surveys utilized in analyses	214 (three national populations had no infant mortality data)			
Number of countries	86			
Number of regions across continents	13			
Number of continents	4			

*p<0.10; **p<0.05; ***p<0.01.

We also assessed whether there were changes in the effects of urban environments on national mortality infant mortality rates among urban dwellers and among rural dwellers, with model estimating rates across continents (Table 9.4) or across regions within continents (Table 9.5). We found that non-significant U-shaped relationship between time period and national infant mortality rates for urban dwellers, with the periods 1995–1999 and 2000–2004 experiencing a receding trend compared with the 1990–1994 and 2005+ periods (the period 1985–1989 being the reference). For rural inhabitants, there seems to be a positive trend over time, although it shows significance only for the period 2005 or later.

As regards the aggregate risk and protective factors, as expected from our conceptual framework, a number of characteristics that tend to distinguish individuals living across ecological settings influence health outcomes and aggregate measures such as infant mortality rates in the national population, including those related to domains of socio-economic status (secondary education or more, electricity in the house), behaviours (exclusive breastfeeding practices, vaccinations taken, reproductive behaviour – fertility) and access to health services (delivery at a health facility).

The risk factors for urban versus rural geographical locations demonstrate that ecological setting influences health: health differences between populations living in urban and rural areas exist in these populations, and the underlying factors that engender discrepancies in middle and low income countries include fertility rates and unmet need for family planning (the higher their levels, the higher the level of infant mortality in urban environments) on the one hand, delivery at a health facility, exclusive breastfeeding, electricity in the house (which are protective factors against infant mortality in urban populations) on the other hand.

Existing research suggests that public health factors such as access to services make living in a city in developing countries advantageous, but the robustness of such association, whether it holds across the entire developing world, why it exists, and whether it will continue to hold into the future are all issues that required further attention, as we noted above. Our study finds that indeed, access to health services (e.g., delivery at a health facility and vaccinations) represent significant protective factors for urban populations. Moreover, the higher the proportion of unmet need for family planning in the urban populations in different countries, the higher their infant mortality rates, even after all controls for measured and unobserved heterogeneities are accounted for. In contrast, rural populations do not seem to show significant differences in vaccination coverage or unmet need for family planning as regards their effects on infant mortality rates in rural environments.

Tables 9.4 and 9.5 also show strong effects of heterogeneity between countries and across surveys within countries, both for urban and rural environments as regards infant mortality rates. This implies that the mechanisms of operation of the influential factors on infant mortality rates in urban environments and rural settings of the low and middle income countries we analyzed are at several levels. This is the case notably at country-level within continent or region within continent, and across waves of surveys for each country in the context of no significant changes in the urban advantage when one exist, above and beyond the compositional effects that remain robust to all controls.

9.7 Conclusion and Discussion

Little is known about health differences between local and national populations living in urban and rural areas and the underlying factors that engender divergent or convergent trends and differentials in health in middle and low income countries. Rates of infant mortality rates are reliable indicators of human and economic development in these countries. The question: 'Why do some individuals have higher risk of death than others?' Could be equally well asked in either of two settings (rural, urban), if in each setting, the individual risks of death vary (proportionately) to about the same extent; and the answers might well be much the same in each instance (that is, genetic variation as well as environmental and behavioral differences). We might achieve a complete understanding of why individuals vary, and yet quite miss the most important public health question, namely: 'Why is risk of death lower in certain urban/rural areas and common in others?' The answer to this question has to do with the determinants of the population mean; what distinguishes the two groups has nothing to do with the characteristics of individuals, it is rather a shift of the whole distribution— a mass influence acting on the population as a whole. To find the determinants of prevalence and incidence rates, we need to study characteristics of populations, not characteristics of individuals.

In most of Africa, Asia and Latin America, the results of Demographic and Health Survey (DHS) data analyzed cross-sectionally indicated that infant and child mortality rates are lower in urban than in rural areas (Montgomery et al. 2003, 127). Moreover, there was a tendency for infant and child mortality rates to be lower in larger urban settlements (Montgomery et al. 2003, 280). This picture looks rather different from the one we found in 18 of the 217 national populations which had infant mortality rates in urban areas higher than the ones found in rural areas, and the evidence from findings from the multilevel models fitted to the repeated cross-sectional data from DHS exploiting multiple waves of data collection per country between 1985 and 2010. We found that unmet need for family planning is a major determinant of urban disadvantage in child survival among urban populations, that infant mortality rates in national urban populations are closely linked to poverty (proxied by education and electricity in the house and access to health services – delivery at a health facility and immunization), that exclusive breastfeeding is a strong protective factor in urban environments whereas it has no significant effects in rural populations, and that there are important and significant variations in urban populations across countries within regions or continents and across waves of surveys within countries. These findings are robust.

Higher than expected national rates of infant mortality in urban populations in low and middle income countries are significantly due to six predictors: (1) high fertility rate; (2) unmet need for family planning; (3) short duration of exclusive breastfeeding; (4) low levels of education; (5) delivery outside a health facility; and incomplete or no vaccination. These predictors are robust above and beyond significant regional influences and unobserved heterogeneities between and within country.

Higher than expected national rates of infant mortality in rural populations in these countries are significantly ascribed to three predictors: (1) high fertility rate, low levels of education and delivery outside of a health facility. These predictors remain robust after all controls for regional influences and unobserved heterogeneities between and within country.

These results indicate that there are public health issues and challenges in urban and rural areas, and the unprecedented demographic shift embodied in the process of urbanization is a public health concern.

How to prevent deaths in urban and non-urban areas during the ongoing demographic and epidemiological changes in countries and regions around the world? The priority of concern should always be the discovery and control of the causes of incidence: this is the attempt to control the determinants of incidence, to lower the mean level of risk factors, to shift the whole distribution of exposure in a favorable direction. In mass prevention each individual has usually only a small expectation of benefit, and this small benefit can easily be outweighed by a small risk. It is important to distinguish three approaches. The first is the restoration of biological normality by the removal of an abnormal exposure (e.g., promoting exclusive breastfeeding for 6 months). The second preventive approach, seeks to interpose additional protective intervention (e.g., immunization). The third is population control through policies and programs to reduce fertility. There has never been a simple planning solution for the inequalities and inequities that we see today in urban settings all over the world. And there is not one policy that will work in every setting, particularly in the context of the complex social processes that create these inequities in different rural and urban areas. In fact, during the latter half of the twentieth century in the low-income countries of Africa, Asia and Latin America, local governments, supported by international agencies, greatly emphasized schemes to support basic needs provision for low-income communities (UN-Habitat 2007, 2011; United Nations 2011). In the 1980s and 1990s these initiatives were widely criticized, civil society groups arguing that such initiatives ignored the upstream socio-cultural context that push people into low-income settlements, and may provide short-term improvements in living conditions and health but do not solve deeper social and structural problems in the communities (Konteh 2009). Many local governments, sometimes with international donor support, developed "slum upgrading" programmes, which commonly comprised a multi-sectoral package of water and sanitation provision, upgraded housing and sometimes primary health care, and local education and employment programmes. This mix of physical service improvement and social service provision had significant impacts on many aspects of health of the low-income communities involved, but still did not change the fundamental issues of inequality (Weeks et al. 2013). In many of these projects to date, wealthier families later moved into the better environment.

Research on urban-rural environment and health arises from several disciplines, including demography, anthropology, urban planning, epidemiology, and sociology, and has focused on assessing differences between and within urban/rural areas. Place of residence has, for centuries, been implicated as a health determinant (Woods 2003; Konteh 2009). In the developed world, differences in urban and rural health go back to medieval times when urban residence was harmful owing to communicable diseases more easily transferred across populations living in cramped and unclean surroundings (Kearns 1988; Landers 1987; Montgomery et al. 2003; Woods 2003). Spatial and ecological settings have long been implicated in a wide variety of health-related behaviours and outcomes at various stages of life and over time, suggesting that location of residence itself is a critical social determinant of health. This is because a number of characteristics that tend to distinguish individuals living across ecological settings influence health outcomes, such as those related to domains of socio-economic status, behaviours, social cohesion and access to health services. Despite the history of research examining the effects of ecological setting on health, surprisingly little is known about health differences between populations living in urban and rural areas and the underlying factors that engender discrepancies in middle and low income countries (Montgomery et al. 2003; UN-Habitat 2011; Stephens 2011). Existing research suggests that public health factors such as access to services and safe water make living in a city in developing countries advantageous. Yet evidence also shows higher risks for lifestyle-related diseases, such as diabetes and cardiovascular disease, beginning to arise in some urban areas in the developing world, and substantial intra-urban variations in health, in the course of the ongoing epidemiological and health changes therein.

Our study found that changes in the characteristics of urban populations can influence health in several ways, and that the mechanisms for doing so should include solutions that have proven efficacious and established here: promoting exclusive breastfeeding in urban populations, meeting the need of these populations for family planning, promoting education, promoting electrification of homes, and promoting full immunization coverage of these populations. The significance of the effects of education for both urban and rural dwellers implies that changes in the knowledge, skills, culture or behaviour of people living in cities or rural areas will also significantly influence health. Although urban and non-urban residents differ, these differences are not inherent within individuals, but are the outcomes of social and economic processes that have distributed people into various urban and non-urban settings. These social processes include housing markets and access to higher education which sort urban residents into different communities and social strata within which the inherent characteristics of individuals interact with the particular social and physical environment to produce an 'urban phenotype' (Galea et al. 2005). As we noted above, ultimately these characteristics of urban residents interact with other dimensions of urban living conditions to influence the health of urban populations. Investing in education of urban and rural dwellers is worth for population health promotion in general and infant mortality reductions in particular in resources-constrained settings of low and middle income countries, both in urban and rural environments.

Reliable urban health statistics are largely unavailable throughout the developing world and particularly in Africa. Disaggregated intra-urban health data for different areas within a city, are even more rare. Data that are available indicate a range of urban health hazards and associated health risks including substandard housing, crowding, air pollution, insufficient or contaminated drinking water, inadequate sanitation and solid waste disposal services, vector-borne diseases, industrial waste, increased motor vehicle traffic, stress associated with poverty and unemployment. There are many challenges of urbanization, and urban health risks and concerns involve many different sectors, including health, environment, housing, energy, transportation, urban planning, and others. Two main policy implications are highlighted: the need for systematic and useful urban health statistics on a disaggregated intra-urban basis and the need for more effective partnering across sectors so as to create healthy and sustainable cities.

As regards future research, most of the research on rural/urban differences in health in developing countries has considered issues that affect non-elderly populations, such as communicable diseases, infant mortality, reproductive health, and traffic-related injuries and deaths. In developing countries, rural/urban discrepancies in health problems typical among older people have been almost completely ignored, and constitute an area of future research that may benefit from the methodology developed for this study.

References

Baltagi, B. H. (2008). *Econometric analysis of panel data* (4th ed.). New York: Wiley.

Basu, A., & Rathouz, P. (2005). Estimating marginal and incremental effects on health outcomes using flexible link and variance function models. *Biostatistics, 6*(1), 93–109.

Bilger, M., & Carrieri, V. (2013). Health in the cities: When the neighborhood matters more than income. *Journal of Health Economics, 32*, 1–11.

Blazer, D. G., Kessler, R. C., McGonagle, K. A., & Swartz, M. S. (1994). The prevalence and distribution of major depression in a national community sample: The national comorbidity survey. *American Journal of Psychiatry, 151*(7), 979–986.

Bocquier, P., Madise, N. J., & Zulu, E. M. (2011). Is there an urban advantage in child survival in sub-Saharan Africa? Evidence from 18 countries in the 1990s. *Demography, 48*, 531–558.

Clayton, D., & Hills, M. (1993). *Statistical models in epidemiology*. Oxford: Oxford University Press.

Collett, D. (2003). *Modelling survival data in medical research*. Boca Raton: CRC press.
Diez-Roux, A. V. (2002). Invited commentary: Places, people, and health. *American Journal Epidemiology, 155*(6), 516–519.
Evans, R. G., & Stoddart, G. L. (1990). Producing health, consuming health care. *Social Science and Medicine, 31*, 1347–1363.
Evans, R. G., & Stoddart, G. L. (2003). Consuming research? Producing policy? *American Journal of Public Health, 93*, 371–379.
Frumkin, H. (2002). Urban sprawl and public health. *Public Health Reports, 117*(3), 201–217.
Galea, S., Freudenberg, N., & Vlahov, D. (2005). Cities and population health. *Social Science and Medicine, 60*, 1017–1033.
Goesling, B. (2001). Changing income inequalities within and between nations: New evidence. *American Sociological Review, 66*(5), 745–761.
Gould, W. T. (1998). African mortality and the new 'urban penalty'. *Health and Place, 4*(2), 171–181.
Green, G. (2012, April). Intersectoral planning for city health development. *Journal Urban Health, 89*(2), 247–257.
Günther, I., & Harttgen, K. (2012). Deadly cities? Inequalities in mortality in sub-Saharan Africa. *Population and Development Review, 38*(3), 469–486.
Henderson, J. V. (2010). Cities and development. *Journal of Regional Science, 50*(1), 515–540.
Hsiao, C. (1986). *Analysis of panel data*. Cambridge: Cambridge University Press.
Jedrychowski, W., Maugeri, U., & Bianchi, I. (1997). Environmental pollution in central and eastern European countries: A basis for cancer epidemiology. *Reviews on Environmental Health, 12*(1), 1–23.
Jerrett, M., Eyles, J., Dufournaud, C., & Birch, S. (2003). Environmental influences on healthcare expenditures: An exploratory analysis from Ontario, Canada. *Journal of Epidemiology and Community Health, 57*(5), 334–338.
Kearns, G. (1988). The urban penalty and the population history of England. In A. Brandstrom & L. Tedebrand (Eds.), *Society, health and population during the demographic transition* (pp. 213–236). Stockholm: Ajmquist and Wiskell International.
Kinsella, K. (2001). Urban and rural dimensions of global population aging: An overview. *Journal of Rural Health, 17*(4), 314–322.
Konteh, F. (2009). Urban sanitation and health in the developing world: Reminiscing the nineteenth century industrial nations. *Health & Place, 15*(1), 69–78.
Kuate Defo, B. (2014). Beyond the "transition" frameworks: The cross-continuum of health, disease and mortality framework. *Global Health Action, 7*, 24804.
Landers, J. (1987). Mortality and metropolis: The case of London 1675–1825. *Population Studies, 41*, 59–76.
MacKinnon, J., White, H., & Davidson, R. (1983). Tests for model specification in the presence of alternative hypotheses: Some further results. *Journal of Econometrics, 21*, 53–70.
Montgomery, M. R., & Hewett, P. C. (2005). Urban poverty and health in developing countries: Household and neighborhood effects. *Demography, 42*(3), 397–425.
Montgomery, M. R., Stern, R., Cohen, B., & Reed, H. E. (Eds.). (2003). *Cities transformed: Demographic change and its implications in the developing world*. Washington, DC: National Academy Press.
Morris, M. (1991). A log-linear modeling framework for selective mixing. *Mathematical Biosciences, 107*(2), 349–377.
Northridge, M. E., Sclar, E. D., & Biswas, P. (2003). Sorting out the connections between the built environment and health: A conceptual framework for navigating pathways and planning healthy cities. *Journal of Urban Health, 80*(4), 556–568.
Paykel, E. S., Abbott, R., Jenkins, R., Burgha, T. S., & Meltzer, H. (2002). Urban-rural mental health differences in Great Britain: Findings from the national morbidity survey. *Psychological Medicine, 30*, 269–280.
Rao, R., & Wu, Y. (1989). A strongly consistent procedure for model selection in a regression problem. *Biometrika, 76*(2), 369–374.

Rodwin, V. G., & Gusmano, M. K. (2002). The world cities project: Rationale, organization, and design for comparison of megacity health systems. *Journal of Urban Health, 79*(4), 445–463.
Rondinelli, D. A. (1986). Extending urban services in developing countries: Policy options and organizational choices. *Public Administration and Development, 6*(1), 1–21.
Ross, C. E. (2000). Walking, exercising, and smoking: Does neighborhood matter? *Social Science and Medicine, 51*, 265–274.
Shima, M., Nitta, Y., Ando, M., & Adachi, M. (2002). Effects of air pollution on the prevalence and incidence of asthma in children. *Achieves of Environmental Health, 57*(6), 529–535.
Stephens, C. (1995). The urban environment, poverty and health in developing countries. *Health Policy and Planning, 10*(2), 109–121.
Stephens, C. (2011). Revisiting urban health and social inequalities: The devil is in the detail and the solution is in all of us. *Environment and Urbanization, 23*(1), 29–40.
Sverdlik, A. (2011). Ill-health and poverty: A literature review on health in informal settlements. *Environment and Urbanization, 23*(1), 123–155.
Takano, T., Nakamura, K., & Watanabe, M. (2002). Urban residential environments and senior citizens' longevity in megacity areas: The importance of walkable green spaces. *Journal of Epidemiology and Community Health, 56*, 913–918.
UN-Habitat. (2007). *State of the world's cities 2006/2007.* New York: United Nations.
UN-Habitat. (2011). *State of the world's cities 2010/2011: Bridging the urban divide.* New York: United Nations.
United Nations. (2011). *Population distribution, urbanization, internal migration and development: An international perspective.* New York: United Nations.
Vlahov, D., Freudenberg, N., Proietti, F., Ompad, D., Quinn, A., Nandi, V., & Galea, S. (2007), Urban as a determinant of health. *Journal of Urban Health, 84*(1). doi:10.1007/s11524-007-9169-3.
Weeks, J. R., Hill, A. G., & Stoler, J. (Eds.). (2013). *Spatial inequalities: Health, poverty, and place in Accra, Ghana.* Dordrecht: Springer Science+Business Media.
Williams, L. M. (2013). *Between health and place: Understanding the built environment.* Toronto: The Wellesley Institute.
Woods, R. (2003). Urban–rural mortality differentials: An unresolved debate. *Population and Development Review, 29*, 29–46.
World Health Organization. (2002). *The World Health Report 2002: Reducing risks, promoting healthy life.* Geneva: World Health Organization.
Xu, H., Logan, J. R., & Short, S. E. (2014). Integrating space with place in health research: A multilevel spatial investigation using child mortality in 1880 Newark, New Jersey. *Demography, 51*, 811–834.
Yamamoto, S., & Watanabe, S. (2001). Geographic characteristics and mortality profiles in the JPHC study. Japan public health center-based prospective study on cancer and cardiovascular diseases. *Journal of Epidemiology, 11*(6 Suppl.), S8–S23.

Chapter 10
Will Urban and Rural Mortality Converge in Africa?

Michel Garenne

10.1 Introduction

The course of the health transition can be partly characterized by mortality changes measured by increase in life expectancy or a decline in age-specific mortality, and in particular in infant and child mortality. The health transition, including changes in both mortality and morbidity, started in the nineteenth century in Europe and in countries of European settlement, and spread all over the world in the twentieth century (Stolnitz 1955, 1965). Even in the most remote areas of Africa, mortality decline has been overwhelming and rapid since 1950 (Hill 1991; Hill and Yazbeck 1994; Ahmad et al. 2000; Garenne and Gakusi 2006a).

One of the features of the health transition in Europe has been the change in urban/rural differences over time. Before and in the early stage of the transition, urban mortality was higher, sometimes much higher, than rural mortality. This is often called the "urban penalty", or the "urban graveyard effect", which has drawn much attention from historians and demographers, including in this volume. Numerous books and articles were devoted to this topic in the United Kingdom (Woods et al. 1988; Woods 2003; Kearns 1988, 1993), in the United States (Haines 2001; Preston and Haines 1991), in Spain (Reher 2001), in the Netherlands (Van der Woude 1982; Van Poppel 1989), in France (Preston and van de Walle 1978) and many other places. The excess mortality in urban areas in the nineteenth century is attributed to a mix of epidemiological, demographic and social factors, which can be summarized as: "the city attracts the poor and the plague". Big cities imply huge

M. Garenne (✉)
Institut de Recherche pour le Développement (IRD), Paris, France

Institut Pasteur, Epidémiologie des Maladies Emergentes, Paris, France

School of Public Health, Witwatersrand University, Johannesburg, South Africa
e-mail: michel.garenne@pasteur.fr

D. Ramiro Fariñas, M. Oris (eds.), *New Approaches to Death in Cities during the Health Transition*, International Studies in Population 12,
DOI 10.1007/978-3-319-43002-7_10

concentrations of human beings, which facilitate the spread and severity of communicable diseases. This applies to airborne diseases (e.g. tuberculosis), to waterborne diseases (e.g. cholera) when the water supply is not clean, as well as to sexually transmitted diseases (e.g. syphilis). The nineteenth century city also concentrated extreme poverty and social disruption, and is often associated with poor nutrition and poor health status (Rosen 1958; Szreter and Mooney 1998). In contrast, with economic development and with the development of modern health systems and health services, the modern city later concentrated wealth (see chapter 7 on Paris in this volume) and medical services, so that the balance shifted in favour of the city, the tipping point being around 1920 in many European countries.

The situation in developing countries is very different, since they started their health transition much later. Cities could benefit from the start from modern health and medical technology, and as a result, by 1950 urban mortality was lower than rural mortality in most developing countries. This situation continued in the later part of the twentieth century in most places, with only a few exceptions (Antoine and Diouf 1988; Timaeus and Lush 1995; Preston 1985; Gilbert and Gugler 1992). Many health programs developed in the past 25 years affected the balance between urban and rural areas, in particular the "primary health care programs", focusing on rural areas; and the "child survival programs" targeting the whole population. These were found to have a rather large effect on mortality trends among young children (Walsh and Warren 1979; Foege and Henderson 1986; Ewbank 1993; Becker et al. 1993; Garenne et al. 2007).

Serious concerns have emerged recently with regard to very rapid urbanization, and with this, the development of new pockets of extreme poverty and very poor hygiene in the slums of the big cities (Harpham et al. 1988; Harpham and Stephen 1991; Harpham and Molyneux 2001; Brockerhoff 1993; Campbell and Campbell 2007; Egunjobi 1991; Fotso 2006; Gracey 2002; Gould 1998; Leon 2008; Montgomery et al. 2004; Montgomery and Ezeh 2005; Montgomery 2009; Patel and Burke 2009; Pryer and Crook 1988; Van de Poel et al. 2007). These subpopulations seem to cumulate all the risks of poor health, and were shown repeatedly to have higher mortality and morbidity than wealthier urban strata, and even occasionally rising mortality and higher mortality than rural areas (APHRC 2002). These effects may be compounded by urban/rural migration, although no clear evidence of these selection factors came out of recent empirical studies (Bocquier et al. 2011). Emerging diseases also posed new problems for developing countries, and in particular HIV/AIDS in Africa. HIV/AIDS became the cause of major mortality increases in Africa since 1990 (Newell et al. 2004; Garenne 2011; Garenne et al. 2011). As with most STI's, HIV/AIDS tends to be more prevalent in cities than in rural areas, and could penalize overall levels of urban mortality.

The aim of this chapter is to document recent changes in the balance between urban and rural under-five mortality in Africa, which means in this case lower mortality in rural areas than in urban areas of the same country. This work is an extension of earlier work of the author on the health transitions and regressions in sub-Saharan Africa since 1950.

10.2 Framework

In this section, we present a broad framework of analysis of health transitions in developing countries, with focus on under-five mortality. Of course, only some of the data that would be needed to fully explain urban/rural differences are in fact available and will be used later. This study focuses on the factors that could account for urban/rural differences, and more importantly on the changes in the balance between both areas of residence. Needless to say, these are complex issues with numerous factors and multiple interactions.

A first array of factors that will be evoked are the classic determinants of health trends, namely: food and nutritional status, hygiene in a broad sense (water, sanitation, food safety, personal cleanliness, etc.), preventive medicine (vaccination, vector control, prevention of STI's, etc.), and curative medicine (physicians, hospitals, medicines, etc.). In general, urban areas enjoy better nutrition, better hygiene, more preventive medicine, and more curative medicine, and most indicators available are in their favour. However, the large gaps between both sectors that prevailed 50 years ago tended to narrow in recent years. In particular, preventive medicine (vaccination, bed nets, prevention of mother to child transmission of HIV, etc.) as well as some specific disease control programs (diarrhoea, acute respiratory infections, treatment of malaria and HIV/aids) now cover rural areas almost as well as urban areas, thanks to large scale health programs, often supported by the international community.

The second array of factors that will be evoked deal with disease dynamics, with the focus on two of the main killers of African children: malaria and HIV. The dynamics of both diseases vary between urban and rural areas. Malaria is usually more frequent and more severe in rural areas, so that programs aimed at controlling the disease can have a stronger demographic impact in rural areas, therefore reducing the urban/rural gap. HIV/AIDS is always more prevalent in urban areas in all countries for which data are available, and until about 2005 HIV/AIDS mortality was rising. So, HIV is likely to have a greater impact in urban areas than in rural areas, therefore reducing the gap between both sectors. If the gap was small originally, and if HIV prevalence differs markedly between urban and rural areas, HIV could by itself reverse the balance in mortality between the two sectors.

A third array of factors that could be evoked is population size and density. With rapid urbanization in Africa, some cities became very large in a short period of time. Large population size and density is associated with faster transmission of communicable diseases, lower age at infection, and potentially higher mortality due to lack of health infrastructure, health personnel and health programs. This was true in the past with respect to airborne diseases (tuberculosis, measles, pertussis, pneumonia etc.) and to waterborne diseases (cholera, typhoid, salmonella, shigella, etc.), and could be true as well in the Third World.

The fourth array of factors that will be investigated are the socio-economic correlates of child mortality, such as wealth (a proxy for income) and education. For instance, if poverty is reduced in rural areas but increases in urban areas, and even possibly by migration of the rural poor to the city, the changing composition of the population could lead to changing the mortality balance between both sectors. Likewise, if education catches up in rural areas, the gap could be reduced, decreasing therefore the mortality gap. Some of these changes could be the result of policies and programs. For instance, the Structural Adjustment Programs (SAP) put in place in the 1980s had, among others, the aim of transferring money from urban to rural areas in order to reduce the gap in wealth between both sectors.

10.3 Data and Methods

Data used for this study were drawn from Demographic and Health Surveys (DHS). These are well standardized, well designed sample surveys conducted all over the world. Some 90 surveys are now available in sub-Saharan Africa, covering a wide range of demographic and health issues. Some of the recent surveys deal specifically with malaria and with HIV/AIDS. More details on the surveys can be found on the DHS web site.

DHS surveys allow one to reconstruct under-five mortality trends, for urban and rural separately. The method of trend reconstruction has been presented elsewhere (Garenne and Gakusi 2004, 2006a). In brief, age specific death rates were calculated by calendar year from maternity histories, and trends were fitted with a linear-logistic model. Periods of monotonic change were studied separately (declining, steady or rising mortality), and only periods of significant changes in slopes were kept for the final analysis. Differences between urban and rural areas are analysed with standard statistical tests given sample size. In the original study, some 37 countries were available, covering more than 90 % of the population of sub-Saharan Africa. These data were made available on the FERDI web site. This study focuses on the three countries for which rural mortality became lower than urban mortality.

DHS surveys provide also a large number of variables that can be used for understanding the factors of urban/rural changes. These include firstly socio-economic factors, in particular level of education and wealth. An absolute wealth index (AWI) was built on a model presented elsewhere (Garenne and Hohmann 2003; Hohmann and Garenne 2011). In brief, this index counts the number of modern goods and amenities available in a household, out of a list of 14 key items. This indicator is linearly correlated with under-five mortality. DHS questionnaires also include a variety of information on health behaviour, and use of health services. Only a few were selected to illustrate this purpose: vaccination coverage, use of bed nets, and treatment of malaria. In addition, we used epidemiologic indicators, namely HIV prevalence and malaria prevalence when available. Here again, the emphasis is not that much on absolute values, but on differences between urban and rural sectors, and on their dynamics over time. Of course, time trends of these indicators are not available, since they are recorded only at the time of survey. But when a country has conducted several surveys (often 3 or 4 surveys conducted every 5 years), one gains some insights into the nature of the urban/rural dynamics.

10.4 Results

Overall Mortality Trends

Figure 10.1 displays the dynamics of urban and rural mortality in sub-Saharan Africa since 1950. The pattern is clearly characteristic of the Third World, and the opposite of the pattern found in nineteenth century Europe at similar levels of mortality. In Europe, urban mortality was first higher, and then crossed over rural mortality around year 1920; later the gap tended to wane reaching low values after 1950. In African countries, under-five mortality declined steadily over the study period (1950–2005). Mortality was lower in urban areas already in 1950, and continued to be so until 2005, the last point available. Mortality decline in rural areas was almost parallel to that of urban areas before 1985, and continued to be sustained thereafter, whereas mortality levels stagnated in urban areas after 1985, reducing the gap between both sectors. Prolonging the 1985–2005 trend suggest that the two curves might cross each other in the future. This has already happened in a few cases discussed below.

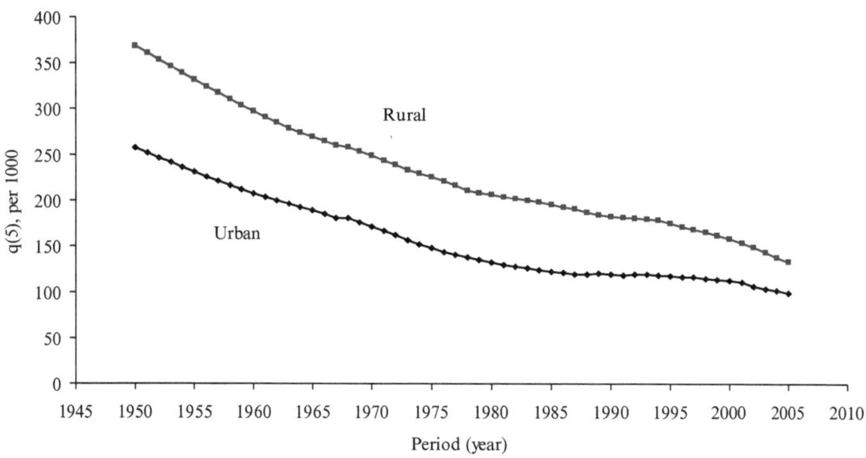

Fig. 10.1 Trends in under-five mortality by area of residence, sub-Saharan Africa (36 countries) (Source: Author's calculation from DHS data)

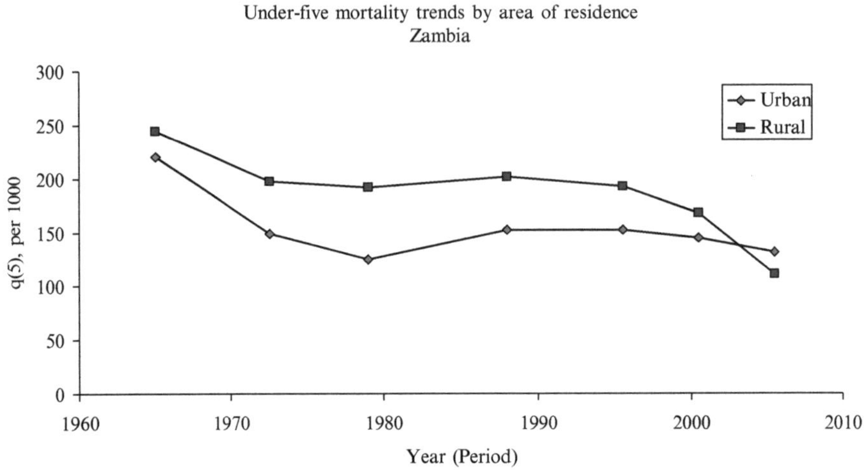

Fig. 10.2 Trends in under-five mortality by area of residence, Zambia (Source: Author's calculation from DHS data)

Countries with Lower Rural Mortality

Among the 37 countries investigated, three exhibited lower rural mortality in the recent years. In Zambia, under-five mortality trends were complex, because of the large impact of the economic crisis caused by the fast decrease in copper prices in 1975, copper being the main export commodity and the main source of state income (see Garenne and Gakusi 2006b for details). With respect to our focus, urban/rural differences were rather moderate in the 1960s, tended to increase during the crisis years because mortality decline stopped in rural areas while it continued in urban areas, then mortality increased in urban areas reducing the gap (Fig. 10.2) (Table 10.1).

In the latest period, after 1992, mortality decline resumed, but was faster in rural areas so that by 2004 rural mortality was below urban mortality, probably for the first time ever, the difference begin statistically significant (P=0.045) (Fig. 10.3).

In Tanzania, mortality also followed erratic trends, although less pronounced than in Zambia. Under-five death rates were declining in parallel until 1980, time after which they started to increase in urban areas up to 1986, where they became almost equivalent to rural death rates. Then they declined again in both areas and faster in urban areas for about 10 years. In the most recent period (1996–2007), mortality decline was faster in rural areas, so that by 2005 rural mortality became apparently lower than urban mortality. The testing of the urban/rural differences was not significant in 2005–2007 (P=0.140), but the ratio of rural to urban mortality changed significantly since the previous 2000–2004 period (P=0.015) which shows that the balance between both areas was altered.

In Sierra Leone, mortality trends were more regular, with the sole exception of the civil war years (1998–2004) during which mortality increased significantly (not

Table 10.1 Changes in urban and rural under-five mortality in selected African countries

Country	Urban		Rural		Comparison urban/rural		Period change
Period	q(5) (per 1000)	Number of deaths	q(5) (per 1000)	Number of deaths	RR	P-value	P-value
Sierra-Leone							
1975–1988	218	155	316	500	1.45	0.000	
1988–1996	186	281	232	785	1.24	0.002	0.185
1997–2004	172	409	194	1257	1.13	0.034	0.279
2005–2008	**156**	**167**	**126**	**364**	**0.81**	**0.021**	**0.002**
Tanzania							
1960–1969	216	101	256	627	1.18	0.114	
1970–1979	149	419	195	2285	1.31	0.000	0.411
1980–1989	151	1001	167	4800	1.10	0.006	0.007
1990–1999	124	955	158	5019	1.28	0.000	0.003
2000–2004	98	279	115	1378	1.17	0.015	0.249
2005–2007	**102**	**82**	**85**	**309**	**0.83**	**0.140**	**0.015**
Zambia							
1960–1969	220	147	244	340	1.11	0.295	
1970–1974	149	218	197	492	1.32	0.001	0.165
1975–1982	125	664	191	1655	1.53	0.000	0.122
1983–1992	152	1783	201	4063	1.32	0.000	0.007
1993–1997	152	782	192	1863	1.27	0.000	0.401
1998–2002	145	480	168	1217	1.16	0.006	0.198
2003–2007	**131**	**211**	**111**	**432**	**0.84**	**0.045**	**0.001**

Source: Author's calculation from DHS surveys

Note: Values in bold are periods of significantly lower rural mortality. The first test compares the value of RR with 1 (higher or lower). The second test compares the changing value of RR from a period to the next

shown). The gap between urban and rural mortality was large (RR = 1.45) at baseline (1975–1988), but decreased steadily over time so that it became lower than one in the most recent period (RR = 0.81 in 2005–2008), all differences being statistically significant. This was simply due to the fact that mortality decline was always faster in rural areas than in urban areas, and to the fact that mortality in urban areas stagnated in the most recent period (Fig. 10.4).

These three case studies, so far unique in Africa, show that in the recent years rural mortality can become lower than urban mortality, mainly because progress was faster in rural areas and to a lesser extent because mortality stagnated or declined little in urban areas. These are new features of the health transition in Africa.

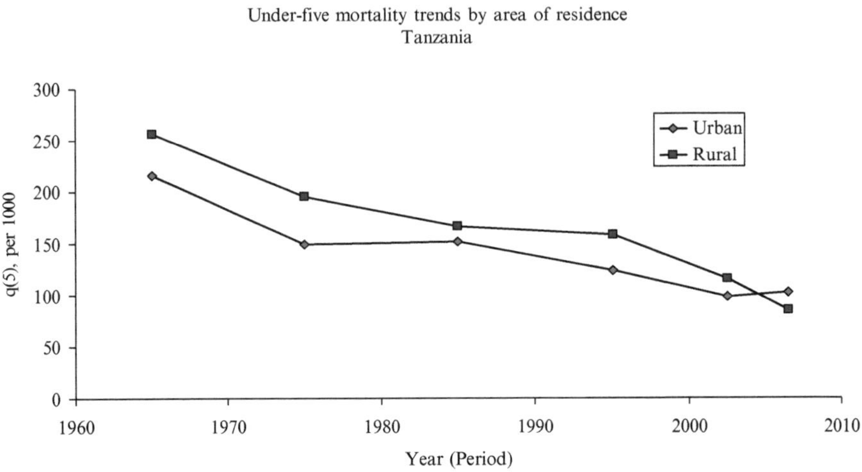

Fig. 10.3 Trends in under-five mortality by area of residence, Tanzania (Source: Author's calculation from DHS data)

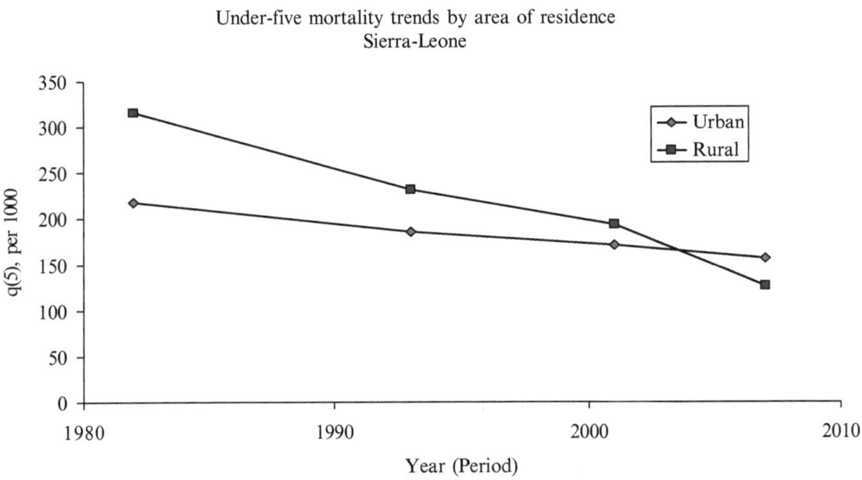

Fig. 10.4 Trends in under-five mortality by area of residence, Sierra-Leone (Source: Author's calculation from DHS data)

Main Determinants

With respect to the main determinants of the health transition (nutrition, hygiene, preventive and curative medicine), it appears that the gap between urban and rural areas was reduced in recent years, but not to an extent to which it could explain lower rural mortality. Nutritional status improved faster in rural areas in Zambia and Tanzania, but was still lower than in urban areas at time of the last survey in all three countries. Access to safe drinking water was markedly different between urban and rural areas in the three countries, and although the gap was somewhat reduced, the urban advantage was still considerable in the last survey available. Vaccination coverage was high in Zambia and Tanzania and moderate in Sierra-Leone, but the gap between urban and rural areas was rather small at last survey, and smaller than before in Zambia, and Tanzania. Vaccination is the only of the four determinants which could reasonably have contributed to narrowing the gap between urban and rural (Table 10.2).

Diseases: Malaria and HIV

The only country for which malaria prevalence was available was Tanzania and as expected, malaria morbidity was much higher in rural areas. However, and surprising compared to studies conducted in the 1970s and 1980s, the gap between urban and rural areas was rather small with respect to prevention and treatment of the disease. The use of bed nets for under-five children was similar in Sierra Leone and in Zambia, and only in Tanzania was the difference more marked. Indoor spraying of insecticides was low, with narrow differences in Tanzania, but more marked in Zambia. More important, presumptive treatment against malaria for mothers during pregnancy and for children during fever episodes was amazingly similar in urban and rural areas in all three countries. This fact, by itself could explain a narrow difference in mortality, whatever the prevalence and the preventive measures.

For HIV/AIDS, the gap was as expected: in all three countries urban HIV prevalence was higher than rural prevalence, differences being large in Zambia (about 10 %), moderate in Tanzania (about 5 %) and small in Sierra-Leone, because much lower level of overall seroprevalence. A 10 % gap in HIV prevalence among mothers could translate into a 20 per 1000 gap in under-five mortality under natural circumstances that prevailed before 2005, that is, before major programs of prevention of mother to child transmission and of treatment with anti-retro-viral therapy (ARV). This difference (20 per 1000) is equivalent to the difference found between urban and rural areas mortality in 2003–2007 in Zambia. DHS surveys do not provide data on prevention and treatment of HIV/AIDS (Table 10.3).

Population Growth and Urbanization

None of the three countries had experienced very rapid urbanization or had very high proportions of population in urban places. Zambia, the most industrialized country, had a fast rise in urbanization between 1950 and 1975, which stopped at the time of the economic crisis, so that the proportion urban remained roughly constant between 1980 and 2010 at around 39 % (range 38–40 % in the four censuses conducted in 1980, 1990, 2000 and 2010). This average hides some local dynamics, but

Table 10.2 Changes in selected determinants of child mortality, three African countries

Year	Survey	Urban	Rural	Difference
Child nutritional status: weight for age Z-score				
	Sierra Leone 2008	–0.6	–1.0	–0.4
	Tanzania 1991–1992	–1.2	–1.3	–0.1
	Tanzania 1996	–1.0	–1.4	–0.4
	Tanzania 1999	–1.0	–1.4	–0.4
	Tanzania 2004–2005	–0.9	–1.2	–0.3
	Tanzania 2010	–0.9	–1.1	–0.2
	Zambia 1992	–1.0	–1.4	–0.4
	Zambia 1996	–1.0	–1.3	–0.3
	Zambia 2001–2002	–1.1	–1.4	–0.3
	Zambia 2007	–0.8	–1.0	–0.2
HIV prevalence (percent)				
	Sierra Leone 2008	2.4	0.9	–1.5
	Tanzania 2003–2004	10.9	5.3	–5.6
	Tanzania 2007–2008	8.7	4.7	–4.0
	Zambia 2001–2002	23.1	10.8	–12.3
	Zambia 2007	19.5	10.3	–9.2
Percent safe drinking water (piped or bottled)				
	Sierra Leone 2008	47.9	8.3	–39.6
	Tanzania 1991–1992	78.7	19.4	–59.3
	Tanzania 1996	78.3	25.3	–53.0
	Tanzania 1999	80.3	22.3	–58.0
	Tanzania 2004–2005	68.9	23.6	–45.3
	Tanzania 2010	61.0	24.1	–36.9
	Zambia 1992	89.3	10.5	–78.8
	Zambia 1996	80.8	7.0	–73.8
	Zambia 2001–2002	81.6	6.5	–75.1
	Zambia 2007	76.9	3.3	–73.6
Vaccination coverage (percent with measles vaccine)				
	Sierra Leone 2008	64.5	58.1	–6.4
	Tanzania 1991–1992	91.6	78.5	–13.1
	Tanzania 1996	94.4	77.7	–16.7
	Tanzania 1999	90.3	75.3	–15.0
	Tanzania 2004–2005	89.7	77.7	–12.0
	Tanzania 2010	92.9	82.5	–10.4
	Zambia 1992	81.3	73.4	–7.9
	Zambia 1996	89.7	84.5	–5.2
	Zambia 2001–2002	85.5	83.9	–1.6
	Zambia 2007	88.5	83.6	–4.9

Source: DHS web site, Statistics Calculator

Table 10.3 Selected indicators of malaria epidemiology, three African countries

		Preventive measures	Treatment		
Country/Survey	Malaria prevalence (%)	Bed net use (%)	Indoor spraying (%)	Pregnancy (%)	Child fever (%)
Sierra-Leone 2008					
Urban		30.9		41.3	25.2
Rural		26.9		31.4	24.4
Tanzania 2007					
Urban	6.8	65.6	5.8	69.9	69.0
Rural	19.9	30.0	3.6	57.3	53.8
Zambia 2008					
Urban		35.0	39.0	93.2	40.3
Rural		32.8	3.2	84.8	37.7

Source: DHS web site, Statistics Calculator

Table 10.4 Selected indicators of HIV/AIDS epidemiology, three African countries

	HIV seroprevalence among adults (%)		
	Urban	Rural	Difference
Sierra Leone 2008	2.4	0.9	−1.5
Tanzania 2003–2004	10.9	5.3	−5.6
Tanzania 2007–2008	8.7	4.7	−4.0
Zambia 2001–2002	23.1	10.8	−12.3
Zambia 2007	19.5	10.3	−9.2

Source: DHS web site, Statistics Calculator

only Lusaka, the capital city, had a marked population growth (4 % a year), and a large size, being the only city with more that one million persons. In Tanzania, the urban population was still moderate in 2002 (23 %), although it has been increasing steadily since the first census conducted in 1967, so that urban growth was only 4.5 % a year in the recent period (1988–2002). Only Dar-es-Salaam had more than one million inhabitants. In Sierra Leone as well, urbanization was moderate and increasing slowly by African standards. The proportion urban was 28 % in 1974 and 37 % in 2004, with a very slow growth in the recent years (2.5 % a year between 1985 and 2004). In summary, none of the three countries seemed to have experienced fast urbanization or contained very large cities, both of which could have a strong negative impact on the health of urban dwellers. However, strong selection for migration still remains a possible explanation: if the most destitute population strata from rural areas moved to the cities, they could affect the balance between urban and rural mortality, but this argument remains purely speculative (Table 10.4).

Table 10.5 Change in selected socio-economic correlates of child mortality, three African countries

Year	Survey	Urban	Rural	Difference
Level of education: percent of women with primary+				
	Sierra Leone 2008	62.5	30.1	–32.4
	Tanzania 1991–1992	67.4	49.9	–17.4
	Tanzania 1996	74.4	53.5	–20.9
	Tanzania 1999	77.1	54.2	–23.0
	Tanzania 2004–2005	82.3	61.5	–20.8
	Tanzania 2010	87.8	68.9	–18.9
	Zambia 1992	88.5	63.5	–25.0
	Zambia 1996	87.2	66.3	–21.0
	Zambia 2001–2002	87.0	68.2	–18.8
	Zambia 2007	90.8	73.1	–17.6
Household poverty (percent very poor = AWI < 3)				
	Sierra Leone 2008	44.4	94.8	50.4
	Tanzania 1991–1992	53.7	93.3	39.6
	Tanzania 1996	42.7	90.6	48.0
	Tanzania 1999	43.7	92.8	49.1
	Tanzania 2004–2005	37.3	87.0	49.7
	Tanzania 2010	34.2	85.2	51.0
	Zambia 1992	29.1	91.9	62.7
	Zambia 1996	30.3	92.5	62.3
	Zambia 2001–2002	30.7	90.9	60.3
	Zambia 2007	25.2	88.5	63.3

Source: Level of education: DHS web site, Statistics Calculator
Poverty: Author's calculation from DHS data

Socio-Economic Correlates

Two socio-economic correlates were investigated: wealth and education. Poverty was defined as the proportion of households with less than 3 modern goods out of a list of 14 items. This proportion was considerably higher in rural areas than in urban areas, as expected. The gap in poverty between both areas ranged from 40–60 %. Even though wealth improved in Zambia and Tanzania, the gap between urban and rural areas tended rather to increase over time and this was visible both for the proportion in poverty and for the average absolute wealth index.

The gap in level of education between urban and rural areas was also very large. Common values of the urban/rural differences in proportions of adults with at least primary level ranged from 20–30 % in the three countries. In Zambia, the gap tended to narrow steadily over the years, reflecting a serious effort in increasing the level in rural areas. In Tanzania, the average level was lower, and it increased in both sectors at about the same speed (Table 10.5).

In summary, trends in socio-economic correlates of health could not explain the convergence of urban and rural mortality, even less the lower rural mortality in the recent years.

10.5 Discussion

This brief analysis focused on a new phenomenon, that of lower under-five mortality in rural areas of three African countries, compared with urban areas. This pattern was unexpected some 10 years ago, even though some countries displayed minor differences between the two sectors in the past (Garenne 2006). What was most surprising in this analysis was the fast mortality decline in rural areas, faster than that in urban areas, which was able to change the balance of mortality between the two sectors. The speed of the changes was also striking and unexpected in two of the three countries investigated.

The reasons for these surprising changes remain to be further explored. This analysis focused on health programs and emerging diseases as a likely explanation. A combination of more efforts in prevention and treatment of infectious diseases in rural areas, bridging the gap for selected diseases such as malaria, measles, tetanus, pertussis, diarrheal diseases, and acute respiratory infections which were the leading causes of children's death, together with the negative effects of HIV/AIDS more prevalent in urban areas could explain the changing balance between urban and rural areas.

This explanation makes sense, and reflects the fact that disease control programs seem to have had a major effect on mortality trends in the past 15 or 20 years. Coverage of prevention and treatment programs is now high enough to have a large effect on mortality levels and trends. Numerous cases of surprising decline in under-five mortality, given minor changes in wealth and education, have been documented in developing countries, and most likely these are due to improvements in health policies and programs. Unfortunately, only a few studies document in detail the impact of child survival programs and disease control programs (Ewbank 1993; Becker et al. 1993; Garenne et al. 2007).

The lack of correlation with socio-economic correlates is notable, and will surprise those who focus on education and wealth as critical factors of mortality trends. This is not to say that these two factors do not play a role on mortality differentials, but only that their dynamics explain almost nothing of the recent changes in the balance between urban and rural mortality.

Before 1985, developing countries seemed to have suffered a "rural penalty", simply because economic development, social change and improving health services were more rapid in cities, implying a real health advantage. We might be facing the opposite situation now, with a new "urban penalty", where the combined effect of emerging diseases, large pockets of poverty and the relatively better situation of rural areas changed the former balance between the two sectors.

The countries examined were the first three cases of lower rural mortality at national level in sub-Saharan Africa. More research is needed to investigate other emerging patterns in the future, since these are likely to occur in other places as well. However, the current negative impact of HIV/AIDS might change in the near future, so that the urban HIV handicap might disappear. Because of increasing prevention of mother to child transmission, and because of wide coverage of ARV treatment, HIV infected children may survive much better in the coming years, so that a gap in HIV prevalence between urban and rural areas will no longer translate into increased urban mortality. This has been documented already in case studies in South Africa, and may occur in other places (Herbst et al. 2009; Garenne et al. 2011).

The saga of urban/rural differences in under-five mortality is not finished, and this study shows how rapid changes may be in response to changing disease environment and disease control. Monitoring these effects is important, and could shed a new light on the impact of health policies and programs.

References

Ahmad, O. B., Lopez, A. D., & Inoue, M. (2000). The decline in child mortality: A reappraisal. *Bulletin of the World Health Organization, 78*(10), 1175–1191.

Antoine, P., & Diouf, P. D. (1988). Urbanisation, scolarisation et mortalité des enfants. *Annales de L'IFORD, 12*(1), 9–24.

APHRC. (2002). *Population and health dynamics in Nairobi's informal settlements* (p. 256). Nairobi: African Population and Health Research Centre.

Becker, S. R., Diop, F., & Thornton, J. N. (1993). Infant and child mortality in two counties of Liberia: Results of a survey in 1988 and trends since 1984. *International Journal of Epidemiology, 22*(Suppl 1), S56–S63.

Bocquier, P., Madise, N. J., & Zulu, E. M. (2011). Is there an urban advantage in child survival in sub-Saharan Africa? Evidence from 18 countries in the 1990s. *Demography, 48*(2), 531–558.

Brockerhoff, M. (1993). *Child survival in big cities: Are the poor disadvantaged?* (Population Council, Research Division Working Papers No 58, 53 p). New York: Population Council, Research Division.

Campbell, T., & Campbell, A. (2007). Emerging disease burdens and the poor in cities of the developing world. *Journal of Urban Health, 84*(Suppl 1), 54–64.

Egunjobi, L. (1991). Tackling Africa's slums. *World Health,* 14–15.

Ewbank, D. C. (1993). Impact of health programmes on child mortality in Africa: Evidence from Zaire and Liberia. *International Journal of Epidemiology, 22*(Suppl 1), S64–S72.

Foege, W. H., & Henderson, D. A. (1986). Selective primary health care. XXV. Management priorities. *Reviews of Infectious Diseases, 8*, 467–475.

Fotso, J. C. (2006). Child health inequities in developing countries: Differences across urban and rural areas. *International Journal for Equity in Health, 5*, 9.

Garenne, M. (2006). Migration, urbanisation and child health: An African perspective. In M. Tienda, S. E. Findley, S. Tollman, & E. Preston-Whyte (Eds.), *Africa on the move: African migration and urbanisation in comparative perspective* (pp. 252–279). Johannesburg: Wits University Press.

Garenne, M. (2011). The impact of HIV/AIDS on the health transition among under-five children in Africa. In G. Letamo (Ed.), *Social and psychological aspects of HIV/AIDS and their ramifications* (pp. 237–248). (Chapter 13). Rijeka: In-Tech Publishers.

Garenne, M., & Gakusi, E. (2004). *Reconstructing under-five mortality trends in Africa from demographic sample surveys* (DHS Working Papers No 26). Calverton: IRD-Macro.

Garenne, M., & Gakusi, E. (2006a). Health transitions in sub-Saharan Africa: Overview of mortality trends in children under-5-years-olds (1950–2000). *Bulletin WHO, 84*(6), 470–478.

Garenne, M., & Gakusi, E. (2006b). Vulnerability and resilience: Determinants of under-five mortality changes in Zambia. *World Development, 34*(10), 1765–1787.

Garenne, M., & Hohmann, S. (2003). A wealth index to screen high risk families: Application to Morocco. *Journal of Health, Population and Nutrition, 21*(3), 235–242.

Garenne, M., Darkaoui, N., Braikat, M., & Azelmat, M. (2007). Changing cause of death profile in Morocco: The impact of child-survival programs. *Journal of Health, Population and Nutrition, 25*(2), 212–220.

Garenne, M., Tollman, S., Kahn, K., & The Agincourt Team. (2011). *Trends in under-five mortality in countries with high HIV prevalence: When will they decline again?* Paper prepared for the UAPS conference (session 23), Ougadougou, Burkina-Faso, 5–9 December 2011.

Gilbert, A., & Gugler, J. (1992). *Cities, poverty and development*. Oxford: Oxford University Press.

Gould, W. T. S. (1998). African mortality and the new urban penalty. *Health and Place, 4*(2), 171–181.

Gracey, M. (2002). Child health in an urbanized world. *Acta Paediatrica, 91*, 1–8.

Haines, M. (2001). The urban mortality transition in the United States, 1800–1940. *Annales de Démographie Historique, 1*, 33–64.

Harpham, T., & Molyneux, C. (2001). Urban health in developing countries: A review. *Progress in Development Studies, 1*, I13–I37.

Harpham, T., & Stephens, C. (1991). Urban health in developing countries: From the shadows into the spotlight. *Tropical Diseases Bulletin, 88*(8), 1–35.

Harpham, T., Lusty, T., & Vaughan, P. (1988). *In the shadow of the city: Community health and the urban poor*. Oxford: Oxford University Press.

Herbst, A., Cooke, G., Bärnighausen, T., KanyKany, A., Tanser, F., & Newell, M. (2009). Adult mortality and antiretroviral treatment roll-out in rural KwaZulu-Natal, South Africa. *Bulletin of the World Health Organization, 87*, 754–762.

Hill, A. (1991). Infant and child mortality: Levels, trends and data deficiencies. In R. Feachem & D. Jamison (Eds.), *Disease and mortality in sub-Saharan Africa* (pp. 37–76). New York: World Bank/Oxford University Press.

Hill, K., & Yazbeck, A. (1994). *Trends in under-five mortality, 1960–90: Estimates for 84 developing countries*. Washington, DC: World Bank.

Hohmann, S., & Garenne, M. (2011). Absolute versus relative measures of poverty. Application to DHS African surveys. *Journal of US-China Public Administration, 8*(7), 748–762.

Kearns, G. (1988). The urban penalty and the population history of England. In A. Brändström & L. G. Telebrad (Eds.), *Society, health and population during the demographic transition* (pp. 231–236). Stockholm: Almqvist & Wiksell International.

Kearns, G. (1993). Le handicap urbain et la baisse de la mortalité en Angleterre et au Pays de Galles 1851–1900. *Annales de Démographie Historique, 1993*, 75–105.

Leon, D. A. (2008). Cities, urbanization and health. *International Journal of Epidemiology, 37*(1), 4–8.

Montgomery, M. R. (2009). Urban poverty and health in developing countries. [Population Reference Bureau]. *Population Bulletin, 64*(2), 20 p.

Montgomery, M. R., & Ezeh, A. C. (2005). The health of urban populations in developing countries. In S. Galea & D. Vlahov (Eds.), *Handbook of urban health: Populations, methods and practice* (pp. 201–222). New York: Springer.

Montgomery, M. R., Stren, R., Cohen, B., & Reed, H. E. (Eds.). (2004). *Cities transformed: Demographic change and its implications in the developing world* (pp. 108–154). London: Earthscan.

Newell, M. L., Brahmbhatt, H., & Ghys, P. D. (2004). Child mortality and HIV infection in Africa: A review. *AIDS, 18*(suppl 2), S27–S34.
Patel, R. B., & Burke, T. F. (2009). Urbanization: An emerging humanitarian disaster. *The New England Journal of Medicine, 361*, 741–743.
Preston, S. H. (1985). Resources, knowledge, and child mortality: A comparison of the US in the late nineteenth century and developing countries today. In *Proceedings of the IUSSP international population conference. Florence. June 5–12, 1985*, *4*, 373–388.
Preston, S. H., & Haines, M. (1991). *Fatal years: Child mortality in the late nineteenth century America*. Princeton: Princeton University Press.
Preston, S. H., & van de Walle, E. (1978). Urban French mortality in the nineteenth century. *Population Studies, 32*(2), 275–297.
Pryer, J. N., & Crook, N. (1988). *Cities of hunger: Urban malnutrition in developing countries*. Oxford: Oxfam.
Reher, D. S. (2001). In search of the urban penalty: Exploring urban and rural mortality patterns in Spain during the demographic transition. *International Journal of Population Geography, 7*, 105–127.
Rosen, G. (1958). *A history of public health*. New York: MD Publications.
Stolnitz, G. (1955). A century of international mortality trends, pt. 1. *Population Studies, 9*(1), 24–55.
Stolnitz, G. J. (1965). Recent mortality trends in Latin America, Asia and Africa: Review and re-interpretation. *Population Studies, 19*(2), 117–138.
Szreter, S., & Mooney, G. (1998). Urbanization, mortality and the standard of living debate: New estimates of the expectation of life at birth in the nineteenth-century British cities. *Economic History Review, 51*, 84–112.
Timaeus, I. M., & Lush, L. (1995). Intra-urban differentials in child health. *Health Transition Review, 5*(2), 163–190.
Van de Poel, A., O'Donnell, O., & van Doorslaer, E. (2007). Are urban children really healthier? Evidence from 47 developing countries. *Social Science & Medicine, 65*, 1986–2003.
Van der Woude, A. D. (1982). Population developments in the northern Netherlands (1500–1800) and the validity of the "urban graveyard effect". *Annales de Démographie Historique, 1982*, 55–75.
Van Poppel, F. (1989). Urban-rural regional differences in demographic behaviour: The Netherlands, 1850–1960. *Journal of Urban History, 15*, 363–398.
Walsh, J. A., & Warren, K. S. (1979). Selective primary health care: An interim strategy for disease control in developing countries. *The New England Journal of Medicine, 301*, 967–974.
Woods, R. (2003). Urban rural mortality differentials: An unresolved debate. *Population and Development Review, 29*, 29–46.
Woods, R. I., Patterson, P. A., & Woodward, J. H. (1988). Mortality decline in England and Wales, 1861–1921. *Population Studies, 42*(3), 343–366.

Chapter 11
Urban Mortality Transitions: The Role of Slums

Günther Fink, Isabel Günther, and Kenneth Hill

11.1 Introduction

From a historical perspective, the relation between urban residence and health outcomes has been mixed, with rather remarkable changes in trends over time. During the nineteenth century, European cities still showed higher mortality rates than rural areas (Williamson 1990; Woods 2003; Cain and Hong 2009). The urban mortality penalty disappeared with the rollout of public health interventions in high income countries at the end of the nineteenth century (Haines 1995), and turned into an urban mortality advantage with the introduction of effective therapeutic interventions in the early twentieth century.

The low and middle income countries (LMICs) of today may have followed a different trajectory. Gould (1998) and Johnson (1964) argue that urban areas in developing countries have had lower mortality than rural areas since the nineteenth century and at least by the end of the twentieth century urban populations typically had lower mortality levels than rural populations in all developing countries. Figure 11.1 summarizes urban to rural mortality ratios in childhood across a large number of nationally-representative household surveys conducted by the Demographic and Health Surveys program in several LMICs starting in the mid-1980s. Three measures of mortality are displayed: the neonatal mortality rate, post-neonatal mortality rate, and the probability of dying between the ages of 1 and 5 years. Since for all

G. Fink (✉) • K. Hill
Global Health and Population, Harvard T.H. Chan School of Public Health, Boston, MA, USA
e-mail: gfink@hsph.harvard.edu; kenneth_hill@harvard.edu

I. Günther
Center for Development and Cooperation, ETH Zürich, Zürich, Switzerland
e-mail: guenther@nadel.ethz.ch

D. Ramiro Fariñas, M. Oris (eds.), *New Approaches to Death in Cities during the Health Transition*, International Studies in Population 12,
DOI 10.1007/978-3-319-43002-7_11

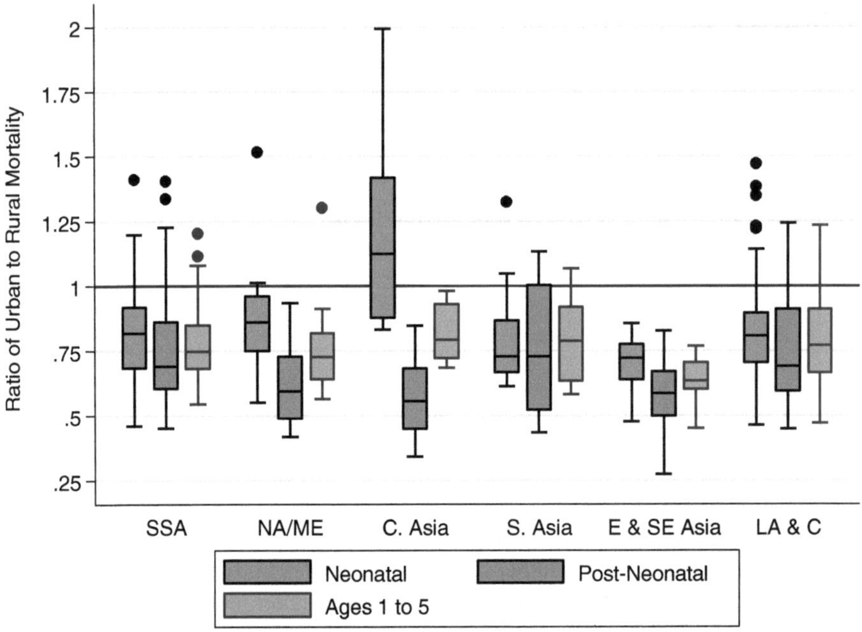

Fig. 11.1 Country-specific ratios of urban to rural child mortality by world region (Note: Data accessed through Statcompiler 18 July 2011. Based on 198 surveys over the period 1985–2010)

(except one) measures and all regions the median ratio is below 1.0, the existence of an urban child mortality advantage seems to be clear.

The ratios presented in Fig. 11.1 – indicating a clear urban mortality advantage – might, however, hide important mortality differentials resulting from the dual nature of LMIC cities, combining low with high mortality urban areas. The increasingly large populations living in, and moving to, LMIC cities have led to the formation of large and rapidly growing informal urban settlements often referred to as "slums" over the past decades. According to the United Nations, more than one billion people, or about 14 % of the total global population live in slum areas today (UN-HABITAT 2007). Outsiders visiting such slums are often repulsed by the sights and smells they encounter, and assume that the health consequences must be disastrous (bringing to mind the nineteenth century concept of miasma in European cities). Given the similarities between these areas and high income country cities in nineteenth century in terms of income, overcrowding and low water and sanitation standards, a mortality disadvantage is generally presumed for urban slums.

Recent analysis has therefore suggested that excess mortality in slums is delaying mortality transitions in LMICs, reminiscent of the history of high income countries in the nineteenth century (see Chaps. 5 and 7 in this volume and Moore, Gouldet et al. 2003; Sclar, Garau et al. 2005; Konteh 2009). However, evidence on mortality differentials and on their potential effects on the mortality transition is scarce and far from conclusive. Montgomery et al.(2003) analyse Demographic and

Health Survey (DHS) data from 56 surveys and document a general mortality childhood mortality risk gap in favour of urban households, while highlighting that specific urban sub-populations can face higher mortality risks than rural populations. In a related study of 85 DHS surveys, Montgomery and Hewett (2005) find that poor households are often spatially intermingled with well-off households in urban areas, but also that areas of concentrated poverty are generally associated with lower rates of health service utilization. Fotso (2007) use DHS data from African cities supplemented with data from demographic surveillance sites to examine trends in urban child mortality. They find that the pace of decline in urban mortality in sub-Saharan Africa has in most countries been below that needed to achieve the target of Millennium Development Goal 4 (to reduce the under-5 mortality rate by two-thirds between 1990 and 2015), and also note the emergence of intra-urban mortality differentials. In a study of 18 African countries, Bocquier et al. (2011) find that after controlling for known demographic and socio-economic correlates of childhood mortality, urban advantages are greatly reduced or indeed reversed. Günther and Harttgen (2012) analyse data from 18 African countries and find that child mortality rates in slum areas are significantly higher than in non-slum urban areas but lower than in rural areas in most countries. Timaeus and Lush (1995) analyse four countries for intra-urban differentials in child health and find that the mortality difference between the urban poor and non-poor is larger than the difference between rural and urban populations.

We build and expand on this literature, investigating both the overall within-urban mortality differentials and their impact on the mortality transition in LMICs. Methodologically, this paper deviates from the existing literature along two dimensions: the use of age-specific mortality measures, and the introduction and application of a community- rather than household-based definition of slums. Given that the urban context is likely to have differential effects on mortality risks at different ages due to the differences in the underlying epidemiology, we separately analyse three age brackets: neonatal mortality, post-neonatal mortality, and mortality 12–36 months. In contrast to previous studies and UN Habitat (2007) – which define a slum household as a household lacking one or more key facilities independent of the household's surroundings – we adopt a community-based definition of slums, classifying only those urban areas where a majority of households lack basic infrastructure as slum neighbourhoods, and further distinguish slum areas within small and large urban settlements.

11.2 Data and Methodology

The data used in this paper are from the Demographic and Health Surveys (DHS). The DHS are population-based nationally representative surveys with a particular focus on fertility and reproductive health. Largely funded by USAID, 188 DHS surveys have been conducted in 76 countries since 1986 and made publicly

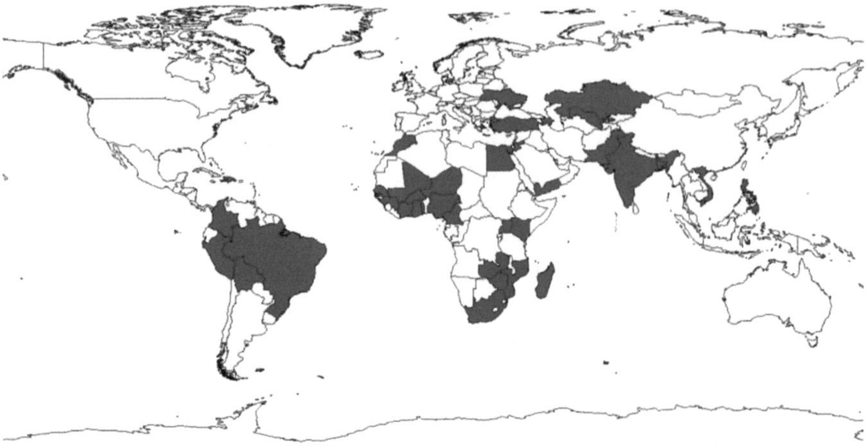

Fig. 11.2 Sample of 37 countries with large cities and available DHS

available.[1] Since we want to distinguish small towns from large urban areas, we limit our analysis to countries with at least one city with a population of one million or larger in 2010, as estimated by the United Nations Population Division (2010). Out of the countries covered by the DHS, 49 countries (and 146 surveys) have at least one such large city in 2010, and thus meet the primary inclusion criterion for this paper. Out of these 146 surveys, 74 surveys do not have information on the household characteristics needed for the slum coding, and thus could not be included, leaving us with a total of 72 surveys across 37 countries. As Fig. 11.2 illustrates, about half of our sample is in sub-Saharan Africa with the rest evenly distributed among Asian and Latin American countries. A full country and year listing is provided in Appendix.

City Classification

The DHS surveys do not provide – at least in the publicly accessible data sets – information on the exact household location. The main geographic information provided by the DHS is the region (administrative unit) the household is located in (DHS standard recode variable hv024). In addition, DHS surveys provide information on the "type" of residence (urban vs. rural, hv025) as well as the "place" of residence, which is divided into rural, small town, and larger city (hv026).

For the purpose of our analysis, households are classified as rural if their "type" of residence is rural (hv025). To investigate whether large urban agglomerations or "cities" as well as their respective slum areas fare differently from smaller urban settlements, we divide urban type of residence (hv025) into "towns" (small urban

[1] 23 August 2011, www.measuredhs.com

areas) and "cities" (urban settlements with a total population estimated to be at least one million in 2009 (UNDP 2011)). Most developing countries have only one or two large cities – in most cases the capital – with the notable exceptions of Brazil and India with over 20 and 40 urban agglomerations above one million inhabitants, respectively (see Appendix).

In order to distinguish towns from cities, we use a combination of spatial variables provided by the DHS. In many cases, large agglomerations, and especially capital areas, constitute separate administrative regions (hv024), in which case the coding is straightforward. To make sure none of the households in these areas are rural settlements at the outskirts of larger urban areas, we check that all of the households placed in these areas are classified as urban according to the "type" of residence (hv025).

For some countries – namely Brazil, Colombia, Egypt, India, Jordan, Morocco, Nigeria, Pakistan, South Africa, Ukraine, Turkey, and Yemen – the regional coding was too coarse to allow a direct mapping from administrative regions into specific urban areas. For these countries we used the DHS variable on "type of place" of residence (hv026), categorizing observations into rural, small town and large city. Given that the DHS definition of "large city" is not necessarily consistent with our one million population threshold, the coding outcomes in these countries are not as precise as the coding in the rest of the sample. We address this issue in a robustness check later in the chapter.

Slum Classification

We are interested in slum mortality relative to mortality in other urban or rural areas. One of the main challenges with this research question lies in the fact that the concept of slums is not clearly defined in general. UN Habitat (UN Habitat 2007) uses a household-based slum definition, and considers any household a slum household if it lacks any one of the following five elements:

- Access to improved water (*access to sufficient amount of water for family use, at an affordable price, available to household members without being subject to extreme effort);*
- Access to improved sanitation (*access to an excreta disposal system, either in the form of a private toilet or a public toilet shared with a reasonable number of people);*
- Durability of housing (*permanent and adequate structure in non-hazardous location)*
- Sufficient living area (*not more than two people sharing the same room)*
- Security of tenure (*evidence of documentation to prove secure tenure status or de facto or perceived protection from evictions*)

While we view each of the five aspects as a good indicator of poor living conditions, the household-based definition of slums appears inconsistent with the more commonly used concept of slums as generally poor areas, i.e. an agglomeration, settlement or neighbourhood of sub-standard housing rather than a single poor house in an otherwise possibly wealthy neighbourhood. For example, Merriam Webster defines a slum as "a densely populated usually urban area marked by crowding, dirty run-down housing, poverty, and social disorganization" (Merriam Webster 2011, http://www.merriam-webster.com/). This distinction appears particularly relevant in the context of health, where a large fraction of health hazards is determined by the household surroundings and environment, and not necessarily by the household itself.

To concur with this general perception of slums we focus on neighbourhoods to define slums in this study. The main unit of analysis for defining slums are the sampling units used by the DHS. DHS surveys are usually carried out applying a two-stage sampling procedure with clusters of about 200 households as a sampling unit, typically representing a single census enumeration area. Prior to the survey, all households are listed, and approximately one in eight households in each area is randomly selected for the interview.

Based on the UN Habitat characteristics listed above, we define a neighbourhood (or, to be precise, a cluster) to be a slum if it is located in an urban area and at least 75 % of households lack at least two of the following characteristics: safe water access, adequate sanitation access, sufficient living space, and solid housing material.[2] The DHS surveys do not collect data on property rights, so that we are unable to address security of tenure as the 5th criterion of slum households as proposed by UN Habitat. While it would have been preferable to include all five UN criteria, security of tenure is extremely hard to define in many developing countries. However, given that all slum measures appear to be highly correlated, adding a fifth dimensions is unlikely to change the classification of households more than marginally.

The use of cluster-level characteristics for the residential coding has important implications for the interpretation of the estimated coefficient on the slum variable. In our definition, households lacking basic facilities but not located in a slum area are hence not defined as slum households. On the other hand, households that are not reported as having poor housing conditions but are located in an area where most other households do lack basic infrastructure are considered as slum households. It is also worth highlighting that our definition is stricter than the UN Habitat's definition in that it requires households to display more than one slum characteristic. The reason for this choice is simply that most households in urban areas of developing countries are deficient of at least one housing characteristic (Günther and Harttgen 2012), so that a majority of households and neighbourhoods would be

[2] Households are considered without access to safe water if the household does not have access to a private or public pipe, bore hole, or a protected well or spring. Households are defined as being deprived of basic sanitation if they either rely on open defecation or use an unimproved pit latrine. Shared sanitation facilities are considered as basic sanitation if they provide access to a flush toilet or ventilated improved pit latrine. A dwelling is considered as overcrowded if there are more than three persons per habitable room. If the floor material of a house is made of earth, dung, sand or wood its structure is considered inadequate.

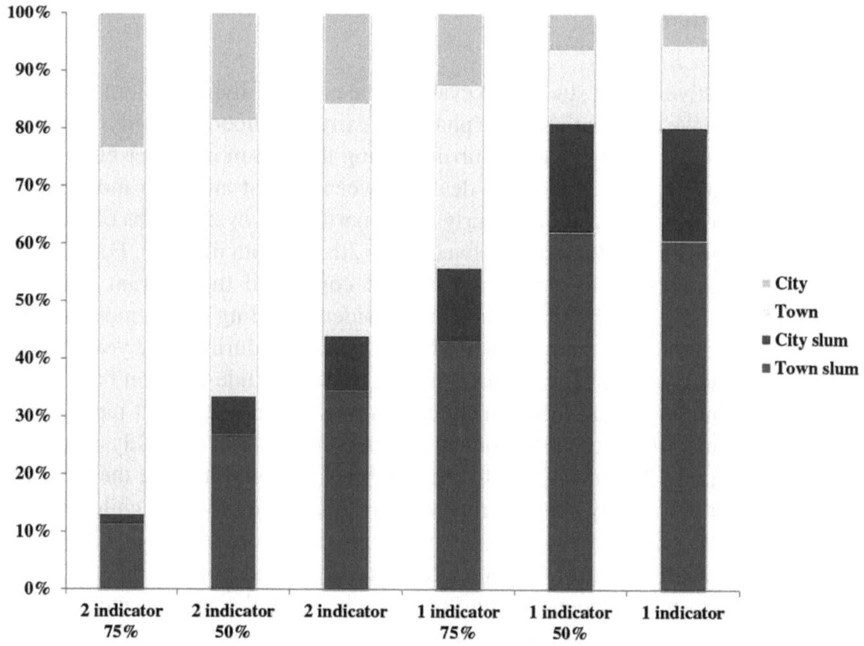

Fig. 11.3 Prevalence of slum households according to different definitions

considered as slums using the standard "one-criterion" cut-off. Similarly, nearly all urban areas would be classified as slums due to the presence of a single household, or small share of households, lacking basic services. Determining a minimum critical threshold for a neighbourhood to be defined as slum is not obvious, and as illustrated in Fig. 11.3, results in largely different fraction of neighbourhoods being defined as slums.

The first column of Fig. 11.3 shows the most restrictive coding, which requires that at least 75 % of households lack basic services. Under this assumption, 13 % of urban households are coded as slums. Under a coding rule relying on a simple majority of deprived households (column 2), 34 % of children would live in areas classified as slums. If a household-based definition was used with 2 indicators, 44 % of households would be defined as slum households (column 3). If a large majority (75 %) of households lacking only at least one basic facility were the criterion for a slum neighbourhood, 56 % of urban households would be considered slum households (column 4). Last, if the UN-Habit definition of households lacking at least one feature were applied – either at the individual or with a simple majority 50 % cut-off at the cluster level – more than 80 % of urban households would be classified as slum households. Since we are mostly interested in the poorest neighbourhoods we use the first definition for our preferred empirical specification, and show results for alternative classification rules later in the robustness check section.

Mortality Outcomes

The main objective of this study is to evaluate the effect of living in slums on early child mortality. We differentiate three phases of early childhood mortality. Neonatal mortality is defined as any death occurring during the first month after birth. Post-neonatal mortality covers children's death between the 1st and 12th months of a child's life, and what we call here "early child mortality" covers deaths of children between the ages of 1 and 3 years (between the 12th and 36th months). For all three measures we analyse only children who have completed the relevant exposure period. In order to keep the risk of incorrect residence coding due to mobility to a minimum, we restrict our analysis to mortality that occurs during the 3 years before the respective survey year. For neonatal mortality, we exclude children born in the month of the interview, and focus on children who were born at least 1 month prior to the survey interview. For post-neonatal mortality, we restrict our analysis to children born at least 12 months prior to the interview, and still alive at the age of 1 month. Similarly, for early child mortality, we restrict our analysis to children born at least 36 month prior to the interview who did not die before the age of 12 months. Accordingly, our measure of "early child mortality" does not correspond to the standard ${}_4q_1$ measure of the probability of dying between the ages of one and five, but rather reflects the cohort-specific probability of dying between the 12th and 36th months.

Figure 11.4 summarize the three mortality variables for rural, town, and city, as well as for slum areas. All figures reflect sample averages, and thus represent unweighted estimates across our entire sample. On average, mortality rates for neonatal, post-neonatal and early child periods are 30, 30, and 26 deaths per 1000, respectively. Towns and cities show substantially lower rates for all three mortality rates. The mortality gap between residential areas appears to be smallest for neonatal mortality, and largest for early child mortality.

Empirical Model

To investigate the effect of residence on child mortality in more detail we estimate a series of empirical models with an increasing set of control variables. The basic logistic model we estimate can be described as follows:

$$\ln\left(\frac{p_{ick}}{1-p_{ick}}\right) = \alpha + \sum_{j=1}^{4} R_j\beta_j + \sum_{k=1}^{71} S_k\delta_k + \varepsilon_{ick}, \tag{11.1}$$

where p_{ik} is the probability of death of child i in cluster c and survey k in the interval of interest, α is a generic constant, R_j are indicator variables for town and city residence, as well as for town and city slums. S_k are survey fixed effects to capture country-period or survey fixed factors affecting all children in a given survey.

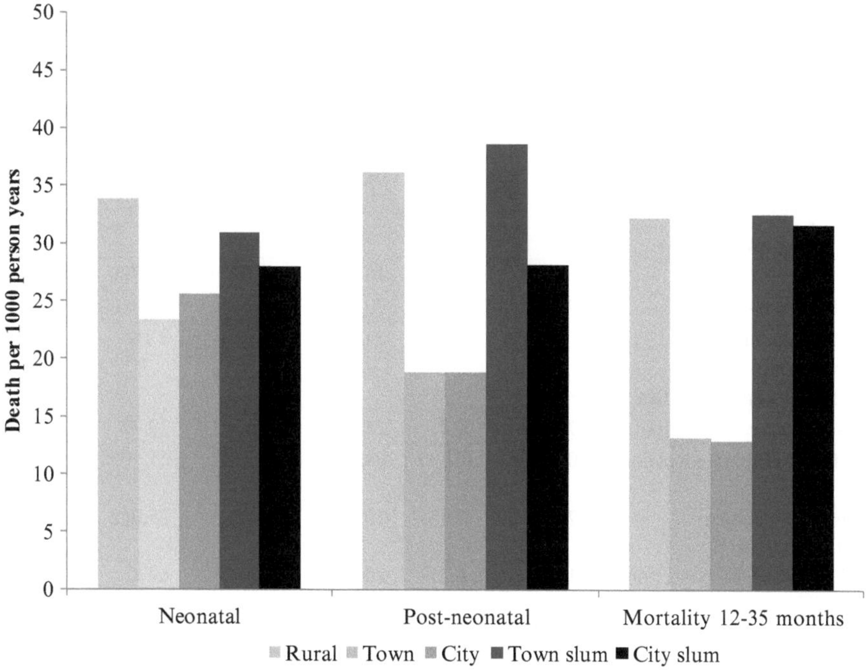

Fig. 11.4 Child mortality by residence (full sample)

Since we want to investigate the total effect of slum residence as well as the effect of slum residence conditional on household characteristics, we show a series of empirical estimates: we control for a varying set of child, mother and family structure characteristics, to allow us to identify the mortality differences directly attributable to local living conditions keeping individual and family characteristics constant.

To see how much our mortality estimates are affected by differences in the underlying population, we start by estimating a basic model without additional controls as described in Eq. (11.1). In model 2, we add a set of child characteristics, including the child's sex, the child's age, and an indicator of whether the child was one of a multiple birth. In Model 3, we control both for child and for mother characteristics, including mother's age, mother's education and mother's marital status. Last, in model 4, we also add controls for the partner's education, household size, and sex of the household head.

11.3 Results

Table 11.1 shows unweighted descriptive statistics for the sample of children used in our analysis. The total sample consists of 510,994 children under the age of 3 observed across 72 surveys in 37 countries. The average age of children in the neonatal death sample is 1.2 years, the average age in the post-neonatal group is 2.1,

Table 11.1 Descriptive statistics

	Neonatal mortality		Post-neonatal mortality		Early child mortality	
	N=*344,984*		*N*=*315,101*		*N*=*101,694*	
Neonatal mortality, *N (%)*	10,512	(3.0)				
Infant mortality			9573	(3.0)		
Early child mortality					2591	(2.5)
Child characteristics						
Female, *N (%)*	169,101	(49.0)	154,647	(49.1)	49,779	(48.9)
Multiple births, *N (%)*	8952	(2.6)	7078	(2.2)	2126	(2.1)
Child age in yeas, *mean (SD)*	1.12	(0.9)	2.08	(0.9)	3.18	(0.4)
Mother characteristics						
Age mother, *mean (SD)*	27.77	(6.7)	28.66	(6.7)	29.72	(6.6)
Mother primary education, *N (%)*	107,967	(31.3)	98,460	(31.2)	31,105	(30.6)
Mother secondary education, *N (%)*	87,239	(25.3)	79,008	(25.1)	25,062	(24.6)
Mother tertiary education, *N (%)*	21,469	(6.2)	20,312	(6.4)	6970	(6.9)
Mother currently married, *N (%)*	258,898	(75.0)	236,728	(75.1)	76,380	(75.1)
Family characteristics						
Partner primary education, *N (%)*	91,625	(26.6)	85,291	(27.1)	27,575	(27.1)
Partner secondary education, *N (%)*	99,776	(28.9)	90,889	(28.8)	29,129	(28.6)
Partner tertiary education, *N (%)*	29,718	(8.6)	28,078	(8.9)	9533	(9.4)
Household size, *mean (SD)*	7.43	(4.5)	7.42	(4.5)	7.54	(4.5)
Household head female, *N (%)*	46,686	(13.5)	42,397	(13.5)	13,386	(13.2)

and the average child in the early child sample is 3.2 years old. The other characteristics look fairly similar across the three subsamples. 49 % of children are female, and about 2.5 % of children are multiple births. The average age of mothers is 28.5 years. Mothers' educational attainment is low on average, with only 6.5 % having pursued higher education, 25 % having attained some secondary, 31 % having attained some primary education, and 38 % of mothers not having received any schooling. Seventy-five percent of mothers are married at the date of the interview, with average education levels of partners only slightly above maternal educational attainment. The average household contains 7.5 members, and 13.4 % of households are headed by a female. In total, 22,767 deaths under the age of 3 are recorded and analysed in our sample.

Residential Differences in Mortality

Tables 11.2, 11.3 and 11.4 show the main results (as odd ratios) for the three mortality variables of interest as well as for the four empirical models described in the previous section. Three main findings emerge from these tables. First, the protective effects of town and city residence are large and statistically significant at all standard confidence intervals. Once we fully control for child, mother and household

Table 11.2 Neonatal Mortality

	Probability of death during first month of life			
Dependent	(1)	(2)	(3)	(4)
Town	0.784***	0.778***	0.859***	0.864***
	(0.0257)	(0.0256)	(0.0286)	(0.0290)
City	0.762***	0.764***	0.860***	0.853***
	(0.0352)	(0.0355)	(0.0409)	(0.0407)
Town slum	0.920	0.916*	0.943	0.957
	(0.0489)	(0.0486)	(0.0501)	(0.0507)
City slum	0.801*	0.795*	0.819	0.811
	(0.102)	(0.103)	(0.107)	(0.106)
Survey fixed effects	Yes	Yes	Yes	Yes
Child controls	No	Yes	Yes	Yes
Mother controls	No	No	Yes	Yes
Household controls	No	No	No	Yes
Observations	344,984	344,984	344,984	344,984

Notes: *Robust z-statistics in parentheses are clustered at the country-cluster level*
Significance: *p<0.1; **p<0.05; ***p<0.01

Table 11.3 Post-neonatal mortality

	Probability of death month 1–11			
Dependent	(1)	(2)	(3)	(4)
Town	0.640***	0.638***	0.762***	0.787***
	(0.0221)	(0.0220)	(0.0270)	(0.0282)
City	0.550***	0.552***	0.678***	0.694***
	(0.0281)	(0.0282)	(0.0351)	(0.0361)
Town slum	0.989	0.984	1.034	1.065
	(0.0485)	(0.0481)	(0.0507)	(0.0522)
City slum	0.805	0.811	0.869	0.877
	(0.116)	(0.118)	(0.124)	(0.125)
Survey fixed effects	Yes	Yes	Yes	Yes
Child controls	No	Yes	Yes	Yes
Mother controls	No	No	Yes	Yes
Household controls	No	No	No	Yes
Observations	315,101	315,101	315,101	315,101

Notes: *Robust z-statistics in parentheses are clustered at the country-cluster level*
Significance: *p<0.1; **p<0.05; ***p<0.01

Table 11.4 Early child mortality (Months 12–35)

	Probability of death age 12–35 months			
Dependent	(1)	(2)	(3)	(4)
Town	0.576***	0.576***	0.695***	0.709***
	(0.0375)	(0.0375)	(0.0469)	(0.0482)
City	0.439***	0.441***	0.545***	0.554***
	(0.0464)	(0.0467)	(0.0582)	(0.0594)
Town slum	0.974	0.971	1.024	1.042
	(0.0902)	(0.0898)	(0.0952)	(0.0974)
City slum	0.924	0.920	0.981	0.979
	(0.230)	(0.231)	(0.242)	(0.244)
Survey fixed effects	Yes	Yes	Yes	Yes
Child controls	No	Yes	Yes	Yes
Mother controls	No	No	Yes	Yes
Household controls	No	No	No	Yes
Observations	101,694	101,694	101,694	101,694

Notes: Robust z-statistics in parentheses are clustered at the country-cluster level. 760 observations are perfectly predicted by the covariates and dropped from analysis
Significance: *$p<0.1$; **$p<0.05$; ***$p<0.01$

structure (column 4), we find that urban residence substantially lowers the odds of neonatal, post-neonatal and early child mortality relative to rural. On average, urban children faces 25–35 % lower odds of mortality, with the largest effect for early child mortality in cities: an estimated odds ratio of 0.554 suggests that all else equal, children living in large cities faces 44.6 % lower odds of dying between age 12 and 36 months. As already suggested by Fig. 11.2, the protective effect of living in urban areas appears smallest for neonatal mortality with estimated protective effects of 13.6 (town) and 14.7 (city) percent, respectively.

Second, and most importantly for the question raised in this paper, we find that children in slums have mortality risks that are not statistically significantly different from those of children in rural areas, but are in general much higher than those of non-slum urban children. While the point estimates reported in Tables 11.2 and 11.3 suggest that slum residents fare on average slightly better than rural residents for neonatal as well as post-neonatal mortality we cannot reject the null that mortality in these areas does not differ from mortality in rural areas once a full set of controls is added. Taking all three age brackets together, the overall risks faced by urban slum dwellers appear to be largely the same as the risks faced by children growing up in rural areas.

With respect to different model specifications, maternal education appears to be the main confounder in the unconditional comparisons between urban and rural, as well as between urban non-slum and slum areas. A basic comparison of the odds ratios presented in columns 2 and 3 of Tables 11.2, 11.3 and 11.4 suggests that controlling for maternal characteristics reduces the observed odds ratios by 10–20 %

across all three age brackets. These differences appear to be mostly driven by differences in maternal education. On average, 48 % of mothers in rural areas have less than primary education, while the same is true only for 18 % of women in towns, and 19 % of women in cities. In the sample analysed, educational attainment of slum dwellers lies nearly perfectly in between these two groups, with 34 % (35 %) of mothers living in town slums (city slums) with less than primary education. Hence, controlling for mothers' education, which is higher in both urban non-slum and slum areas than in rural areas, the urban mortality advantage decreases (in relation to rural areas), but, as Tables 11.2, 11.3 and 11.4 suggest, does not disappear.

Robustness Checks

One of the main challenges faced during the data coding for this study was the proper classification of households into residential categories. As discussed in Sect. 11.2, in some surveys classification of urban households into "town" or "city" residence was not obvious, raising concerns regarding the quality of the coding as well as the potential biases induced by measurement error. To ensure that this type of measurement error does not affect our main results, we have run a series of auxiliary regressions, where we re-estimate column 4 of Tables 11.2, 11.3 and 11.4 for a subsample of surveys where the urban coding is unambiguous. The comparison of columns 1–3 (full sample) with columns 4–6 (high quality sample) of Table 11.5 shows that no major differences between the full and the restricted (high-quality) sample can be detected. The only notable change is a slightly lower odds-ratio for neonatal

Table 11.5 Robustness check 1: urban coding quality

	Full sample			High quality coding sample		
	Neonatal	Post-neonatal	Early child mortality	Neonatal	Post-neonatal	Early child mortality
Dependent	(1)	(2)	(3)	(4)	(5)	(6)
Town	0.864***	0.787***	0.709***	0.850***	0.788***	0.760***
	(0.0290)	(0.0282)	(0.0482)	(0.0349)	(0.0316)	(0.0601)
City	0.853***	0.694***	0.554***	0.859***	0.685***	0.591***
	(0.0407)	(0.0361)	(0.0594)	(0.0503)	(0.0407)	(0.0681)
Town slum	0.957	1.065	1.042	0.883**	1.068	1.141
	(0.0507)	(0.0522)	(0.0974)	(0.0527)	(0.0564)	(0.114)
City slum	0.811	0.877	0.979	0.836	0.745	0.885
	(0.106)	(0.125)	(0.244)	(0.130)	(0.135)	(0.265)
Observations	344,984	315,101	101,694	257,090	231,068	71,439

Notes: All specifications include a complete set of child, mother and household characteristics as well survey fixed effects. Robust z-statistics in parentheses are clustered at the country-cluster level. The sample used in columns 4–6 exclude Brazil, Colombia, Egypt, India, Jordan, Morocco, Nigeria, Pakistan, South Africa, Turkey, Ukraine and Yemen

Significance: *p<0.1; **p<0.05; ***p<0.01

Table 11.6 Robustness check 2: relevance of slum definition

	Cluster definition			UN habitat definition		
	Neonatal	Post-neonatal	Early child mortality	Neonatal	Post-neonatal	Early child mortality
Dependent	(1)	(2)	(3)	(4)	(5)	(6)
Town	0.864***	0.787***	0.709***	1.025	0.741***	0.686***
	(0.0290)	(0.0282)	(0.0482)	(0.0655)	(0.0577)	(0.0629)
City	0.853***	0.694***	0.554***	0.923	0.682***	0.615**
	(0.0407)	(0.0361)	(0.0594)	(0.0900)	(0.0728)	(0.129)
Town slum	0.957	1.065	1.042	0.859***	0.872***	1.064
	(0.0507)	(0.0522)	(0.0974)	(0.0265)	(0.0269)	(0.0837)
City slum	0.811	0.877	0.979	0.841***	0.717***	0.611***
	(0.106)	(0.125)	(0.244)	(0.0404)	(0.0380)	(0.0667)
Observations	344,984	315,101	101,694	344,935	314,926	101,488

Notes: All specifications include a complete set of child, mother and household characteristics as well survey fixed effects. Robust z-statistics in parentheses
Significance: *p<0.1; **p<0.05; ***p<0.01

mortality in town slums; however, the difference between the estimated coefficients in columns 1 and 4 is however not significantly different from zero at standard confidence intervals.

To address any concerns with regard to the validity of our slum definition, we compare our main results to a set of regression estimates based on the much wider household-based slum definition suggested by UN Habitat in Table 11.6. Similar to the structure in Table 11.5, we show the results from our preferred specification in columns 1–3 of Table 11.6, and then show the results based on the alternative model in columns 4–6. While the estimated coefficients continue to highlight a general urban mortality advantage, the results for slums change under the UN Habitat definition, suggesting a substantial and statistically significant mortality gap in favour of urban slum dwellers relative to their rural counterpart for infant and post-neonatal mortality. It is important to stress here that these estimates cannot be directly compared. Given that 80 % of urban children are considered slum dwellers under this definition as illustrated in Fig. 11.3, the results displayed in columns 4–6 of Table 11.6 simply show that (i) the average urban child fares betters than the average rural child, and that (ii) the top quintile of urban children (those not classified as slums) fare better than the rest of urban children only with respect to post-neonatal and early child mortality.

Mortality Transitions

In order to investigate changes in childhood mortality by residence over time, we divide our sample into observations pre- and post-2000, and repeat the regressions displayed in Tables 11.2, 11.3 and 11.4, interacting the residential indicators with a dummy variable which marks observations based on surveys conducted in 2000 or later. We carry out this analysis using both ordinary least squares regression (OLS) to show absolute differences in mortality probabilities and using logistic regression to estimate relative change (odds ratios). In order to avoid compositional bias, we restrict our analysis to countries with at least one survey before 2000 and after 2000, and include country fixed effects in all of our specifications.[3] Table 11.7 shows the results of this estimation: the first three columns show results using standard OLS models; columns 4–6 show odds ratios estimated in standard logistic models.

The most striking result emerging from Table 11.7 is the rather remarkable progress in child mortality made between the 1990s and the early 2000s. The estimated coefficient on the post-indicator suggests that on average neonatal, post-neonatal and child mortality declined by 8, 15 and 18 deaths per 1000 children in rural areas (columns 1–3), which translates into 23, 35 and 47 % lower odds of death in the respective age groups. Urban children appear to have on average experienced slightly smaller improvements relative to rural children with respect to post-neonatal mortality. Estimated coefficients of 0.005 and 0.007 suggest that urban areas experienced approximately only half the mortality improvements experienced by rural children in this age range. Town slums appear to have improved more than rural areas with respect to early child mortality; no such patterns can be detected for the two other mortality categories as well as for city slums, suggesting that overall the improvements in mortality experienced in slum is fairly similar to the improvements seen in rural areas, and slightly above the improvements in urban areas. In terms of relative improvement, the differences across residential areas appear even smaller, with all areas experiencing unconditional improvements in mortality rates of approximately 20 % relative to the pre 2000 period.

11.4 Discussion and Conclusion

The results presented in the previous section of this paper demonstrate that children in non-slum urban settlements experience up to 15 % lower odds of neonatal, 30 % lower odds of post-neonatal, and up to 45 % lower odds of early child mortality compared to children in rural areas, but that no systematic mortality differences exist between rural children and children residing in the most deprived slum neighbourhoods. Moreover, child mortality changes over time do not seem to appear slower in urban slum areas than among rural households. Given the rapid pace of urbanization observed over the past decades in developing countries (Bloom et al. 2010), this raises the question of how urbanization in general, and the formation of urban slums in particular, have affected mortality rates and changes at the country level.

---

[3] In order to be able to estimate pre-post differences, survey-fixed effects cannot be included in the empirical model.

Table 11.7 Changes in mortality 1990–2000s

Model	Absolute changes (OLS)		Relative changes (Logistic model, odds-ratios)			
	Neonatal	Post-neonatal	Early child mortality	Neonatal	Post-neonatal	Early child mortality
Dependent	(1)	(2)	(3)	(4)	(5)	(6)
Town	−0.00632***	−0.00827***	−0.0104***	0.794***	0.810***	0.740**
	(0.00145)	(0.00162)	(0.00269)	(0.0472)	(0.0503)	(0.0891)
City	−0.00382	−0.0122***	−0.0128***	0.893	0.712***	0.699**
	(0.00244)	(0.00228)	(0.00410)	(0.0840)	(0.0664)	(0.119)
Town slum	−0.00437*	0.00297	0.0109*	0.863*	1.075	1.396**
	(0.00233)	(0.00301)	(0.00567)	(0.0695)	(0.0750)	(0.195)
City slum	−0.00430	−0.00595	−0.00325	0.857	0.874	0.871
	(0.00630)	(0.00774)	(0.0159)	(0.194)	(0.192)	(0.354)
Post	−0.00751***	−0.0148***	−0.0176***	0.772***	0.645***	0.525***
	(0.00109)	(0.00125)	(0.00234)	(0.0275)	(0.0228)	(0.0382)
Town x post	0.00252	0.00509***	0.00447	1.070	0.982	0.907
	(0.00181)	(0.00190)	(0.00307)	(0.0828)	(0.0828)	(0.137)
City x post	−0.000432	0.00680**	−0.00306	0.961	1.180	0.706
	(0.00345)	(0.00341)	(0.00523)	(0.133)	(0.169)	(0.190)
Town slum x post	0.00415	−0.00459	−0.0186***	1.170	0.901	0.565***
	(0.00370)	(0.00414)	(0.00713)	(0.150)	(0.106)	(0.117)
City slum x post	−0.00112	0.00810	0.00666	0.996	1.279	1.372
	(0.0100)	(0.0125)	(0.0255)	(0.368)	(0.479)	(0.856)
Observations	221,109	202,146	65,386	221,109	202,146	65,386
R-squared	0.020	0.015	0.025			

Notes: All specifications include a complete set of child, mother and household characteristics as well country fixed effects. Robust standard errors in parenthesis are clustered at the sample cluster level. Countries analysed are Bangladesh, Dominican Republic, Ghana, Haiti, Jordan, Kenya, Madagascar, Mali, Niger, Nigeria, Peru, Philippines, Senegal, Uganda, Vietnam, Zambia, Zimbabwe

Significance: *p<0.1; **p<0.05; ***p<0.01

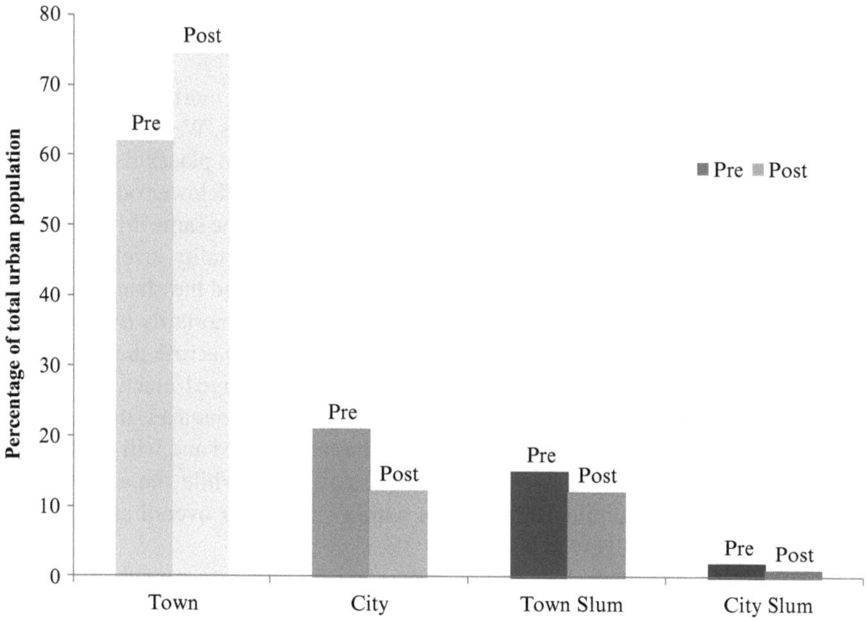

Fig. 11.5 Urban trends: pre and post 2000

In order to provide some sense of how large a shift in the population distribution occurred over the sample period, we use data from the World Population Prospect (UNDP 2011) to compute the fraction of the population living in urban areas. Restricting the data to our sample of 37 countries, we find that the fraction of the population living in areas classified as urban increased from 35.6 to 40.3 % between the 1990 and the 2005.

Given the overall urban mortality advantages documented in Tables 11.2, 11.3, 11.4, and 11.5, the conclusion that the overall changes in residential distribution has been accelerating, rather than slowing down the mortality transition appears tempting. This conclusion, however, is only true if most, or at least some, of the urban growth occurred in the better-off urban areas rather than in the slum areas more similar in terms of child mortality to rural areas.

To investigate this, we plot the division of the urban population in our sample before and after 2000 in Fig. 11.5 above. To make sure the observed patterns do not reflect differences in sample composition, we restrict this comparison to countries with at least one survey pre, and one survey post 2000 (the results look highly similar without this restriction). As Fig. 11.5 shows, there is no evidence of particularly large growth in slum areas; on average, the percentage of town slum residents declined from 15.0 to 12.2 %, while the percentage of urban residents residing in city slums declined from 1.9 to 1.1 %. Overall, this suggests that urban growth is not particularly strong in slum areas, but, if anything most pronounced in small urban centres.

11.5 Conclusions

In this chapter, we have analysed the relation between child mortality and type of place of residence across 37 low and middle income countries. We have shown that the average childhood mortality gap between rural and urban places remains sizeable, with urban children experiencing on average about 25 % lower odds of death in the first 3 years of life relative to their rural counterparts. The same differences do not, however, apply to urban slum areas, where we find mortality levels generally very similar to those observed in rural areas. We also analysed the changes in relative mortality over time. The overall improvements in child mortality over the past 10 years are rather remarkable and the average mortality gap across the residential areas analysed in this chapter does not appear to have changed much. Given the rapid pace of urbanization experienced in most developing countries, this suggests that the overall shifts in residential distribution has contributed and will continue to contribute positively to the overall mortality transitions. While the existence of slums implies large mortality differentials within cities, their overall effect on the mortality transition is likely to be small.

Appendix: Countries and Urban 1 Mill. Agglomerations

Country	Year(s)	Urban agglomerations above 1 mill. Inhabitants in 2000
Azerbaijan	2006	Baku
Bangladesh	1993, 2008	Chittagong, Dhaka Khulna
Bolivia	1993, 1998	La Pay, Santa Cruz
Brazil	1991, 1996	20 cities
Burkina Faso	1992, 1998	Ouagadougou
Cameroon	1991, 1998	Douala, Yaounde
Colombia	1990, 1995	Barrangquilla, Bogota, Bucaramanga, Cali, Medellin
Cote d'Ivoire	1994, 1998	Abidjan
Dominican Rep.	1991, 1996, 2007	Santo Domingo
Egypt, Arab Rep.	1992, 1995	Cairo, Alexandria
Ghana	1993, 1998, 2008	Accra, Kumasi
Guinea	1999	Conakry
Haiti	1994, 2005	Port-au-Prince
India	2005	43 cities
Jordan	1997, 2007	Amman
Kazakhstan	1995	Almaty
Kenya	1993, 1998, 2008	Nairobi

(continued)

Country	Year(s)	Urban agglomerations above 1 mill. Inhabitants in 2000
Madagascar	1992, 1997, 2008	Antananarivo
Mali	1995, 2006	Bamako
Morocco	1992	Casablanca, Fes, Rabat
Mozambique	1997	Maputo
Niger	1992, 1998, 2006	Niamey
Nigeria	1999, 2008	Abuja, Benin City, Ibadan Kaduna, Kano, Lagos, Ogbomosho, Port Harcourt
Pakistan	2006	Faisalabad, Gujranwala, Hyderabad, Karachi, Lahore, Multan, Peshawar, Rawalpindi
Peru	1991, 1996, 2003	Lima
Philippines	1993, 1998, 2008	Davao, Manila
Senegal	1992, 1997, 2006, 2008	Dakar
South Africa	1998	Cape Town, Durban, East Rand, Johannesburg, Port Elizabeth, Pretoria, Vereeniging
Togo	1998	Lome
Turkey	1993, 1998	Adana, Ankara, Bursa, Gaziantep, Istanbul, Izmir
Uganda	1995, 2006	Kampala
Ukraine	2007	Dnipropetrovsk, Kharkiv, Kiev, Odesa
Uzbekistan	1996	Tashkent
Vietnam	1997, 2000	Ha Noi, Hai Phong, Ho Chi Minh City
Yemen, Rep.	1991	Sanaa
Zambia	1992, 1996, 2007	Lusaka
Zimbabwe	1994, 2005	Harare

Source: Population Division of the Department of Economic and Social Affairs of the United Nations Secretariat; World Population Prospects: The 2008 Revision; World Urbanization Prospects: The 2009 Revision

References

Bloom, D. E., Canning, D., et al. (2010). Urban settlement: Data, measures, and trends. In J. Beall, B. Guha-Khasnobis, & R. Kanbur (Eds.), *Urbanization and development: Multidisciplinary perspectives*. Oxford: Oxford University Press.

Bocquier, P., Madise, N. J., et al. (2011). Is there an urban advantage in child survival in sub-Saharan Africa? Evidence from 18 countries in the 1990s. *Demography, 48*, 531–558.

Cain, L., & Hong, S. (2009). Survival in 19th century cities: The larger the city, the smaller your chances. *Explorations in Economic History, 46*(4), 450–463.

Fotso, J. C. (2007). Urban-rural differentials in child malnutrition: Trends and socioeconomic correlates in sub-Saharan Africa. *Health & Place, 13*(1), 205–223.

Gould, W. T. (1998). African mortality and the new 'urban penalty'. *Health & Place, 4*(2), 171–181.

Günther, I., & Harttgen, K. (2012). Deadly cities? Inequalities in mortality in Sub-Saharan Africa. *Population and Development Review, 38*, 469–486.

Haines, M. R. (1995). Socio-economic differentials in infant and child mortality during mortality decline: England and Wales, 1890–1911. *Population Studies, 49*(2), 297–315.

Johnson, G. (1964). Health conditions in rural and urban areas of developing countries. *Population Studies, 17*, 293–309.

Konteh, F. (2009). Urban sanitation and health in the developing world: Reminiscing the nineteenth century industrial nations. *Health & Place, 15*(1), 69–78.

Montgomery, M. R., & Hewett, P. C. (2005). Urban poverty and health in developing countries: Household and neighborhood effects. *Demography, 42*(3), 397–425.

Montgomery, M. R., Stren, R., et al. (Eds.). (2003). *Cities transformed: Demographic change and its implications in the developing world*. Washington, DC: National Academies Press.

Moore, M., Gouldet, P., et al. (2003). Global urbanization and impact on health. *International Journal of Hygiene and Environmental Health Affairs, 206*, 269–278.

Sclar, E., Garau, P., et al. (2005). The 21st century health challenge of slums and cities. *Lancet Infectious Diseases, 365*(9462), 901–903.

Timaeus, I. M., & Lush, L. (1995). Intra-urban differentials in child health. *Health Transition Review, 5*(2), 163–190.

UNDP. (2011). *World urbanization prospects: The 2009 revision*. United Nations Population Division. Accessed online at: http://esa.un.org/unpd/wup/index.htm

UN–HABITAT. (2007). *State of the world's cities 2006/7*. London: Earthscan Publications.

Williamson, J. G. (1990). *Coping with city growth during the British industrial revolution*. Cambridge: Cambridge University Press.

Woods, R. (2003). Urban-Rural mortality differentials: An unresolved debate. *Population and Development Review, 29*(1), 29–46.

Chapter 12
Health Disparities on the Periphery of Ouagadougou

Clémentine Rossier, Abdramane Bassiahi Soura, Bruno Lankoande, and Roch Modeste Millogo

12.1 Introduction

Until recently, Sub-Saharan African cities held little interest for health researchers and program designers, because, on average, urban areas boast better socio-economic and health indicators than rural ones (Brockerhoff and Brennan 1998). In Burkina Faso, for instance, according to the 2006 census, life expectancy at birth is 67 in the Centre Region (which roughly corresponds to the capital city of Ouagadougou), and only 57 in the country as a whole (Baya et al. 2009). Furthermore, while in rural areas, 53 % of the population lives below the poverty line, this number is only 19 % is urban areas (INSD 2009). But despite the concentration of wealth in urban areas, poor African city dwellers may be worse off than average rural residents. They tend to live in slums, with recent studies showing that people living in informal urban settlements can experience worse health conditions than rural residents because of high population density and lack of public services (APHRC 2002; Magadi et al. 2003; Hacker and Ryan 2003). In Ouagadougou, informal urban settlements encircle the city almost entirely and house an estimated 30 % of the city's population (Boyer and Delaunay 2009).

C. Rossier (✉)
Institute of Demography and Socioeconomics, University of Geneva, Geneva, Switzerland

Institut National d'Etudes Démographiques, Paris, France

Institut Supérieur des Sciences de la Population, University of Ouagadougou, Ouagadougou, Burkina Faso
e-mail: clementine.rossier@ined.fr

A.B. Soura • B. Lankoande • R.M. Millogo
Institut Supérieur des Sciences de la Population, University of Ouagadougou, Ouagadougou, Burkina Faso
e-mail: asoura@issp.bf; blankoande@issp.bf; rmillogo@issp.bf

D. Ramiro Fariñas, M. Oris (eds.), *New Approaches to Death in Cities during the Health Transition*, International Studies in Population 12,
DOI 10.1007/978-3-319-43002-7_12

Because of rural-urban migration and population growth, African city dwellers are becoming a more numerically significant group by the day. In Burkina Faso, 3.1 million people lived in cities in 2006 (26 % of the national population), but by 2030, this number is expected to reach 11.6 million (40 % of the national population) (Guengant 2009). In this context of rapid urbanization, the Institut Supérieur des Sciences de la Population at the University of Ouagadougou launched the Ouagadougou Health and Demographic Surveillance System (Ouaga HDSS) in 2008. The research platform aims to provide a greater understanding of the health and development challenges facing urban populations in West Africa, and ultimately, to provide African policy makers and programme designers the information they need to create interventions and systems adapted to the urban context.

Some rural African populations still face health challenges characteristic of the period preceding the epidemiologic transition: most individuals die from communicable diseases, perinatal and maternal conditions, or malnutrition (Murray et Lopez 1996; WHO 2008). These illnesses are strongly correlated with poverty and failing public institutions (inadequate health system, poor sanitation, etc.), and affect children the most. Life expectancy at birth is very low in these pre-transitional contexts. On the other hand, African cities, whose populations are, on average, in the middle-income range, have begun the epidemiological transition. Middle-income populations see the burden of communicable disease diminish (but not disappear altogether) but they face additional, health challenges that primarily concern adults, such as non-communicable diseases, and accidents or other violent causes of ill health. Because people in middle-income populations die less often as children and more often as adults, life expectancy is higher, but, premature adult deaths nevertheless remain common. This situation has been described as a "double burden of disease" (communicable and non-communicable diseases), or as one of a "triple burden of disease", when counting accidents and other violent deaths as a third burden. HIV/AIDS constitutes an additional burden which weighs heavily on adult mortality in certain African countries, and is sometimes envisioned as a separate, "fourth" burden of disease. By contrast, in the world's richest populations, infectious diseases (including HIV/AIDS) and accidents/violence, cause few deaths. At the end of the epidemiological transition, most people die from a single burden: that of non–communicable diseases, often at an advanced age, causing life expectancy to reach very high levels.

Preliminary results from the Ouaga HDSS show that Ouagadougou today seems to face a quadruple burden of disease. In the neighbourhoods surveyed, the most common cause of death for children under age five is still infectious disease,[1] while for adults 15–59, the most frequent causes of deaths are AIDS, cardiovascular disease and accidents (Duthé and Soura 2011). In this analysis, we explore how these

[1] At 26 per 1000, the infant mortality rate in the Ouaga HDSS is lower compared to the four HDSS located in rural Burkina Faso: Nouna, Kaya, Nanoro, Sapone (*First comparative workshop for the Burkinane HDSS*, April 2–7 2012, Ouagadougou, Institut Supérieur des Sciences de la Population, Université de Ouagadougou).

four different urban health burdens affect different socio-economic groups within the city. Almost everywhere in the world, and at most times throughout history, wealthier individuals have been advantaged in terms of health (Victoria et al. 2003; Gwatkin et al. 2007; Marmot 2007). While this (almost) universal rule is likely to hold for children (infectious diseases certainly affect the poorest urban children disproportionately), the adverse health events that affect adults (HIV, cardiovascular disease and accidents) may more heavily concern the most affluent. Indeed, wealthier individuals are more likely to engage in risky practices associated with improved economic status (for example drive with a motorcycle instead of a bicycle). In a population that has just entered the epidemiological transition, a generalized lack of prevention may characterize these new types of behaviours (for example, people seldom wear helmets when driving motorcycles). Moreover, there may be a lack of affordable medical care for these illnesses, which are only now starting to pose a significant health burden. In such a context, wealthier adults may take greater health risks and end up in worse health, despite their greater ability to afford medical care.

In this analysis, we take different dimensions of socio-economic status into account (Carr 2004; Montgomery 2009): household wealth, education level of the head of household, and type of neighbourhood in which the household is situated (formal or informal). We first calculate, in a bivariate analysis, age-specific mortality rates (data 2009–2010) as a function of these three variables. To understand the observed mortality differences, we then use multi-variate techniques to investigate differences in a number of health behaviours, using data from a survey performed in 2010 in the Ouaga HDSS, supplemented by data from the 2003 Demographic and Health Survey. For children under five, we examine socio-economic differences in the risk factors associated with infectious diseases (malnutrition, use of mosquito nets), in morbidity and access to health care. For adults 15–59, we analyse how socio-economic status is related to the risk factors associated with HIV/AIDS (risky sexual behaviour, condom use), risk factors associated with cardiovascular diseases (excess weight, hypertension) and with accidents. We also examine social differentials in adults' access to health care. These morbidity and health behaviour data help us propose, in conclusion, a number of hypotheses to explain the observed social differentials in child and adult mortality in Ouagadougou.

12.2 Data and Methods

The Context

The Ouaga HDSS was created at the end of 2008 in five neighbourhoods at the northern periphery of the city (Fig. 12.1). The population followed by the Ouaga HDSS numbers approximately 80,000 individuals, divided among two official neighbourhoods (Kilwin and Tanghin) and three unplanned informal settlements (called "*non loti*" or "unlotted" in the local jargon), Nonghin, Polesgo and Nioko 2.

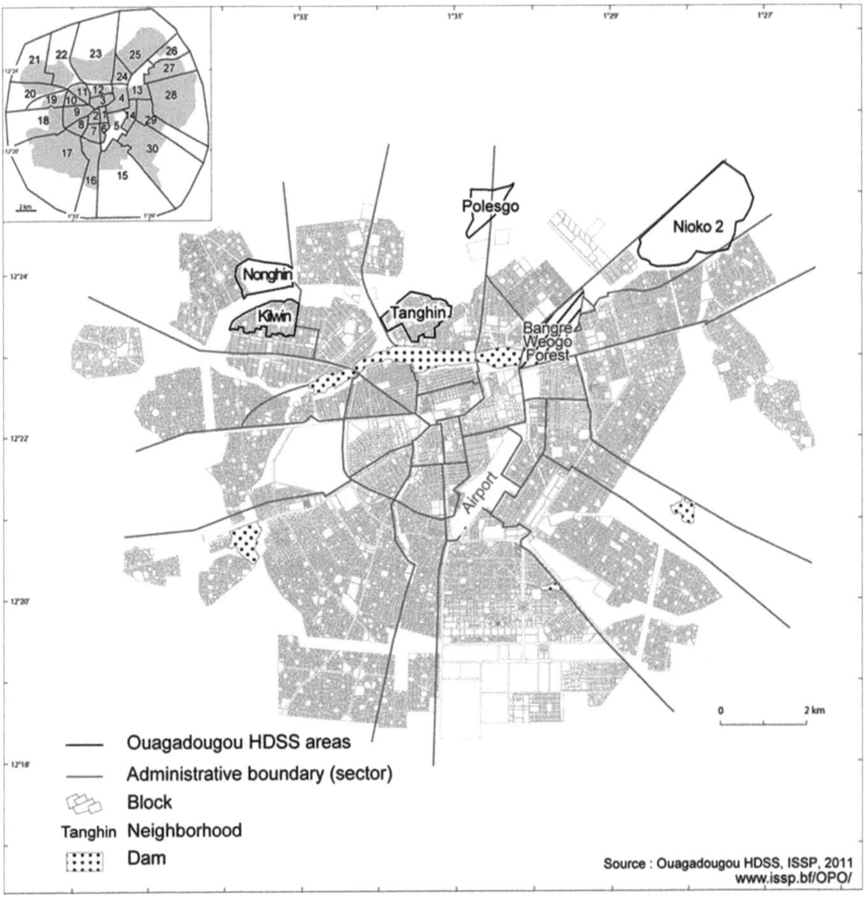

Fig. 12.1 Location of zones studied by the Ouagadougou Demographic Surveillance System

The "lotting" or division of new land is conducted by municipal authorities; this operation consists of dividing the land (which used to belong to local traditional leaders), recording the parcels in the official land registry, and then distributing the parcels, giving priority to those who were already there. The state then proceeds to equip the area with the standard utilities and public institutions (electricity, running water, waste management, streets, schools, health centres, etc.).

The unlotted settlements are considered illegal and are almost entirely deprived of these types of state-run services. Accordingly, households living in the informal areas of the Ouaga HDSS are characterized by poor sanitation facilities (water, waste management, latrines) (Djourdebbe et al. 2011; Dos Santos et al. 2011). The informal neighbourhoods of the Ouaga HDSS are essentially populated by migrants, with only 20 % of their inhabitants 15 and older born in Ouagadougou, 64 % born in rural areas, and 16 % in other cities or countries (Rossier et al. 2011a). This trend is similar, though less pronounced, in the formal neighbourhoods followed at the city's periphery, where 36 % of adults were born in Ouagadougou and 41 % in rural areas. An analysis with Ouaga HDSS data shows that migrant status does not seem to be related to children's health; among adults, migrants seem to have certain advantages (they are less likely to be overweight and less often depressed) and certain disadvantages (more often hypertensive and less familiar with health services when they arrive) (Rossier et al. 2011b; Nikiema et al. 2011). Overall, migrants have mortality rates comparable to non-migrants. In this analysis, we will systematically control for the place of birth and length of time since arrival in the city in the multivariate analyses, so that we can focus on the effects of wealth, education and type of neighbourhood on the health of children and adults.

The Demographic Surveillance System

After an initial census (Round 0) of the Ouaga HDSS neighbourhoods (including the name, sex, age, ethnic group, and marital status of each individual), an exhaustive list of dwellings and their residents has been updated approximately every 8 months. A brief life history, including migration, marital and reproductive history, is collected for each new resident. At each new passage, field agents collect information on demographic events that have taken place since the last passage (new arrivals, departures, births, deaths, changes in marital status, etc.) Each death is followed by a verbal autopsy which is then diagnosed by a team of eight local doctors. In this analysis, we will use the mortality data collected through the first two passages and cover a period from October 2008 through November 2010, during which time 426 deaths were recorded; 78 % of recorded deaths (333) were assigned a definite cause. While urban neonatal and post neonatal mortality exhibit comparable levels in the 2003 Demographic and Health Survey, the neonatal mortality rate recorded in the Ouaga HDSS is lower compared to post-neonatal mortality (Duthe and Soura 2011). The reason for this difference remains to be understood, since HDSS fieldworkers are as competent as DHS fieldworkers, and the period since the event is much shorter in HDSS. Every two passages, field agents collect information on the living standard of each household (household goods and characteristics of the home), and the characteristics of residents (education level, economic activities, etc.) A complete description of the Ouaga HDSS can be found in Rossier et al. 2012.

Proxy for Living Standards

We have created a first proxy for living standard as means to compare poverty within the Ouaga HDSS areas with the rest of the city and country. We chose to include the possession of a television, refrigerator, motorcycle or car in this first indicator of wealth, because information on these goods were also collected the national Comprehensive Survey on Household Life Conditions (EICVM as it known by its

French initials) which was conducted in 2007 and which allows us to compare our areas with the rest of the country. Adopting a Principle Component Analysis (Filmer et Pritchett 1999, 2001; Lachaud 2001), we first dichotomized the scores and then retained the first component to create the proxy. The weight that this axis carries may seem weak (50.4 % of variance explained) but the standard of living indicator is correlated with the head of household's education level[2] (Filmer and Pritchett 2001). The factorial coefficients were estimated using EICVM data. These coefficients were then applied to the Ouaga HDSS households that responded to the survey on household goods during the first re-questioning in 2010 (n = 15,929), in order to estimate their standard of living scores. Conforming to the PCA principle, the variables are aggregated linearly for each household as presented in Eq. 12.1.

$$score_i = \sum_j \alpha_0 + \alpha_{ij}\text{variable}_{ij} \tag{12.1}$$

Based on these scores, but also on a reasoned approach (many households had similar scores and it was impossible to divide them evenly into quartiles), the households were classified in three categories ranging from the lowest standard of living to the highest. The household at the low end of the spectrum do not have televisions, refrigerators, cars or motorbikes. They get around on bicycles or on foot. These households are the most common in our population and are classified are "poor." In what we are identifying as "middle class," households have a television and nearly 9 out of 10 of them have a motorbike for transportation, but refrigerators and cars are still rare in this group. In what we identify as the most affluent group, almost all households have televisions, 8 out of 10 have refrigerators and the primary means of transport is equally divided between motorbike and car.

The informal neighbourhoods studied by the Ouaga HDSS are, on average, poorer than the rest of the city: 66 % of households there are "poor", compared to 24 % in the city as a whole. The formal neighbourhoods studied (27 % of households are poor) are comparable to the city average. The informal neighbourhoods studied by the Ouaga HDSS are more affluent on average than rural areas where 73 % of households are poor according to our definition. The exception to this is the Ouaga HDSS neighbourhood of Polesgo, which is a village that has recently been subsumed into the city, and where the rate of poverty is comparable to the rural average (75 % of households are "poor").

The poverty line in Burkina Faso was estimated at 82,672 CFA Francs per person per year (126.20 euros) in 2009. The National Institute of Statistics and Demography (INSD by its French initials) estimates that 52.3 % of the rural population lives below this poverty level, compared to 19.9 % of the urban population (INSD 2009).

[2] Almost half (46 %) of residents 15 and older in the Ouaga HDSS neighbourhoods have never been to school, and the proportion is lower in the formal neighbourhoods (36 %) than in the formal neighbourhoods (59 %). While educational level and wealth are associated, the relation is far from systematic, since an important part of the economy remains informal; rich illiterates are common, as are jobless graduates.

Our poverty indicator (calculated in 2010) gives us an urban poverty rate in Ouagadougou of 24 %, which is only slightly above the INSD's urban poverty rate. Our indicator, however, clearly overestimates poverty in rural areas, where wealth is invested in different goods, like livestock. Another limitation of this first indicator is that is does not distinguish between the poorest of the poor: 50 % of the population in the ODSS's neighbourhoods is "poor". To introduce greater sensitivity into the poverty measure, we repeated the same procedure introducing supplementary criteria: the average number of mobile telephones per household and home ownership, distinguishing formal and informal home ownership. With these additional criteria, we were able to classify households into poverty quartiles: the 25 % poorest, the 25 % fairly poor, the 25 % fairly affluent and the 25 % most affluent.[3]

The Health Survey

Between February and June 2010, a quantitative survey (called the health survey) was conducted among 1700 Ouaga HDSS households (a sampling rate of 11.4 %) to collect data about health status and access to health care in case of illness. These households were randomly selected to ensure that they were representative of the study area. The population of interest consisted of children aged less than 5 years and adults aged 15 years and over, with an oversample of adults aged 50 and more. We interviewed the parents of 950 children 0–4 years of age, 1371 adults 15–49, and 986 adults older than 50 (n = 3307 individuals). The survey was implemented simultaneously in the informal and formal neighbourhoods so that there would be no seasonality bias (the rainy season in Burkina Faso, associated with a peak in malaria cases, goes from June to October).

12.3 The Health of Children Under 5 Years of Age

Weight and height were measured for each selected child, which allowed us to calculate whether children under 5 were underweight (weight/age); children with a Z score less than two were identified as suffering from malnutrition. Preventive behaviours are captured through a question about use of mosquito nets for children 5 and under the night prior to the survey (yes/no).[4] For each child, a series of question was asked regarding the occurrence of fever, diarrhoea and cough over the previous

[3] We tested two additional poverty indicators, but did not keep them in the final analyses. An indicator of household food insecurity (questions provided by J. M. Prevel and his team at the Institut de Recherche pour le Développement) proved not sensitive enough, with 70 % of households reporting severe food insecurity. Second, households headed by widowed/separated/divorced women were not associated with poorer health outcomes, even though women in general have less ability to generate revenue; economically successful women are probably over-represented in these households.

[4] Useable vaccination data were collected for children only at the third re-enumeration.

2 weeks; this series finished with a question regarding the presence of others symptoms over the past 2 weeks. We added here these symptoms together to define the population of children who experienced an episode of illness over the previous 2 weeks. For this group, a series of follow-up questions was asked regarding whether care was sought at a health centre (yes/no).

12.4 The Health of Adults Aged 15 and Over

Although HIV is the largest cause of death among adults (aged 15–59) in the Ouaga HDSS neighbourhoods (Duthé and Soura 2011),[5] we did not collect data regarding HIV risk factors, nor did we measure HIV status of the respondents. In this analysis, we use the published DHS data from 2003 (only the preliminary results were available for the 2010 DHS at the time of analysis), to explore the risk factors of HIV/AIDS (engage in non-marital sexual behaviour, and condom use at last non-marital sexual encounter). We measured two risk factors for cardiovascular disease: being overweight and arterial hypertension. To determine whether a respondent was overweight, we calculated their Body Mass Index (with a BMI>25 signalling an overweight person) and an indicator of abdominal obesity. Abdominal obesity was defined as a waist circumference of 102 cm for men and 88 cm for women. Only adults 20 and older were screened for excess weight. Both diastolic and systolic blood pressures were measured three times for all respondents 15 and older at the end of each interview. We calculated the average of these three measures and defined a hypertensive person as someone with a systolic blood pressure >=140 and a diastolic blood pressure >=90. Accidents were measured with the following question: "Over the past 12 months, have you had one or more than one accident that incited you to seek the services of a doctor, nurse or health centre?" (Yes/no). Finally, a question allowed us to identify adults who experienced an illness over the past: "Did you have a health problem during the last 30 days?" (yes/no). Those identified by this question were then asked whether they sought care in a health centre. A complete description of the health survey can be found in Rossier et al. 2012.

12.5 Methods

We first calculated the age-specific mortality rate for poor and non-poor households (first proxy), for households whose head went to school compared to those who did not go to school, and for households living in informal versus formal neighbourhoods, using the deaths collected over the first two passages. The relatively low

[5] During the two first years of data collection we report on here, causes of death were defined by a group of local doctors. Later, the Ouaga HDSS used a software to determine the causes of death: using that approach, over the 2009–2012 period and for adults aged 35 and over, AIDS is only the 7th causes of death (Rossier et al. 2014).

number of deaths collected by the time of this analysis (n=426 in 2 years) did not allow to us to go further than a bivariate analysis for mortality. The relationships between household and individual characteristics (or, for certain variables, the mother of the individual), and the different health indicators described above are explored through a series of logistic regressions.

12.6 Results

Health Disparities Among Children

In the neighbourhoods covered by the Ouaga HDSS, the infant mortality rate is 26.3 per 1000, as opposed to 97.9 per 1000 nationally, according to 2006 census data (Baya et al. 2009). The mortality rate between ages 1 and 4 is 7.9 per 1000 in the Ouaga HDSS neighbourhoods, versus 14.3 at the national level. According to census data, mortality rates in the Centre region (which more or less corresponds to the capital) are half as low as in the country as a whole (Baya et al. 2009, p. 51). If the child mortality rate in the Ouaga HDSS neighbourhoods in 2009–2010 matches the results from the 2006 census, the mortality of those under 1 year of age is about half of what can be expected from census data; this difference remains to be interpreted.[6] Most deaths of small children in the Ouaga HDSS neighbourhoods are due to communicable diseases and therefore largely preventable (Fig. 12.2): most die from intestinal infections and malaria (Duthé and Soura 2011).

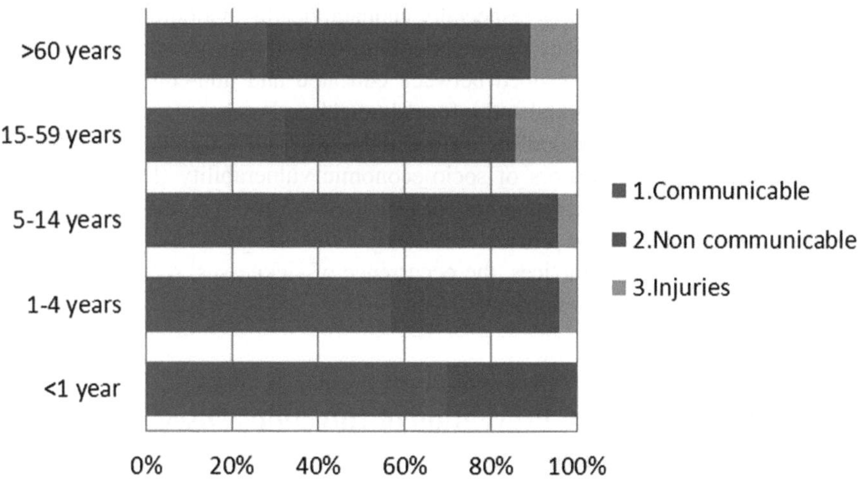

Fig. 12.2 Major causes of deaths, by age group, Ouaga DSS, 2009–2010

[6] Reporting of children's deaths, while a problem during the first years of surveillance, appears to have become complete later on (Lankoande et al. 2016).

Table 12.1 Mortality rate per 1000 $_5m_x$ before age 5 by different indicators of vulnerability, Ouaga HDSS 2009–2010

	Less than 1 year			1–4 years		
	Rate	[95 % Conf. Interval]		Rate	[95 % Conf. Interval]	
Poverty level						
Poor	34.47	26.98	44.04	11.17	9.01	13.85
Non poor	23.49	17.94	30.74	6.06	4.65	7.90
Type of area						
Formal	17.26	12.14	24.54	5.15	3.78	7.02
Informal	31.95	26.05	39.20	9.99	8.25	12.09
Education hh						
No schooling	32.85	26.12	41.32	10.36	8.46	12.68
Went to school	22.50	16.50	30.67	5.26	3.79	7.29
All	26.31	22.05	31.39	7.93	6.74	9.33

We see (Table 12.1) that the mortality rate before age one in poor families is about one-third higher than that of middle or upper class families. Differences of a similar order of magnitude are found between families with educated heads of household and those in which the head of household has never been to school. Differences are even stronger between families with infants who live in "official" neighbourhoods, as compared to those who live in informal settlements, who are almost twice as likely to die.

Socio-economic differences in mortality rates are more pronounced in children aged 1–4 years, which is to be expected since the death of youngest infants is more often related to genetic causes (especially neonatal deaths). Children aged 1–4 are twice as likely to die if they are born to poor families as if they are born to rich families, a phenomenon again echoed between educated and non-educated heads of household, and between formal and informal neighbourhoods.

To understand these mortality differentials, we will examine the relations between these three indicators of socio-economic vulnerability (living standard, educational level, type of neighbourhood: formal or informal) on the one hand, and different dimensions of the process sustaining a child in good health on the other hand: preventive health practices, the occurrence of sicknesses, recourse to health care, and the child's nutritional status.

12.7 Disparity in the Prevention of Infectious Diseases Among Children

The most basic way for children to avoid dying from these disease is to avoid getting sick in the first place. To approach disparities in preventive health practices for children, we will examine here the use of mosquito nets in the Ouaga HDSS

Table 12.2 Probability of using a mosquito net during the last 15 days, children <5 years, logistic regression (1 = used, 0 = not used)

Variables	Odds ratio	P.value
Sex (base: boy)	1.18	0.301
Age of the Child	**0.85**	**0.017**
Standard of Living (base: 1st quartile)		
2nd quartile	0.96	0.860
3rd quartile	1.38	0.160
4th quartile	**2.29**	**0.002**
Mother's level of education (base: none)		
Primary	0.98	0.939
Secondary and higher	1.33	0.217
Type of neighbourhood (base: formal)	1.04	0.824

Control variables: mother's ethnicity, place of birth and duration since first arrival I the city

neighbourhoods (Table 12.2).[7] 34.6 % of children surveyed slept under a mosquito net the previous night. The household wealth indicator is significantly correlated to the probability of children sleeping under the nets, with wealthier people more likely to use them. Mosquito nets remain indeed relatively expensive in Burkina Faso, and periodic national mosquito net giveaways are organized periodically to increase coverage; the most recent of these campaigns took place in 2011, just after this survey was carried out. There is some evidence of the expected relationship between a mother's education level and the use of mosquito nets, but this relationship is not statistically significant, indicating that knowledge of mosquito nets' utility is widespread.

All other things being equal, the inhabitants of the informal settlements do not seem to use mosquito nets for their children less than others do. This finding holds true for other health prevention behaviours across the Ouaga HDSS neighbourhoods. No matter the behaviour, be it the use of contraception (Rossier and Ortiz 2011) or prenatal care (Soura 2009), the simple fact of living in the informal settlements does not have its own independent effect on the use of preventative health services.

12.8 Disparity in the Occurrence of Sicknesses Among Children

Despite parent's best efforts at prevention, children often get sick. A majority (70.1 %) of children under 5 years of age in the survey showed a symptom of illness during the previous 2 weeks. Mothers with more education and wealthier households did not report significantly fewer illnesses among their children. As already

[7] Data on children's vaccination in the Ouaga HDSS are available only from the third enumeration on.

Table 12.3 Likelihood of experiencing an episode of illness during the last 15 days, children <5 years, logistic regression (1 = had a health problem, 0 = did not have a health problem)

Variables	Odds ratio	P.value
Sex (base: girl)	**2.44**	**0.076**
Age of the Child	**0.59**	**0.004**
Standard of Living (base: 1st quartile)		
2nd quartile	0.84	0.834
3rd quartile	0.95	0.945
4th quartile	0.93	0.927
Mother's level of education (base: none)		
Primary	0.59	0.343
Secondary and higher	0.50	0.308
Type of neighbourhood (base: formal)	**8.86**	**0**

Control variables: mother's ethnicity, mother's age, place of birth, duration since in Ouaga, distance from a health centre

said, questions seeking information about the respondents' recent illnesses (or those of his family members) may reflect only partially the objective health conditions of these individuals. Indeed, a person with fewer means to seek formal health care or who thinks a symptom can be taken care of with traditional medicine will be less likely to conceptualize the symptom as "an illness", and will be less likely to declare it as such in a survey. We saw that children born in poorer households and whose head of household is uneducated have a greater chance of dying before age five than children born in wealthier households. It is therefore almost sure that children living in poorer households with less educated families actually do get sicker more often than their wealthier, more-educated counterparts, and that the lack of observed relationship is due to a reporting bias (poorer household reporting only the most serious illnesses). As a matter of fact, we see that, all other things being equal, parents of children living far from a health care provider tend to report fewer illnesses for their children, highlighting the extent to which this question is subject to interpretation (Table 12.3).

But despite this bias, many of the differences in reported morbidity do indeed seem to be real. Thus, we see that boys are more often sick than girls and that older children get sick less than younger ones (both tendencies are confirmed by differentials in mortality). One particularly interesting result is the extremely high incidence of illness in young children living in informal neighbourhoods. When all else is equal, these children have nine times the reported incidence of disease as their counterparts living in formal neighbourhoods, a result that is corroborated by the differential in mortality rates between the two groups. This morbidity specific to the children of the periphery remains significant even after controlling for socio-economic status. In other words, a child born to a family that is relatively well-off and has educated parents is much more likely to be sick if s/he lives in an informal neighbourhood on the periphery than if s/he lives in an official neighbourhood. This phenomenon seems to be explained by poor the sanitation that characterizes these areas (Djourdebbe et al. 2011, Dos Santos et al. 2011).

12.9 Disparity in Access to Health Care Among Children

An analysis of the characteristics related to care-seeking behaviour for children (Table 12.4) shows that the younger a child is, the more likely the parents are to seek medical care. Moreover, all things being equal, parents in wealthier households (two upper quartiles) are more likely to seek medical care, as are parents in the poorest quartile. This finding may seem counter-intuitive but should be interpreted as the product of a reporting bias: very poor parents tend to only to report the most serious episodes which are, by definition, those that require medical attention. Education level has the expected effect on the likelihood of accessing care, though the relationship is not statistically significant; more educated mothers are more likely to identify the symptoms of an illness in their children and to report them, a fact which hides their propensity to seek care more often. It is also worth noting that parents who live farther from a health centre do not consult less often, however, these parents report less illness among their children, and thus, access care less often in reality.

Finally, living in informal areas is not linked to a lower propensity of seeking care compared to individuals living in legal neighbourhoods. However, further anal-

Table 12.4 Accessing care among children, logistic regression (1 = sought care, 0 = did not seek care)

Variables	Odds ratio	P.value
Sex (base: girl)	1.30	0.451
Child's Age	**0.545**	**0.000**
Distance from a Health Clinic (base: 25–500 m)		
501–1000 m	0.74	0.194
>1000 m	0.35	0.430
Standard of Living (base: 1st quartile)		
2nd quartile	**0.43**	**0.085**
3rd quartile	0.93	0.89
4th quartile	1.47	0.548
Mother's level of education (base: none)		
Primary	1.53	0.342
Secondary and higher	2.46	0.152
Type of neighbourhood (base: formal)	0.98	0.967

Control Variable: Child's ethnicity, mother's age, place of birth, duration since in Ouaga

ysis on access to care (Nikiema et al. 2011) shows that parents in the informal areas seek more often care for their children in hospitals (though not for themselves). This finding indicates that these parents report "illness" among their children as a more serious condition than their counterparts in the formal neighbourhoods, and thus are underestimating (and under-reporting) illness among their children, perhaps because childhood illnesses are so common in this unhealthful environment.

12.10 Disparity in the Nutritional Status Among Children

Regardless of the prevention activities and frequency of illness and care-seeking practices, the nutritional status of children plays an important role in the exacerbation of an illness. Malnutrition can be the aggravating factor that causes a sick child to die. In the neighbourhoods surveyed, 20.5 % of children suffer from malnutrition, while 5.1 % experience severe malnutrition; we show here only the results for malnutrition (Table 12.5). Our data suggest that malnutrition (whatever its level) is not dependent on the living standard of a child's parents or on their education level. However, malnutrition is more pronounced in the informal neighbourhoods, especially severe malnutrition, which is 2.4 times more common there. This phenomenon, which is independent of the poverty differential of those living in the informal neighbourhoods, may be explained by the higher incidence of disease among children in these neighbourhoods, which weaken them from a nutritional point of view. Malnourished children are in turn more likely to contract infectious diseases, and to die from them.

To summarize this analysis of health inequalities among children, we can say that in the Ouaga HDSS neighbourhoods, the poorest children and children with less educated parents are more likely to die than children with more affluent parents, with the risk doubling for children 1–4 years old. The differences are also pronounced for children under 1 year of age. The higher mortality of poor children is

Table 12.5 Malnutrition (Z score < −2), Children < 5 years, logistic regression (1 = malnourished; 0 = non malnourished)

Variables	Odds ratio	P.value
Sex (base: boy)	0.94	0.737
Child's Age	**0.61**	**0.000**
Standard of Living (base: 1st quartile)		
2nd quartile	0.98	0.951
3rd quartile	1.00	0.991
4th quartile	0.77	0.431
Mother's level of education (base: none)		
Primary	0.95	0.826
Secondary and higher	0.93	0.805
Type of neighbourhood (base: formal)	**1.63**	**0.037**

Control Variable: Mother's Ethnicity, mother's age, place of birth, duration since in Ouaga

explained by a difference in use of preventative measures (represented here by the use of mosquito netting) and in care-seeking behaviours (the evidence of which is masked in our regressions by under-reporting of illness among the poor). In contrast, children of poorer and less educated parents are not more malnourished than their counterparts. A second result is that the elevated mortality of children in informal neighbourhoods does not seem to be explained by the composition of the population – poorer households headed by less educated parents. Rather, the context of the informal neighbourhoods themselves, with more unhealthful living environments, seems to cause more illness among the children who live there. These frequent illnesses have two main consequences, which in turn have health consequences of their own. First, controlling for other factors, children in informal neighbourhoods are more often malnourished, which increases susceptibility to disease. Second, the inhabitants of the informal neighbourhoods tend to seek medical care for their children less often (a result which is clear when looking at the type of health facilities visited: more often hospitals). Perhaps more accustomed to children's illnesses, reluctant to spend money each time a child gets sick because it happens very often, familiar with the treatments offered in primary health centres, these families seem to prefer to use self-medication and to wait some time before seeking care.

Adult Health Disparities

The mortality rate for adults between 15 and 59 is 2.3 per 1000 in the Ouaga HDSS neighbourhoods (Table 12.6). At the country level, the mortality rate for the same age group is 3.7 per 1000 (Baya et al. 2009), which is 1.6 times higher. The mortality rates measured for adults in the ODSS are plausible because the mortality rate for the Centre region (which roughly corresponds to Ouagadougou) is about two times less than national rates.

Table 12.6 Mortality rates by different indicators of vulnerability, adults aged 15–59, Ouaga HDSS 2009–2010

	Rate	[95 % Conf. Interval]	
Poverty level			
Poor	2.31	1.83	2.93
Non-poor	2.44	2.02	2.93
Type of area			
Formal	2.60	2.18	3.11
Informal	1.89	1.50	2.39
Education hh			
No schooling	2.65	2.19	3.21
Went to school	1.91	1.49	2.43
All	2.29	1.99	2.63

There is a difference in premature adult mortality according to the household's education level. Adults living in families where the head of household never went to school have a mortality rate 1.4 times as high as those who live in families with an educated head of household. In contrast, the risk of dying before 60 years of age among adults is similar between poor and non-poor households. Adult residents of the formal neighbourhoods have a mortality rate 1.6 times higher than residents of informal neighbourhoods; recall here that the residents of the formal neighbourhoods are, on average, wealthier and better educated.

To understand these mortality differentials, we will examine the socio-demographic characteristics related to the principle risk factors for death in this age group. The three principal causes of premature death among adults 15–59 in the Ouaga HDSS neighbourhoods (in order of magnitude) are HIV, cardiovascular and accidents (of which approximately half are road accidents) (Duthé and Soura 2011). (see previous note on that point). With the help of the 2003 DHS results (INSD and Macro 2004), we examine the social inequalities that characterise risky sexual behaviours. We will then examine the socio-economic inequalities as they relate to excess weight and blood pressure (two risk factors for deaths from cardiovascular disease), and then finally the differentials in accident risk (a risk factor in deaths from accident). We will end with a description of the differential in access to health care in case of illness among adults.

12.11 Disparity in HIV Risk Among Adults

We use nationwide published data from the 2003 DHS to explore the relation between HIV risk factors among adults 15–49 and standards of living (which the DHS calculates from their household goods and home characteristics, given in quintiles). The first risk factor for HIV is "high-risk" sexual activity, which is defined here as activity with a person with whom one is neither married nor cohabitating. Let us first note a great difference as a function of place or residence, with Ouagadougou residents much more likely to have had sex outside of a union over the past 12 months (5.4 % of women and 30.7 % of men). Some 25.6 % of women in the richest quintile report such a high-risk activity over the last 12 months, compared to 4.7 % of women in the lowest quintile. 57.9 % of men in the richest quintile report high-risk sexual behaviours compared to 26.7 % among the poorest quintile. Differences are even wider by education, with 42.1 % of high school-educated women reporting high-risk sexual behaviours compared to 5.5 % among women who have never been to school. Among men, 64.6 % of those who have been to high school report high-risk sexual activity over the past 14 months compared to 28.8 % of those who have no formal education.

The second risk factor for HIV is high-risk sexual activity without condom use. Generally, the populations who most often have sex outside of a union also tend to use condoms more. Those living in Ouagadougou report higher condom use at last high-risk sex than those living in rural areas (68.5 % compared to 33.5 % of women;

93.1 % compared to 52.4 % of men). The wealthiest group tends to report more condom use at last high-risk sex than the poorest group (65.1 % compared to 34.1 % among women; 88.6 % compared to 35.6 % among men). Those with a secondary education or higher use report higher condom use at last high-risk sex than those with no education (75.5 % compared to 34.7 % among women; 89.6 % compared to 51.6 % among men). Though well-educated women tend to protect themselves against HIV better than wealthy women, these findings suggest that well-educated men and wealthy men report similar rates of condom use. Other findings, however, suggest that wealthy men do not protect themselves from STIs as well as well-educated men, echoing the findings for women. Wealthy men do not have as good a grasp on knowledge of prevention, with only 58.5 % of the wealthiest men rejecting incorrect information about HIV transmission, compared to 70.5 % of the most educated men.

The differences in HIV prevalence in Burkina Faso reflect mainly differences in sexual behaviours (the probability of engaging in high risk sex). The HIV prevalence is highest in the richest quintile, with 3.1 % of the most affluent individuals HIV+ compared to 1.1 % of the least affluent individuals. Differences are equally as pronounced between rural and urban areas, with 4.2 % of people between 15 and 49 in Ouagadougou HIV+, compared to 1.3 % of people in rural areas. These differences persist but are less pronounced between the well-educated and non-educated groups, with 2.8 % of those who have a secondary education HIV+, compared to 1.6 % of those with no education. The differences between the educated and the non-educated in terms of HIV prevalence are less pronounced than the difference between the wealthiest and the poorest, because although both the richest and the most educated engage more in risky sexual behaviours, the latter protect themselves better.

12.12 Disparities in Risk-Factors for Cardiovascular Disease Among Adults

Being overweight is an important risk factor for cardiovascular disease. In our sample, nearly one quarter of adults (23.3 %) are overweight (with a Body Mass Index higher than 25). Women are nearly three times more often overweight than men in Ouagadougou (see also Zeba et al. 2012) (Table 12.7). Being overweight becomes more common with age. Being overweight is strongly correlated with a high standard of living, with the most affluent people 2.5 times more likely to be overweight than the least affluent people. Once living standard is controlled for, neither education level nor neighbourhood of residence (formal or informal) is related to being overweight.

The same results appear when we examine waist size (Table 12.8). The most affluent are two times as likely to manifest abdominal obesity as the least affluent. No other socio-economic characteristics are related to waist size.

Table 12.7 Probability of being overweight, adults, logistic regression (1 = BMI >= 25; 0 = BI < 25)

Variables	Odds ratio	P.value
Sex (base: man)	**2.81**	**0**
Age (base: 20–24 years)		
25–34 years	**3.45**	**0**
35–44 years	**5.21**	**0**
45–54 years	**5.91**	**0**
55 and +	**2.61**	**0**
Standard of Living (base: 1st quartile)		
2nd quartile	**1.69**	**0.019**
3rd quartile	**1.98**	**0.001**
4th quartile	**2.54**	**0**
Level of Education (base: none)		
Primary	1.12	0.548
Secondary and higher	1.14	0.505
Type of Neighbourhood (base: formal)	0.79	0.130

Control Variables: ethnicity, place of birth and length of time in city

Table 12.8 Probability of abdominal obesity, adults, logistic regression (1 = abdominal obesity; 0 = none)

Variables	Odds ratio	P.value
Sex (base: man)	**12.92**	**0.000**
Age (base: 20–24 years)		
25–34 years	**1.66**	**0.084**
35–44 years	**3.22**	**0.000**
45–54 years	**2.94**	**0.001**
55 and +	**2.16**	**0.017**
Standard of Living (base: 1st quartile)		
2nd quartile	**2.31**	**0.003**
3rd quartile	**1.88**	**0.020**
4th quartile	**2.38**	**0.002**
Level of Education (base: none)		
Primary	1.14	0.569
Secondary and higher	0.85	0.546
Type of Neighbourhood (base: formal)	0.76	0.155

Control Variables: ethnicity, place of birth and length of time in city

Hypertension is another important risk factor for cardiovascular disease. In the health survey, 15.1 % of adults were hypertensive. We see (Table 12.9) that age is strongly related to the probability of being hypertensive. After age 55, an individual has 29.8 times the likelihood of high blood pressure as a younger person (between 15 and 24 years old). No other factors examined here are related to hypertension.

Table 12.9 Probability of hypertension, adults, logistic regression (1 = hypertensive; 0 = not)

Variables	Odds ratio	P.value
Sex (base: man)	1.21	0.212
Age (base: 20–24 years)		
25–34 years	**2.13**	**0.046**
35–44 years	**8.46**	**0.000**
45–54 years	**13.86**	**0.000**
55 and +	**29.79**	**0.000**
Standard of Living (base: 1st quartile)		
2nd quartile	1.39	0.143
3rd quartile	1.09	0.732
4th quartile	1.38	0.162
Level of Education (base: none)		
Primary	0.97	0.869
Secondary and higher	0.91	0.735
Type of Neighbourhood (base: formal)	1.01	0.976

Control Variables: ethnicity, place of birth and length of time in city

12.13 Disparities in Accident Risk Among Adults

The third largest cause of premature death among adults in the Ouaga HDSS neighbourhoods is accidents. In the 2012 health survey, 9 % of adults reported having had an accident severe enough that it caused them to seek health care over the past year. Half of these accidents took place on public streets and can be attributed to road traffic.

Table 12.10 shows that women had more accidents, perhaps because they are exposed both to domestic accidents and road accidents. Respondents reported more accidents in the informal neighbourhoods of the Ouaga HDSS, which may be attributed to the undeveloped status of the neighbourhood (no proper roads, holes due to digging to make mud bricks, etc.). Finally, those who are better educated report many more accidents, probably because they move more around the city more (more often employed in formal jobs) thus are more exposed to road accidents.

12.14 Disparities in Access to Care Among Adults

In order to measure access to health care, one must first collect data on recent illness. Overall, 19.9 % of adults 15 and old who took the health survey reported having been ill over the past month (Table 12.11).

The best educated and the wealthiest adults did not report significantly fewer illnesses than others. As already discussed for children, it is likely however that illness

Table 12.10 Probability of having had an accident, last 12 months, adults, ODSS health survey, 2010 (1 = had an accidence; 0 = did not have an accident)

Variables	Odds ratio	P.value
Sex (base: man)	**1.72**	**0.005**
Age (base: 20–24 years)		
25–34 years	1.06	0.808
35–44 years	0.98	0.953
45–54 years	0.87	0.691
55 and +	0.64	0.195
Standard of Living (base: 1st quartile)		
2nd quartile	0.99	0.968
3rd quartile	1.23	0.429
4th quartile	1.20	0.552
Level of Education (base: none)		
Primary	**1.59**	**0.056**
Secondary and higher	**1.89**	**0.020**
Type of Neighbourhood (base: formal)	**1.84**	**0.009**

Control Variables: ethnicity, place of birth and length of time in city

Table 12.11 Probability of having an illness over the past month, adults, logistic regression (1 = have an health issue; 0 = no health issue)

Variables	Odds ratio	P.value
Sex (base: woman)	**0.62**	**0.036**
Age (base: 15–24 years)		
25–34 years	1.43	0.215
35–44 years	**2.43**	**0.006**
>=45 years	**1.84**	**0.074**
Distance from a health clinic (base: 25–500 m)		
501–1000 m	1.11	0.708
1000 and more	**0.89**	**0.021**
Standard of living (base: 1st quartile)		
2nd quartile	1.57	0.189
3rd quartile	1.07	0.828
4th quartile	0.82	0.589
Level of education (base: none)		
Primary	0.82	0.508
Secondary and higher	0.80	0.470
Type of neighbourhood (base: formal)	1.22	0.468

Control Variables: ethnicity, place of birth and length of time in city

is actually more common for those living in households where the adults are poorer and less educated, because these groups tend to report only the most serious illness. In fact, further analyses show that poorer adults tend to go to hospitals more often: they report indeed only severe episodes of sickness (Nikiema et al. 2011). As for children, those who live farther from a health clinic report fewer illnesses, a result which highlights the degree to which this question is open to interpretation (the more difficult it is to access care, the less one perceives him/herself to be ill). Adult women are ill more often, which may also be due to reporting bias (women may find it easier to report a state of weakness).

Despite the interpretative nature if this variable, some of the results illustrate real healthdifferentials. For example, we see than the frequency of reported illness increases with age, certainly an expected result. Finally, adults who live in informal neighbourhoods are not more often ill than those who live in formal neighbourhoods, another result which is likely to be true.

Among adults who report an illness, 51.1 % sought care in a health centre. The probability of seeking care among adults does not depend on the distance to the closest health centre (Table 12.12). When other factors are controlled for, household wealth does not seem to have an effect on care-seeking behaviours either. Yet, health care is actually less often accessed in these two subgroups, because, as showed above, they report fewer illnesses.

The frequency of care-seeking behaviour among adults is the same in formal and informal neighbourhoods, when all else is equal. This result is plausible because we do not have any reason to believe that adults in informal neighbourhoods are under-

Table 12.12 Seeking health care, adults, logistic regression (1 = sought care; 0 = did not seek care)

Variables	Odds ratio	P.value
Sex (base: woman)	0.93	0.869
Age (base: 15–24 years)		
25–34 years	1.14	0.826
35–44 years	2.82	0.203
45–54 years	3.25	0.243
55 years and more	2.21	0.348
Distance from a health clinic (base: 25–500 m)		
501–1000 m	2.06	0.216
1000 and more	0.91	0.877
Standard of living (base: 1st quartile)		
2nd quartile	0.74	0.662
3rd quartile	0.58	0.462
4th quartile	0.53	0.418
Level of education (base: none)		
Primary	1.81	0.251
Secondary and higher	**8.35**	**0.000**
Type of neighbourhood (base: formal)	0.77	0.582

Control Variables: ethnicity, place of birth and length of time in city

reporting their illnesses. The only individual characteristic that is significantly related to the likelihood of seeking care is education level, which is very strongly correlated: those with a high school education are eight times more likely to seek care than those who have not been to school.

Overall, the wealthiest adults in Ouagadougou seem to be in worse health than the poorest adults: they are far more often HIV+, and are also much more likely to be overweight, putting them at higher risk of cardiovascular disease. Although the more affluent seek medical care more often (a finding that is masked in our regressions by under-reporting of less severe illnesses among the poor), this difference does not seem to help them avoid significant excess premature mortality.

Further analyses showed that this excess mortality in formal neighbourhood is actually due to migrants dying more often in formal neighbourhoods, either because families there host rural family members who need healthcare, or because people who have come to the city during their life time and have moved to the informal areas retreat back to their extended family (in the center of the city or in the village) when seriously ill (Rossier et al. 2014a).

When all else is equal, better educated people face certain health challenges: they have more accidents (due to their greater mobility) and, because they are more likely to have sex outside of marriage, a higher prevalence of HIV. However, educated individuals, everything else being constant, are more aware of the importance of prevention (for example: they seem to do a better job at HIV prevention). Furthermore, the better educated tend to access health care much more, which gives them a health advantage. More in-depth analyses show that not only do the better educated tend to seek care more often, but they tend to do so at non-profit clinics (associated with NGOs) which generally offer a higher quality of care at prices that the middle class can afford (Nikiema et al. 2011).

12.15 Conclusion

One of the most interesting findings of this analysis is the contrasting mortality rates between adults and children living in informal neighbourhoods. Children living in informal neighbourhoods have higher mortality rates than their counterparts in the formal neighbourhoods, while adults in these same neighbourhoods have lower mortality rates. The higher mortality among children 1–4 in the informal neighbourhoods does not seem to be explained simply by the demographic population of the neighbourhood, but rather by an independent effect of the neighbourhood itself. Though the parents of the children in informal neighbourhoods are certainly often poorer and less educated (which means that they are less likely to use preventative measures and to seek health care), the excess childhood mortality appears to be due to the high incidence of infectious diseases in these areas, likely because of the unsanitary conditions there (Djourdebbe et al. 2011; Dos Santos et al. 2011). This affects all children in the informal neighbourhoods, regardless of the relative wealth or education of their parents. Because illness is so common in this population, parents tend to wait longer before seeking health care for their children, resulting in a greater likelihood in going to hospitals (a phenomenon that is not apparent in adult care-seeking patterns). Another important impact of frequent illness on children's health is a high prevalence of malnutrition.

In contrast, the wealthier adults seem to have certain health disadvantages in Ouagadougou. Although they seek health care more often when they are ill, they have a higher prevalence of HIV and of risk-factors for cardiovascular disease (like being overweight), compared to poorer adults. Altogether, adult mortality is higher in formal areas, but once we control for migration status, better-off adults live longer, as expected (Rossier et al. 2014b).

Until recently, most African countries faced only the single burden of infectious disease, and constructed their health systems primarily to address this challenge. Their populations have benefited from prevention techniques for infectious diseases (like bed net campaigns for malaria and national vaccination campaigns) and have gained access to treatments (through generic medicines, etc.). As prevention and treatment for infectious disease became available, they first benefited the upper-classes which have the means, knowledge and wherewithal to access them, and slowly filtered down through the middle classes to the poor. This historical process helps to explain why our results show poorer health outcomes for children of lower socio-economic status.

Although the African continent has remained mostly rural, poor and dominated by infectious disease for a long time, it is now undergoing rapid urbanization. Cities, the epicentres of economic development, are richer than rural areas and the urban environment is now characterized by new epidemiologic burdens that are tied to development and its subsequent health challenges: chronic disease, (road) accidents, and HIV infection. All of these health problems affect adults prematurely and cause many preventable deaths. At a micro level, morbidity and mortality among adults are important contributors to poverty. The problems of accidents and chronic diseases in African have received only scant attention from health policy makers, both at the local and international levels. Prevention techniques and treatments exist for these health problems, but are often not (yet) available at the local level, even for the better-off, who are the first to suffer from this burden of disease. Furthermore, despite concerted HIV campaigns over the last 20 years, prevention practices are still not widespread enough, which disproportionately affects the more affluent, which is the group more likely to engage in high-risk sexual activity.

These findings have several important programmatic implications. First, it is important to continue the health education and facilitation of access to care for urban children, since large differences are found between the children of rich and poor, educated and uneducated. Moreover, it is urgent to improve sanitary conditions in the informal neighbourhoods, where many small children live (Rossier et al. 2011c), with an emphasis on immediate solutions instead of waiting for official "lotting." Thirdly, it is important to create and test chronic disease and accident prevention programs at a local level and work at the international level to bring affordable treatments for chronic diseases to the countries of the South. Fourth, we must continue to promote effective prevention strategies for high-risk sexual activity and adapt these strategies to the local context. As the countries continue to urbanize, the premature deaths of urban adults will also continue to grow. Decision makers must act today to control the epidemics of tomorrow.

References

African Population and Health Research Centre. (2002). *Population and health dynamics in Nairobi informal settlements*. Nairobi: African Population and Health Research Centre.

Baya, B., Zida, H., & Bonkoungou, Z. (2009). *Recensement général de la population et de l'habitation 2006 (RGPH 2006)*. Rapport d'analyse des données du RPGH 2006. Thème 07: La mortalité. Ouagadougou: Institut National de la Statistique et de la Démographie.

Boyer, F., & Delaunay, D. (2009). *Ouaga 2009, Peuplement de Ouagadougou et développement urbain*. Rapport provisoire (pp. 250). Ouagadougou: IRD.

Brockerhoff, M., & Brennan, E. (1998). The poverty of cities in developing countries. *Population and Development Review, 24*, 75–114.

Carr, D. (2004). *Improving the health of the world's poorest people* (Health bulletin n°1). Washington, DC: Population Reference Bureau.

Djourdebbé, F. B., LeGrand, T., Dos Santos, S., Soura, A., & Nikiéma, A. (2011). *Effet de l'environnement immédiat sur la survenue de la fièvre chez les enfants de moins de 5 ans à Ouagadougou*. Paper presented at the conference of the Union for African Population Studies, 5–9 december 2011, Ouagadougou.

Dos Santos, S., Djourdebbé, F. B., Nikiéma, A., Peumi, J.-P., & Soura, A. (2011). *Risques environnementaux et santé des enfants. Caractérisation des populations et des quartiers à risque à Ouagadougou*. Poster presented at the conference of the Union for African Population Studies, 5–9 December 2011, Ouagadougou.

Duthé, G., & Soura, A. (2011). *La mortalité dans les zones de l'ODSS*. Atelier des chercheurs de l'ODSS, 18–20 juillet 2011, Ouagadougou: ISSP.

Filmer, D., & Pritchett, L. (1999). The effect of household wealth on educational attainment: Evidence from 35 countries. *Population and Development Review, 25*(1), 85–120.

Filmer, D., & Pritchett, L. (2001). Estimating wealth effects without expenditure data – or tears: An application to educational enrollments in states India. *Demography, 28*(1), 115–132.

Guengant, J. P. (2009). Evolution passée et future de la ville de Ouagadougou. dans Boyer et Delaunay, Peuplement de Ouagadougou et développement urbain. Rapport provisoire (pp. 42–49). Ouagadougou: IRD.

Gwatkin, D. R., Rutstein, S., Johnson, K., et al. (2007). Socio-economic differences in health, nutrition and population within developing countries: An overview. *Nigerian Journal of Clinical Practice, 10*(4), 272–282.

Hacker, A., & Ryan, C. (2003). Prevalence of infant stunting in an urban Kenyan population: Comparison to the 1998 Kenyan health and demographic survey and the 2000 CDC growth grids. *Nutritional Research, 23*, 1643–1649.

INSD. (2009). *Annuaire statistique* (2008th ed.). Ouagadougou: INSD, Burkina Faso.

INSD and Macro International. (2004). *Enquête Démographique et de Santé du Burkina Faso 2003*. Ouagadougou/Calverton: INSD/ORC Macro.

Lachaud, J.-P. (2001). Dynamique de pauvreté et inégalité de la mortalité des enfants au Burkina Faso, *Centre d'Economie du développement,* Document de travail n°66, Université Bordeaux-Montesquieu IV, 2001.

Lankoande, B., Soura, A., Millogo, R., Compaoré, Y., & Rossier, C. (2016). Surmortalité des enfants dans les quartiers informels de Ouagadougou: Effet de composition ou effet de contexte? *African Population Studies, 30*(1), 2192–2202.

Magadi, M., Zulu, E., & Brockerhoff, M. (2003). The inequality of maternal health care in urban sub-Saharan Africa in the 1990s. *Population Studies, 57*, 347–366.
Marmot, M., & Commission on Social Determinants of Health. (2007). Achieving health equity: From root causes to fair outcomes. *Lancet, 370*(9593), 1153–1163.
Montgomery, M. (2009, juin). Urban poverty and health in developing countries. *Population Reference Bureau, 64*(2).
Murray, C. J., & Lopez, A. D. (1996). *The global burden of disease: A comprehensive assessment of mortality and disability from diseases, injuries and risk factors in 1990 and projected to 2020* (Global burden of diseases and injury series, Vol. 1). Boston: Harvard School of Public Health.
Nikiema, A., Millogo, R., Rossier, C., & Ridde, V. (2011). *Inégalités de l'accès aux soins en milieu urbain africain: le cas de la périphérie nord de Ouagadougou.* Paper presented at the conference of the Union for African Population Studies, 5–9 december 2011, Ouagadougou.
Rossier, C., & Ortiz, I. (2011). *Unmet needs for contraception in formal and informal neighbourhoods of Ouagadougou.* Paper presented at the conference of the Union for African Population Studies, Ouagadougou, December 5–9 2011.
Rossier, C., Soura, A., Lankoande, B., & Millogo, R. (2011a). *Observatoire de Population de Ouagadougou.* Données du R0, R1 et R2: rapport descriptif. www.isssp.bf/ODSS
Rossier, C., Soura, A., & Lankoande, B. (2011b). *Migration, pauvreté et santé à la périphérie de Ouagadougou.* Paper presented at the Chaire Quételet, Louvain-la-Neuve, November 16–18 2011.
Rossier, C., Lankoande, B., & Ortiz, I. (2011c). *Fertility differentials in formal and informal neighbourhoods of Ouagadougou?* Paper presented at the conference of the Union for African Population Studies, Ouagadougou, December 5–9 2011.
Rossier, C., Soura, A., Baya, B., & The ODSS Group. (2012). The Ouagadougou health and demographic surveillance system. *International Journal of Epidemiology.* doi:10.1093/ije/dys090.
Rossier, C., Soura, A., Duthé, G., & Findley, S. (2014a). Non-communicable diseases mortality and risk factors in formal and informal neighborhoods, Ouagadougou, Burkina Faso: Evidence from a health and demographic surveillance system. *PloS one, 9*(12), e113780.
Rossier, C., Soura, A., Duthé, G., Lankoande, B., & Millogo, R. (2014b). Are the urban poor always worse off? Socioeconomic differentials in adult cause specific mortality at the periphery of Ouagadougou, Burkina Faso. *Revue Quételet, 2*(2), 61–80. doi:10.14428/rqj2014.02.02.03.
Soura, B. A. (2009). Disparités spatiales de mortalité infanto-juvénile à Ouagadougou: niveaux, tendances et facteurs explicatifs. *Espace, Populations, Sociétés, 1*, 159–174.
Victora, C. G., Wagstaff, A., Schellenberg, J. A., et al. (2003). Applying an equity lens to child health and mortality: More of the same is not enough. *Lancet, 19: 362*(9379), 233–241.
World Health Organization. (2008). *The global burden of disease.* 2004 Update. Geneva: World Health Organization.
Zeba, A., Delisle, H., Renier, G., Savadogo, B., & Baya, B. (2012). The double burden of malnutrition and cardio-metabolic risk widens the gender and socio-economicsocio-economic health gap: A study among adults in Burkina Faso (West Africa). Pub Health Nut [FirstView Article]. March 30 2012; 1–10. Available from: http://dx.doi.org/10.1017/S1368980012000729

MIX
Papier aus verantwortungsvollen Quellen
Paper from responsible sources
FSC® C105338

If you have any concerns about our products,
you can contact us on
ProductSafety@springernature.com

In case Publisher is established outside the EU,
the EU authorized representative is:
Springer Nature Customer Service Center GmbH
Europaplatz 3, 69115 Heidelberg, Germany

Printed by Libri Plureos GmbH
in Hamburg, Germany